URBAN HEALTH
AND SOCIETY

URBAN HEALTH AND SOCIETY

Interdisciplinary Approaches to Research and Practice

NICHOLAS FREUDENBERG

SUSAN KLITZMAN

SUSAN SAEGERT

Editors

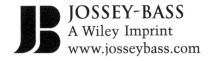

JOSSEY-BASS
A Wiley Imprint
www.josseybass.com

Published by Jossey-Bass
A Wiley Imprint
989 Market Street, San Francisco, CA 94103-1741—www.josseybass.com

Readers should be aware that Internet Web sites offered as citations and/or sources for further information may have changed or disappeared between the time this was written and when it is read.

Limit of Liability/Disclaimer of Warranty: While the publisher and author have used their best efforts in preparing this book, they make no representations or warranties with respect to the accuracy or completeness of the contents of this book and specifically disclaim any implied warranties of merchantability or fitness for a particular purpose. No warranty may be created or extended by sales representatives or written sales materials. The advice and strategies contained herein may not be suitable for your situation. You should consult with a professional where appropriate. Neither the publisher nor author shall be liable for any loss of profit or any other commercial damages, including but not limited to special, incidental, consequential, or other damages.

Jossey-Bass books and products are available through most bookstores. To contact Jossey-Bass directly call our Customer Care Department within the U.S. at 800-956-7739, outside the U.S. at 317-572-3986, or fax 317-572-4002.

Jossey-Bass also publishes its books in a variety of electronic formats. Some content that appears in print may not be available in electronic books.

Library of Congress Cataloging-in-Publication Data

Urban health and society: interdisciplinary approaches to research and practice/
Nicholas Freudenberg, Susan Klitzman, Susan Saegert, editors.
    p. ; cm
Includes bibliographical references and index.

ISBN 978-0-470-38366-7 (pbk.)

1. Urban health.   2. Interdisciplinary research.   I. Freudenberg, Nicholas.   II. Klitzman, Susan.
III. Saegert, Susan. [DNLM: 1. Urban Health.   2. Healthcare Disparities.
3. Socioeconomic Factors. WA 380 U7157 2009]

RA566.7.U735 2009

362.1'042—dc22

2009013922

Printed in the United States of America
FIRST EDITION

PB Printing   10 9 8 7 6 5 4 3 2 1

CONTENTS

Preface   xi

The Contributors   xiii

PART ONE
INTRODUCTION   1

**1   FRAMEWORKS FOR INTERDISCIPLINARY URBAN
     HEALTH RESEARCH AND PRACTICE**   3

Nicholas Freudenberg, Susan Klitzman, Susan Saegert

Introduction   4

The Implications of Urban Life for Health   6

Levels and Types of Interdisciplinarity   8

Conundrums in Interdisciplinarity   10

Interdisciplinarity and Theories of Knowledge   11

Methodological Challenges and Approaches to Interdisciplinarity   12

Interdisciplinarity: Which Disciplines When?   12

Role Definitions in Interdisciplinary Research and Practice   13

Multiple Levels of Intervention   14

Summary   15

**2   ENVIRONMENTAL JUSTICE PRAXIS: IMPLICATIONS FOR
     INTERDISCIPLINARY URBAN PUBLIC HEALTH**   19

Tom Angotti, Julie Sze

Environmental Justice and Public Health   22

The Built Environment, Urban Planning, and Urban Public Health   23

Environmental and Social Justice, Interdisciplinarity, and the
     Politics of Knowledge   26

Asthma and the Environmental Justice Campaign for a Solid
Waste Plan in New York City   29

Asian Immigrant and Refugee Organizing for Environmental
Health and Housing in the Bay Area   34

Conclusion   37

Summary   38

PART TWO
INTERDISCIPLINARY APPROACHES TO STUDYING CAUSES OF URBAN HEALTH PROBLEMS   43

3 INTERDISCIPLINARY, PARTICIPATORY RESEARCH ON URBAN FOOD ENVIRONMENTS AND DIETARY BEHAVIORS   45

*Shannon N. Zenk, Amy J. Schulz, Angela M. Odoms-Young,
Murlisa Lockett*

Introduction   46

Determinants of Retail Food Environments in Cities   47

Using CBPR to Understand the Health Implications of Detroit's
Food Environment   48

Directions for Future Research   54

Summary   56

4 AN ECOLOGICAL MODEL OF URBAN CHILD HEALTH   63

Kim T. Ferguson, Pilyoung Kim, James R. Dunn, Gary W. Evans

Introduction   64

An Ecological Model   64

Bronfenbrenner's Bioecological Model   65

Influences on Children's Health in the Urban Context   68

Research Across Multiple Levels   76

Agenda for Future Research and Practice   78

Summary   80

5 GEOGRAPHIC INFORMATION SYSTEMS, ENVIRONMENTAL
JUSTICE, AND HEALTH DISPARITIES 93

Juliana Maantay, Andrew R. Maroko,

Carlos Alicea, A. H. Strelnick

Introduction 94

Community-Based Participatory Research 95

Multilevel Models of Causation 96

Role of Geographic Information Systems 96

Environmental Justice and Health in the Bronx 97

Methods 101

Findings 110

Implications of Findings 111

Lessons on Interdisciplinary Approaches to Urban Health Research 117

Conclusion 119

Summary 119

6 RACIAL INEQUALITY IN HEALTH AND THE POLICY-INDUCED
BREAKDOWN OF AFRICAN AMERICAN COMMUNITIES 127

Arline T. Geronimus, J. Phillip Thompson

Introduction 128

Racialized Ideologies: Developmentalism, Economism,
and the American Creed 131

Implications for Public Policy 138

Building a Movement for Policy Reform 144

Summary 148

7 AN INTERDISCIPLINARY AND SOCIAL-ECOLOGICAL
ANALYSIS OF THE U.S. FORECLOSURE CRISIS AS IT
RELATES TO HEALTH 161

Susan Saegert, Kimberly Libman, Desiree Fields

Housing and Health: What's the Connection? 162

The Social Ecology of Foreclosure 164

The Research and Its Context 166

Focus Group Analysis and the Emergence of Health as an Issue 170

Foreclosure and Public Health   173

Neoliberalism, the Foreclosure Crisis, and Health Consequences   174

Conclusion   176

Summary   178

PART THREE
INTERDISCIPLINARY APPROACHES TO
INTERVENTIONS TO PROMOTE URBAN HEALTH   183

8   TRANSDISCIPLINARY ACTION RESEARCH
    ON TEEN SMOKING PREVENTION   185
    Juliana Fuqua, Daniel Stokols, Richard Harvey,
    Atusa Baghery, Larry Jamner
    Introduction   186
    Review of Transdisciplinary Action Research   186
    Transdisciplinary Action Research Cycle   187
    Translating Transdisciplinary Research into Community
        Intervention and Policy   189
    Factors Facilitating or Impeding Collaboration Among
        TPC Members   196
    Implications and Additional Lessons Learned from
        the TPC Study   205
    Future Directions   207
    Summary   211

9   HOW VULNERABILITIES AND CAPACITIES SHAPE
    POPULATION HEALTH AFTER DISASTERS   217
    Craig Hadley, Sasha Rudenstine, Sandro Galea
    Social and Economic Determinants of Health After Disasters   218
    Humanitarian Crises in Angola and the Balkans   223
    Hurricane Katrina   224
    September 11, 2001, Terrorist Attacks on New York City   226
    Implications for Prevention and Intervention   229
    Summary   231

10 IMMIGRANTS AND URBAN AGING: TOWARD A POLICY FRAMEWORK   **239**

Marianne Fahs, Anahí Viladrich, Nina S. Parikh

The New Urban Demography: Baby Boomers and Immigrants   240

Economic and Social Influences on Aging and Health Policy   242

Social and Environmental Considerations   246

Toward a Conceptual Framework   254

A Public Health Research and Policy Agenda   255

Summary   258

11 REVERSING THE TIDE OF TYPE 2 DIABETES AMONG AFRICAN AMERICANS THROUGH INTERDISCIPLINARY RESEARCH   **271**

Hollie Jones, Leandris C. Liburd

A Dialogue Between Two Disciplines: Psychology and
Medical Anthropology   273

Ethnic Identity and the Experience of Being African American
with Type 2 Diabetes   278

Interdisciplinary Research Methods   281

Integrating Social Psychology and Medical Anthropology
to Reduce the Burden of Diabetes   284

Summary   285

PART FOUR
PUTTING INTERDISCIPLINARY APPROACHES INTO PRACTICE   293

12 USING INTERDISCIPLINARY APPROACHES TO STRENGTHEN URBAN HEALTH RESEARCH AND PRACTICE   **295**

Nicholas Freudenberg, Susan Klitzman, Susan Saegert

Doing Interdisciplinary Research and Practice   296

Defining the Problem   299

Creating a Process for Interdisciplinary Work   302

Choosing Institutional and Community Partners 305

Influencing Policy and Practice 309

Evaluating Impact 311

Wanted: Interdisciplinary Researchers and Practitioners 312

Summary 314

GLOSSARY 319

INDEX 325

PREFACE

In this volume, we seek to bring together two emerging fields of study. The first, urban health, asks how city living shapes health and how researchers, policymakers, health professionals, and others can contribute to healthier cities around the world. The second, interdisciplinary research, seeks to transcend the limitations of research approaches informed by a single discipline. As more of the world's populations move to cities and as urban areas face more complex health problems, improving the health of urban populations has become a central challenge for public health professionals, government officials, researchers, and urban dwellers. More than ever, understanding and solving problems like obesity, depression, diabetes, heart disease, pollution-related diseases, violence, and infant mortality will require researchers who can investigate health at individual, family, community, and policy levels and integrate theories, methods, and analytic techniques from a variety of disciplines.

We wrote and edited *Urban Health and Society: Interdisciplinary Approaches to Research and Practice* to prepare researchers and practitioners to be better equipped to meet the challenges of improving the health of urban populations in the coming decades. Our intended audience is researchers and graduate students in public health, social sciences, nursing, social work, and other related fields. In Part One of the book (Chapters One and Two), we introduce the central themes of the book and highlight the connections between population health and social justice. In Part Two (Chapters Three through Seven), interdisciplinary researchers who have studied food access in low-income urban neighborhoods, child development and poverty, asthma and air pollution in New York City, the impact of social policy on the health of African Americans, and the health consequences of the recent housing foreclosure crisis explain how they studied the causes of these problems using a variety of disciplinary, conceptual, and methodological approaches. Part Three (Chapters Eight to Eleven) focuses on creating interventions to solve urban health problems. In each chapter, authors from two or more disciplines analyze the contributions their approach offers to solving a particular problem, including teen tobacco use, responses to natural and human-origin disasters, healthy aging for immigrants in urban areas, and reducing the epidemic of diabetes in African American communities. In Part Four (Chapter Twelve), we suggest how readers can use the insights from previous chapters to bring interdisciplinary approaches to research and intervention into their own work settings.

To assist faculty and students who use this book in graduate courses, we have included objectives and discussion questions at the end of each chapter and, in the back of the book, a glossary that defines the key concepts the authors discuss.

Our work as teachers, researchers, and policy advocates motivated us to compile this book. At City University of New York, we have worked together to develop interdisciplinary approaches to teaching and research, created new courses on interdisciplinary approaches to urban health for masters and doctoral students in public health and the social sciences, and collaborated on research projects aimed at understanding how housing policies and practices influence the health of urban populations. Separately, we have each worked for decades in university, municipal government, and community settings to study and develop interventions to reduce a variety of urban health problems. While we have benefited from the growing body of literature on the theoretical foundations of interdisciplinary approaches to health research, our focus is more practical. We want to help our colleagues and students to use these methods to improve their work and increase its relevance to improving the health of urban populations.

We were fortunate to have the support of numerous individuals and organizations to complete this volume. A Collaborative Incentive Grant from the Chancellor's Office of City University of New York (CUNY) helped us get started on this work. A Roadmap Curriculum Development Award to Nicholas Freudenberg from the National Institute of General Medical Sciences (1 K07 GM72947) supported our work on creating an interdisciplinary doctoral curriculum in urban health at CUNY and supported some of the authors of the chapters in this volume. This award also supported a faculty seminar on interdisciplinary research that served as a valuable forum for developing this volume. In June 2006, we convened a workshop of faculty from eight U.S. and Canadian universities to discuss research and teaching in urban health. These discussions informed this volume and especially our observations in Chapters One and Twelve.

Many colleagues were kind enough to read chapters and provide helpful suggestions to authors and editors. These include Tom Angotti, Mimi Fahs, Sandro Galea, Mary Clare Lennon, Shirley Lindenbaum, and Amy Schulz. Several students also helped to compile literature reviews, prepare manuscripts, and assist in other ways. We thank Tracy Chu, Zoe Meleo Erwin, Lauren Evans, and Rachel Verni. At Jossey-Bass, Andrew Pasternack and Seth Schwartz provided encouragement and helpful suggestions for improving the manuscript. Finally, we thank our students and our community and municipal agency partners in research, who continually challenge, amplify, and enrich our understanding of urban health, interdisciplinary research, and the links between public health and social justice. We gratefully acknowledge the help we have received from all these sources but of course accept full responsibility for the content of this volume.

New York City
Nicholas Freudenberg
Susan Klitzman
Susan Saegert
February 2009

THE CONTRIBUTORS

Angotti, Tom, PhD
Professor of Urban Planning and
  Director
Center for Community Planning and
  Development
Hunter College, City University of
  New York
New York, N.Y.

Alicea, Carlos
President
For a Better Bronx
Bronx, N.Y.

Baghery, Atusa
School of Social Ecology
University of California, Irvine
Irvine, Cal.

Dunn, James R., PhD
Research Scientist, Center for Research
  on Inner City Health
St. Michael's Hospital; Associate Professor
University of Toronto, Dalla Lana School
  of Public Health
Toronto, Canada

Evans, Gary W., PhD
Elizabeth Lee Vincent Professor
  of Human Ecology
Departments of Design and
  Environmental Analysis and of
  Human Development
Cornell University
Ithaca, N.Y.

Fahs, Marianne, PhD, MPH
Professor, Urban Public Health
Co-Director, Brookdale Center for
  Healthy Aging & Longevity
Hunter College, City University of
  New York
New York, N.Y.

Ferguson, Kim T., PhD
Psychology Program
Sarah Lawrence College
Bronxville, N.Y.

Fields, Desiree
PhD student in Environmental
  Psychology
Graduate Center
City University of New York
New York, N.Y.

Freudenberg, Nicholas, DrPH
Distinguished Professor of Public
  Health and Social/Personality
  Psychology
Hunter College and The
  Graduate Center, City University
  of New York
New York, N.Y.

Fuqua, Juliana, PhD
Assistant Professor
Department of Psychology and
  Sociology, California State
  Polytechnic University, Pomona
Pomona, Cal.

Galea, Sandro, MD, DrPH, MPH
Professor of Epidemiology
University of Michigan, School of Public
    Health
Ann Arbor, Mich.

Geronimus, Arline T., ScD
Professor of Health Behavior & Health
    Education
University of Michigan, School of Public
    Health
Ann Arbor, Mich.

Hadley, Craig, PhD
Assistant Professor of Anthropology
Emory University
Atlanta, Ga.

Harvey, Richard, PhD
Assistant Professor of Health Education
Department of Health Education
San Francisco State University
San Francisco, Cal.

Jamner, Larry, PhD
Professor of Psychology and Social
    Behavior
School of Social Ecology
University of California, Irvine
Irvine, Cal.

Jones, Hollie, PhD
Assistant Professor of Psychology
Medgar Evers College
City University of New York
New York, N.Y.

Kim, Pilyoung, MEd
Doctoral student
Department of Human Development
Cornell University
Ithaca, N.Y.

Klitzman, Susan, DrPH, MPH
Professor and Director, Urban Public
    Health Program
Hunter College, City University of
    New York
New York, N.Y.

Libman, Kimberly
PhD student in Environmental
    Psychology, CUNY Graduate Center
    and MPH student, Hunter College
City University of New York
New York, N.Y.

Liburd, Leandris C., PhD, MPH
Branch Chief, Community Health and
    Program Services Branch, Division of
    Adult and Community Health,
    National Center for Chronic Disease
    Prevention and Health Promotion,
    Centers for Disease Control and
    Prevention
Atlanta, Ga.

Lockett, Murlisa, MA
Detroit Department of Health and
    Wellness Promotion
Detroit, Mich.

Maantay, Juliana, PhD, MUP
Associate Professor of Urban
    Environmental Geography
Department of Environmental,
    Geographic & Geological Sciences
Lehman College, City University of
    New York, Bronx, N.Y.
Director of Geographic Information
    Science Program
Doctoral Program in Earth and
    Environmental Sciences, City University
    of New York Graduate Center
New York, N.Y.

Maroko, Andrew R.,
Ph.D. student in Earth and
   Environmental Science
Lehman College and Graduate Center,
   City University of New York
Bronx, N.Y.

Odoms-Young, Angela M., PhD
Assistant Professor of Public Health and
   Health Education
Northern Illinois University School of
   Nursing & Health Studies
DeKalb, Ill.

Parikh, Nina S., PhD, MPH
Senior Research Associate
Brookdale Center for Healthy Aging &
   Longevity
Hunter College, City University of
   New York
New York, N.Y.

Rudenstine, Sasha
Site Coordinator
Disaster Research Education and
   Mentoring Center (DREM)
University of Michigan, School of Public
   Health
Ann Arbor, Mich.

Saegert, Susan, PhD
Professor of Community Psychology
Vanderbilt University
Nashville, Tenn.

Schulz, Amy J., PhD
Research Associate Professor, Health
   Behavior & Health Education;
   Associate Director, CRECH
   Research Associate Professor, Institute
   for Research on Women and Gender

University of Michigan, School of Public
   Health
Ann Arbor, Mich.

Stokols, Daniel, PhD
Chancellor's Professor of Planning,
   Policy & Design
School of Social Ecology, University of
   California, Irvine
Irvine, Cal.

Strelnick, A. H., MD
Professor of Clinical Family & Social
   Medicine
Director, The Bronx Center to Reduce
   and Eliminate Ethnic and Racial
   Health Disparities
Albert Einstein College of Medicine,
   Montefiore Medical Center
Bronx, N.Y.

Sze, Julie, BA, PhD
Associate Professor of American Studies
University of California, Davis
Davis, Cal.

Thompson, J. Phillip, PhD
Associate Professor of Urban Politics
Massachusetts Institute of Technology
Cambridge, Mass.

Viladrich, Anahí, PhD
Associate Professor
Urban Public Health Program
Hunter College, City University of New York
New York, N.Y.

Zenk, Shannon N., PhD, MPH, RN
Assistant Professor
Department of Health Systems Science
University of Illinois at Chicago College
   of Nursing

URBAN HEALTH AND SOCIETY

PART

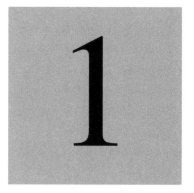

INTRODUCTION

CHAPTER

FRAMEWORKS FOR INTERDISCIPLINARY URBAN HEALTH RESEARCH AND PRACTICE

NICHOLAS FREUDENBERG, SUSAN KLITZMAN, SUSAN SAEGERT

LEARNING OBJECTIVES

- Offer three reasons why interdisciplinary research approaches are especially suitable for investigation of urban health problems.

- Explain the characteristics of cities that affect the public health challenges they face and that make urban health problems particularly appropriate for interdisciplinary study.

- Compare and contrast unidisciplinary and interdisciplinary research from the point of view of both substance and the processes involved, as well as the challenges inherent in interdisciplinary research.

- Describe approaches to overcoming interdisciplinary challenges related to assumptions, methods, institutional settings, and the focus of interventions.

INTRODUCTION

For the past two centuries, cities and urbanization have been a dominant influence on health and disease, and today, more of the world's population lives in cities than ever before. In 2007, half of the world's population lived in urban areas, and by 2030, three-quarters will live in cities.[1,2] For health researchers and practitioners, understanding how the urban environment influences health and well-being will determine how successful we are in caring for individuals and families, in promoting population health, and in achieving local, national, and global health goals.

More broadly, as the United Nations *State of the World's Cities* report noted in 2001, "For better or worse, the development of contemporary societies will depend largely on understanding and managing the growth of cities. The city will increasingly become the test bed for the adequacy of political institutions, for the performance of government agencies, and for the effectiveness of programmes to combat social exclusion, to protect and repair the environment and to promote human development."[3]

As the urban population grows and as cities become more diverse and complex, it becomes increasingly difficult for any single individual, academic discipline, profession, institution, or agency to develop the insights and skills needed to improve the health of urban populations or to create healthier cities. Despite the growing recognition that only interdisciplinary research and practice can solve the health challenges facing cities today, most universities still train health researchers and professionals in a single discipline, teach them only a few research methods, and do not acquaint their students with the growing literature on interdisciplinary approaches to health. In this volume, we seek to remedy this problem by introducing students, researchers, and practitioners in public health, medicine, social work, nursing, sociology, anthropology, psychology, urban planning, geography, and other disciplines to the concepts of interdisciplinary approaches to urban health research and practice. Our goals are to familiarize readers with the emerging concepts and principles that characterize interdisciplinary urban health research, to provide case studies of interdisciplinary health research within cities, and to prepare readers to work more effectively within interdisciplinary research and intervention teams.

This volume grows out of our own experiences as researchers and teachers, from our reading of several bodies of literature, and from recent calls for more emphasis on interdisciplinary education and research. Since the early 1980s, we have separately and together studied, developed, directed, and evaluated interventions to address several quintessential urban social, health, and environmental problems: childhood lead poisoning, asthma, deteriorated housing, HIV infection, reentry from jail, violence and crime, mothers' and children's mental health problems, and obesity and diabetes. In each of these cases, our efforts to understand and reduce the health problems facing urban neighborhoods forced us to transcend the disciplinary boundaries of our professional training and to learn new languages, concepts, and methods.

As teachers at City University of New York (CUNY), the largest urban public university in the nation, and Vanderbilt University, we also bumped against disciplinary boundaries. Our graduate students in psychology, public health, environmental health, health education, nursing, public policy, and sociology—many of them working in the health field during the day—wanted to take courses, learn skills, and integrate methods from different disciplines to succeed in solving the problems they faced in their own research and in jobs at the municipal health department, in voluntary health agencies, or with community organizations. Too often, however, the requirements of accrediting agencies, the curriculum or departmental structure of our universities, or our own limitations as disciplinary researchers made it difficult for our students to achieve their interdisciplinary objectives. Recently, we have worked to develop at CUNY a variety of interdisciplinary approaches to graduate education for social science and public health students interested in urban health. These experiences have reinforced our view of both the potential and the obstacles facing interdisciplinary study.

As social scientists and health researchers, we are influenced by several emerging bodies of literature on urban health, on social determinants of health, on social support and health, on health inequities and disparities, on various participatory research methods, and on human rights, social justice, and health. Each of these fields has been developed by investigators from several disciplines, and each has begun to establish an interdisciplinary foundation that can guide future research and intervention. Although these new developments have informed our research and teaching, we have also been frustrated with the difficulty of developing for ourselves and our students a user-friendly synthesis of these emerging principles, theories, and methods that can guide research and practice. Once again, our own and our colleagues' disciplinary roots make it difficult to integrate new scholarship across levels and disciplines.

Finally, this book is a response to several recent calls for more attention to interdisciplinary research and education. In its report *The Future of the Public's Health in the 21st Century,*[4] the National Academies Press emphasized the importance of interdisciplinary education in health. It called on universities to "increase integrated interdisciplinary learning opportunities for students in public health and other related health science professions . . . and interdisciplinary education and appropriate incentives for faculty to undertake such activities." The 2003 National Academies Press report *Who Will Keep the Public Healthy?*[5] also stressed the need for more interdisciplinary education for biomedical and social science researchers. In its 2005 report *Facilitating Interdisciplinary Research,*[6] the National Academies Press suggested that graduate students should explore ways to broaden their experience by gaining "requisite" knowledge in one or more fields in addition to their primary field. They also suggested that researchers and faculty members desiring to work on interdisciplinary research, education, and training projects should immerse themselves in the languages, cultures, and knowledge of their collaborators.

In its effort to chart a "road map" for medical research in the twenty-first century, the National Institutes of Health observed that "the scale and complexity of today's biomedical research problems increasingly demand that scientists move beyond the confines of their own discipline and explore new organizational models for team science."[7] As urban health researchers and teachers, we support these calls for new paradigms but note the lack of practical tools for achieving these ambitious aims. We hope this volume will help to fill this gap.

Finally, the Institute of Medicine, the Council on Education for Public Health, and other bodies have called on schools of public health to strengthen preparation of students in interdisciplinary collaboration and communication. Most faculty and researchers agree in principle with this call, but few have developed practical strategies for meeting this new mandate or found ways to equip students with the competencies to defuse the land mines one encounters when crossing disciplinary boundaries. This book hopes to meet that need.

In sum, we hope this collection of essays will help to educate health professionals and researchers who can transcend the limitations we have faced. By introducing students early in their careers to the concepts and methods of other disciplines, by describing the benefits but also the real-world challenges that interdisciplinary researchers face, and by presenting case studies from the interdisciplinary front lines of public health and social science research and practice, we hope today's students will be better prepared to accept interdisciplinary approaches as the norm rather than the exception. In this chapter, we introduce several themes that are developed in subsequent chapters.

THE IMPLICATIONS OF URBAN LIFE FOR HEALTH

One recurring theme is that interdisciplinary research and the field of urban health are good partners for a lasting relationship. What makes the health of urban populations especially suitable for these interdisciplinary approaches?

First, like coral reefs or tropical rain forests, cities are complex biological, social, and physical systems in which organisms (in this case, humans are our main interest) interact with each other and their environment at the molecular, local, and global levels. No single discipline can capture the complexity of these interactions, and only interdisciplinary methods can consider these dynamics at several levels simultaneously.[8, 9]

Second, cities have diverse populations. Population heterogeneity sets the stage for a variety of biological, cultural, political, and social encounters among and within the various subpopulations. For example, understanding the health implications of the food practices of urban ethnic groups and their varying interactions with the urban food system requires nutritional, anthropological, sociological, and psychological expertise,[10] as Zenk and her colleagues describe in Chapter Three.

Third, cities have dense populations. Sociologists, economists, and biologists have studied the consequences of population density for more than 200 years, and more recently, epidemiologists and psychologists have also taken on this issue. Some research suggests that density contributes to negative effects on physical and mental health, but other studies document increased access to health services, close knit subcultures, and greater freedom of choice and personal development. By integrating the findings on density from these various disciplines, it may be possible to develop a more nuanced view of the various ways that density influences health. More pragmatically, understanding the complex ways that density affects health can assist urban planners to design cities and neighborhoods that better promote well-being. In Chapter Nine, Hadley and colleagues examine how urban density shapes the health consequences of disasters such as earthquakes, tsunamis, or terrorist attacks.

Fourth, because most cities are characterized by high levels of inequality, interventions—even beneficial ones—run the risk of reinforcing or even widening disparities in health.[11] Thus, opening new municipal fitness centers may exacerbate the gap in physical activity levels between the poor and the better off unless the poor have what Paul Farmer has called a "preferential option" for the new services.[12] What is beneficial at the individual level may be harmful to population health and to social justice. To avoid this unintended effect, urban public health planners need to define disparity reduction as an explicit goal. This requires thinking across levels and considering technical and ethical concerns; both tasks are suited to interdisciplinary research. In Chapter Six, Geronimus and Thompson examine the multiple pathways by which public policies have often undermined the health of African American communities.

Fifth, most cities organize the municipal services that affect health in sectoral programs: education, health care, sanitation, water, or housing. Each sector has its own experts, and rarely do policymakers or researchers consider the impact of developments in one sector (e.g., increasing rates of high school dropout) on outcomes in another (e.g., longevity or premature death). For urban residents, however, it is the totality of their environment and the services available to them that shape their living conditions. Interdisciplinary research can begin to examine these intersections across levels and sectors and analyze their impact on health. Saegert and her colleagues provide such an example in Chapter Seven in their analysis of the health consequences of housing foreclosures.

Sixth, compared to other areas, cities have a rich array of social and human resources—dense social networks, many community-based organizations, and diverse formal and informal service providers. These human resources and the social capital inherent within them constitute key assets for urban health promotion, and effective public health programs use these resources both to root interventions in a specific urban context and to reduce the need for external resources.[13–15] Recent work on social capital in psychology, sociology, and public health demonstrates the potential for both theory and research in this area and the value of investigating the dynamic interactions among different social levels.[16–18] For example, in Chapter Ten, Fahs and her colleagues assess the contributions that immigrant urban communities can bring to healthy aging, and in Chapter Eleven, Jones and Liburd describe some of the assets that African American communities can bring to the task of reversing the diabetes epidemic. Finding the right assets, mobilizing them, and ensuring their sustainability are important tasks for urban health interventionists.

Seventh, the development of modern cities and their impact on the health and well-being of their inhabitants are dynamic across time and place. For example, although many cities in North America and Europe began experiencing unprecedented population expansion during the latter half of the nineteenth century, it was not until a century later that many of their southern counterparts in Asia, Africa, and Latin America did so. Temporal and geographic differences are also manifest in disease patterns: Many northern cities have experienced significant overall declines in infectious diseases and subsequent increases in longevity, although these diseases continue to burden disproportionately disadvantaged subgroups in the population. Now, developed world cities are battling noninfectious diseases like cancer, diabetes, heart disease, and Alzheimer's disease that are associated with cumulative exposures, aging, and long latency periods. Meanwhile, in many developing world cities, infectious diseases like HIV/AIDS, tuberculosis, malaria, and dengue fever are still raging, shortening life spans, and imposing misery. To understand the growth and character of cities and their impact on health requires that we consider a myriad of historical, geographic, economic, political, and social forces. No single discipline possesses the framework and tools for such an analysis.

In sum, we seek to show that the *methods* of interdisciplinary research can help to understand better the outcome of the health of urban populations. The complex health conditions facing cities have determinants and consequences at multiple levels of biological and social organization, and they vary significantly across time and place. In addition, they often need to effectively address simultaneous changes in behavioral, community, organizational, and policy domains. No single discipline can provide the tools needed to operate in these many dimensions.

LEVELS AND TYPES OF INTERDISCIPLINARITY

Our second theme is that interdisciplinarity is best considered a continuum rather than a polarity with disciplinary approaches. In our view, any specific research project, intervention, or program in urban health can be located along a continuum that begins with disciplinary approaches, proceeds to multidisciplinary, then to interdisciplinary, and finally to transdisciplinary. Examples of disciplinary approaches to the study of urban health abound in the peer-reviewed and popular literature—sociological studies of urban crime, psychological studies of population density and crowding, environmental health studies of urban noise, air pollution, or childhood lead poisoning, and clinical studies of anti-hypertension, cholesterol, or malarial drugs.

Multidisciplinary research joins investigators from different fields to bring their own methods and concepts to a common problem. As Stokols and others have noted,[19] fields such as public health and urban planning are inherently multidisciplinary in that they encompass several different disciplines whose perspectives are combined in analyses of complex topics, such as population health and urban development. For example, epidemiologists, environmental health researchers, pediatricians, housing specialists, and psychologists have studied the epidemic of childhood asthma in U.S. cities. Each researcher uses his or her analytic methods and concepts to examine the role of, say, air pollution, quality of medical care, housing characteristics, diet, or parental management in the prevalence of asthma or the severity of symptoms. And as Fuqua and her colleagues show in Chapter Eight, reducing the toll from tobacco has forced researchers from many disciplines to form innovative research collaboratives. Occasionally, these investigators work together, and such efforts have led to a better understanding of asthma. Too often, however, multidisciplinary research resembles more the parallel play of toddlers than the collaborative work of a single team. Differences in language, methods, scale, and outcome make it difficult to integrate findings across disciplines and to develop science-based multilevel interventions to improve urban health.

The National Academies Press has defined *interdisciplinary research* as "a mode of research by teams or individuals that integrates information, data, techniques, tools, perspectives, concepts, and/or theories from two or more disciplines or bodies of specialized knowledge to advance fundamental understanding or to solve problems whose solutions are beyond the scope of a single discipline or field of research practice."[6] The operative distinction with multidisciplinary approaches is the *integration* of perspectives from two or more disciplines. Several chapters illustrate this process, including Angotti and Sze in Chapter Two, who integrate urban planning with historical and environmental health approaches to the study of urban environmental hazards and Maantay and her colleagues, who in Chapter Five synthesize geographic and medical perspectives to better understand childhood asthma.

More recently, Stokols and others have proposed the term "transdisciplinary research," which is characterized by a deliberate integration of concepts and methods from several fields to address a common problem. It results in "collaborative products" that "reflect an integration of conceptual and/or methodological perspectives drawn from two or more fields."[19] Their work on tobacco control,[19] recent studies of the obesity epidemic,[20–22] and studies of child development in urban settings, described by Ferguson and colleagues in Chapter Four, illustrate transdisciplinary approaches. In some cases, transdisciplinary approaches lead to the creation of new discipline that integrates previously separate ones. For example, the new field of "cognitive science" brings together researchers and methods and concepts from anthropology, artificial intelligence, neuroscience, education, linguistics, psychology, and philosophy.[6] In Chapter Twelve, we consider the advantages and disadvantages of viewing urban health as a new transdisciplinary field.

To help readers locate their own efforts and the cases described in this volume on the disciplinarity continuum, it may be helpful to describe some of the characteristics that distinguished more unidisciplinary research from interdisciplinary research (IR). First, the starting point for IR is often a problem rather than a single hypothesis about the relationship between two variables. Second, IR often struggles to define a common language and concepts, a task not usually needed in disciplinary research. Third, IR often works at two or more levels of organization, requiring more sophisticated methods to account for the influences of one level on another. Fourth, IR is less often guided by theory, in part because theories often describe only one analytic level or are bounded by a single discipline. Finally, compared to the frequently incremental approach of disciplinary research, in which each research finding contributes a small addition to a fuller picture of the question of interest, IR may take a more dynamic approach. Integrating findings across levels may lead to a reformulation of basic concepts and a reframing of research questions.

In our view, the important task is not so much how to create precise definitions that distinguish among the points on the disciplinarity continuum but rather to help researchers decide where to locate their own efforts. Our own experience and the chapters in this volume suggest that this decision is based on the nature of the problem under study and the specific research questions that drive this decision and not on inherent characteristics of the different degrees of disciplinarity. Although we appreciate the distinction between interdisciplinary and transdisciplinary research, in this volume, we generally use the more common term *interdisciplinary* for clarity and simplicity.

CONUNDRUMS IN INTERDISCIPLINARITY

A third theme that emerges from this book is that interdisciplinary research is difficult. We resist the effort to paint it as the ideal solution to all complex problems and argue instead that researchers need to have a clear rationale for its use in any specific situation.

What makes interdisciplinary research so challenging? First, the value of disciplines— part of the reason they emerged—is to help focus attention on a defined set of variables, usually at a single analytic level and informed by a small number of relevant theories. Once researchers give up the disciplinary lens, they can be dizzied by choices—like looking through a microscope, binoculars, and a telescope simultaneously. And interdisciplinary approaches offer not only multiple ways of framing the problem but also multiple methods of collecting and analyzing data. Choosing this path significantly expands the number of choices a researcher needs to make.

A related challenge is integrating methods and theories from different analytic levels or different levels of social organization. In some cases, methodologies such as multilevel statistical models or structural equation modeling provide a framework for explaining the relationship among different levels, but the simplified assumptions these models require may limit the insights they can offer. In childhood lead poisoning, for example, the child's nutritional status, behavioral patterns, interactions with parents, and access to health care, as well as the living conditions inside the household, the building, the block, the neighborhood, and the policies of the city, state, and national government all influence the individual and population prevalence of elevated lead levels. How do we integrate findings from these different levels to develop more effective lead poisoning prevention policies and interventions? The practical difficulty explains why researchers often choose to focus on a single level using data and theories from a single discipline—even if such studies are of limited use in the development of effective prevention policies.

Another difficulty for the researcher considering interdisciplinary approaches is the sheer volume of knowledge needed to be effective in this task. The unread journals that pile up in our own offices show how hard it is to keep up with new findings and new methods in our own field. Imagine having to stay on top of two or three fields to stay current. Learning what you do—and do not—need to know to move beyond your own discipline is a critical skill for interdisciplinary researchers. The chapters in this volume suggest some of the strategies these authors have used, including the value of interdisciplinary colleagues as sources of guidance and information.

Institutional obstacles also hamper interdisciplinary research. As we have discussed interdisciplinary approaches with our colleagues, we heard several stories from faculty members who had been warned by their departmental chairs not to stray too far from their own discipline. Tenure and promotion, they were told, depended on publishing in their disciplinary journals and using methods and theories with which their colleagues were familiar. In our own university, while administrators were supportive of our development of interdisciplinary approaches to urban health research and teaching, the practical questions of who gets overhead, release time, and teaching credit arose with every effort. Like others, we often found that disciplinary approaches elicited fewer questions and concerns, forcing us to consider whether the extra effort our interdisciplinary initiatives required was worth the benefits. In the final chapter, we review some of the methods the authors of these chapters have used to overcome the challenges posed by their choice of interdisciplinary approaches.

INTERDISCIPLINARITY AND THEORIES OF KNOWLEDGE

A fourth theme that several authors consider is the intersection between interdisciplinary and social constructivist perspectives. Social constructivists believe that reality is produced and reproduced by people acting on their *interpretations* and their *knowledge* of the world.[23] In disciplines like anthropology, history, and some schools of thought in political science and sociology, scholars point out that the answers to the question of how, for example, city living affects health are not univocal but depend on the geographic, cultural, socioeconomic, religious, and other statuses of the analyst. Although interdisciplinary approaches also acknowledge the value of different voices, there is no inherent belief that all knowledge is "constructed" or that essential truths do not exist.

Bringing together interdisciplinary teams that include both constructivists and essentialists may be something like asking atheists and devout believers to write scriptures together. However, failing to include these two fundamental approaches to modern scholarship may limit researchers' ability to understand phenomena of interest. For public health researchers, the most useful perspective may be a pragmatic one. Not all points of view are equally effective in reducing threats to health, so perhaps the utility of any given perspective depends on its value to fulfilling the public health mission of promoting health and preventing disease. This perspective is further discussed by Angotti and Sze in Chapter Two.

To give an example, the HIV epidemic has evoked numerous analyses from both constructivists and essentialists.[24, 25] Most (but not all) researchers now agree that the human immunodeficiency virus has been established as the proximate cause of HIV infection beyond any reasonable doubt, and this analysis has led to the development of antiretroviral treatments that have substantially reduced morbidity and mortality—but not HIV incidence—around the world. However, the effectiveness of HIV prevention campaigns depends almost wholly on the perceptions of their recipients, who construct meaning for the messages based on their socioeconomic status, culture, nationality, gender, sexual orientation, and so on. From this pragmatic perspective, the essentialist framework has contributed a tool to treat the infection, and the constructivist approach yields insights for prevention and disease management. The more general point is that only research teams that appreciate the differences between and respective value of each approach can make informed decisions about research and intervention priorities. In Chapter Eleven, Jones and Liburd apply this insight to their discussion of the cultural dimensions of diabetes.

METHODOLOGICAL CHALLENGES AND APPROACHES TO INTERDISCIPLINARITY

A fifth theme is that interdisciplinary researchers need to become familiar with a wide range of new and old methods for data collection and analysis. New methodological technologies that have merged in the last decade or two are DNA sequencing, geographic information systems (GIS), network analysis, community-based participatory research, multilevel and structural equation modeling, and software for textual analysis. In some cases, these new technologies have enabled new interdisciplinary research questions. For example, infectious disease researchers used polymerase chain reaction methods to sequence the genotype of *Mycobacterium tuberculosis* in a cluster of patients in New Jersey and then mapped cases using GIS. This analysis led to new insights into the transmission of various strains of tuberculosis in urban neighborhoods and suggested tuberculosis control strategies.[26] Similarly, in Chapter Five, Maantay and her colleagues map asthma cases identified by the health care system and levels of environmental pollutants assessed by the city environmental agency to analyze the distribution of asthma hospitalizations.

Some observers have emphasized the high concept dimensions of interdisciplinary research: integrating findings from different levels of analysis, synthesizing theories from different disciplines, or framing new paradigms. We have been equally impressed by the practical and operational questions of mastering new methods, learning new languages, integrating databases collected by different agencies, and creating appropriate organizational structures to support interdisciplinary research.

INTERDISCIPLINARITY: WHICH DISCIPLINES WHEN?

For urban health researchers, *interdisciplinary* may include more players than two or more academic disciplines, a sixth theme that recurs in this book. Among the other participants in the cases described in the following chapters are other professions like urban planning, law, architecture, and engineering; representatives of other sectors such as education, housing, criminal justice, and transportation; social movements and activists from environmental justice, women's health, food justice, occupational safety and health, and human rights; policymakers from local, state, national, and global governance bodies; and residents of the communities most affected by health problems. Each of these stakeholders has a role to play in conceptualizing, implementing, interpreting, and disseminating research studies.

Of course, not all interdisciplinary research includes all these players, but knowing who to invite to the table, when to make the invitation, what to serve to bring and keep guests at the table, and how to prevent food fights at the banquet are critical skills for interdisciplinary urban health researchers. The growing body of literature on community-based participatory research[27-29] can help researchers identify some of the tasks, but in our view, this literature often underestimates the difficulties of this approach and pays inadequate attention to the importance and methods of bringing in nonacademic participants from social movements to policymakers and businesses. In Chapter Two, Angotti and Sze discuss some of the issues that arise when environmental justice activists interact with researchers to apply research methods to policy questions.

ROLE DEFINITIONS IN INTERDISCIPLINARY RESEARCH AND PRACTICE

Seventh, the chapters in this book suggest that strengthening the capacity for IR in urban health will require redefining the roles of various participants in the research enterprise. Both new and experienced researchers will need the ability to communicate with researchers from other disciplines. They will need to have an appreciation of their own discipline and its contributions but also an understanding of its limitations, especially in regard to the particular problem under investigation. No single researcher will be able to master all the disciplines and methods needed to understand a particular problem, but they will need to have a methodology for learning new content and also for identifying the unique contributions of other disciplines and methods. In their analysis of the "policy-induced breakdown" of health in African American communities in Chapter Six, Geronimus and Thompson show some of the benefits of integrating biological, social science, public health, and historical perspectives but also the complexity of synthesizing findings across levels and disciplines.

Students also will need to learn new skills. Researchers debate whether it is better to introduce students to other disciplines and the value of IR before, during, or after they have mastered their own discipline.[30, 31] In our view, the more important question is what are the IR competencies that students need and how can we best assure those competencies are achieved by the end of training.

Universities, too, will need to take on new roles. Already, many institutions have created new units to study urban health, and often, these units reflect an interdisciplinary perspective. For example, the doctoral program in public health at the University of California, Los Angeles, requires students to choose both a major and minor area of concentration.[32] And at City University of New York, we have created a variety of pathways by which public health and social science graduate students interested in urban health can study across disciplines.[33]

MULTIPLE LEVELS OF INTERVENTION

The eighth and final theme we highlight is the value of interdisciplinary approaches to integrating and reconciling research and practice that aims to improve population health and that seeks to promote social justice. Modern public health research emerged in the nineteenth century as reformers and scientists, first in Europe then in the United States and elsewhere, joined forces to document the adverse impact of urban living conditions on the health of residents. They then acted to improve urban conditions such as housing, water, nutrition, working conditions, and sanitation.[34] In the past century, however, public health research became increasingly divorced from its roots in social justice and focused more on documenting individual-level risk factors and studying the impact of various techniques for financing and delivering medical care.

In this century, social movements such as the women's movement, the labor movement, the environmental movement, and more recently, movements for living wages and food justice, more than health researchers, have followed the tradition of linking health improvements with social justice. Several chapters in this volume describe the contributions these social movements have made to improvements in urban health.

Interdisciplinary researchers can contribute to the reintegration of these two concerns by studying the linkages among allocation of power, political and social processes, and health outcomes. For example, researchers from several fields, including psychology, biology, immunology, and public health, have documented a range of adverse health effects associated with higher levels of social stress.[35–38] At the same time, social scientists have shown that social processes and conditions such as racism, stigma, poverty, and unemployment produce high levels of stress at the individual and population levels. One interpretation of these findings is to develop interventions to help individuals better manage their response to stress;[39] another is to identify changes in social structures or conditions that could reduce levels of stress, as Geronimus and Thompson describe in Chapter Six. Only researchers who can consider and understand the range of evidence on these questions can compare the relative efficacy of these two approaches.

Undoubtedly, cities in both the developed and developing world will continue to grow throughout this century. What will this growth mean for the health of urban populations? Morbidity and mortality patterns suggest that the urban environment and the complexity of factors that contribute to the growth of cities can have both a positive and negative impact on health. Urban health researchers face a formidable challenge in sorting out how the urban environment influences health and well-being. We hope this volume will contribute to knowledge that can be translated into policies and practices to improve the health of urban communities.

SUMMARY

In this chapter, we have examined the unique contributions that interdisciplinary approaches to research and practice can make to improving population health in cities. We have described the growing interest of funders, researchers, and health professionals in interdisciplinary perspectives and identified common themes that will emerge in the chapters that follow. These themes include the importance of considering the impact of different levels of organization on health in order to develop multilevel interventions, the methodological and practical challenges that confront interdisciplinary researchers, the process of deciding which disciplines to include in a specific research project, and the importance of defining appropriate roles for the various participants in interdisciplinary urban health research. Ultimately, the approaches to research and practice described in this volume will help health professionals strengthen the health-promoting features of urban environments and to mitigate those factors that damage health.

DISCUSSION QUESTIONS

1. Identify what you believe to be the most pressing urban health problems in the United States and globally. What do you think are the characteristics of urban health problems that warrant interdisciplinary approaches to research and intervention?

2. What insights might be lost if these problems were addressed from within a single discipline?

3. Pick an area of urban health that you think requires an interdisciplinary approach and explain (a) why it requires an interdisciplinary approach, (b) the criteria you would have for selecting the disciplines to engage, and (c) the processes you would use to pull together a well-functioning interdisciplinary team.

4. Using the example from question 3, what challenges would you face and what you would do to overcome them?

NOTES

1. United Nations Population Division. *World Urbanization Prospects: The 1999 Revision.* New York: United Nations Population Division, 2002.

2. Gelbard, A., Haub, C., and Kent, M. World population beyond six billion. *Population Bulletin,* 54, no. 1 (1999): 3–40.

3. United Nations Centre for Human Settlements, *State of the World's Cities, 2001.* Nairobi, Kenya: United Nations, 2001.

4. Committee on Assuring the Health of the Public in the 21st Century. *The Future of the Public's Health in the 21st Century.* Washington, D.C.: National Academies Press, 2003.

5. Committee on Educating Public Health Professionals for the 21st Century. *Who Will Keep the Public Healthy? Educating Public Health Professionals for the 21st Century.* Washington, D.C.: National Academies Press, 2003.

6. Committee on Facilitating Interdisciplinary Research. *Facilitating Interdisciplinary Research.* Washington, D.C.: National Academies Press, 2005.

7. Zerhouni, E. The NIH roadmap. *Science,* 302 (2003): 63–65.

8. Freudenberg, N., Galea, S., and Vlahov, D., eds. *Cities and the Health of the Public.* Nashville, Tenn.: Vanderbilt University Press, 2006.

9. Dye, C. Health and urban living. *Science,* 319 (2008): 766–769.

10. Yeh, M-C., and Katz, D. L. Food, nutrition and the health of urban populations. In N. Freudenberg, S. Galea, and D. Vlahov, eds., *Cities and the Health of the Public,* pp. 106–125. Nashville, Tenn.: Vanderbilt University Press, 2006.

11. Link, B. G., and Phelan, J. Social conditions as fundamental causes of disease. *Journal of Health and Social Behavior,* 35, Special issue (1995): 80–94.

12. Farmer, P. *Pathologies of Power.* Berkeley: University of California Press, 2003.

13. Kretzmann, J. P., and McKnight, J. L. *Building Communities from the Inside Out: A Path Towards Finding and Mobilizing Community Assets.* Chicago: ACTA, 1993.

14. James, S. A., Schultz, A. J., and van Olphen, J. Social capital, poverty, and community health. In S. Saegert, P. Thompson, and M. Warren, eds., *Building Social Capital in Urban Communities,* pp. 165–188. Thousand Oaks, Cal.: Sage, 2001.

15. Schulz, A. J., Parker, E. A., Israel, B. A., Allen, A., Decarlo, M., and Lockett, M. Addressing social determinants of health through community-based participatory research: The East Side Village Health Worker Partnership. *Health Education and Behavior,* 29, no. 3 (June 2002): 326–341.

16. Almedom, A. M. Social capital and mental health: An interdisciplinary review of primary evidence. *Social Science and Medicine,* 61, no. 5 (2005): 943–964.

17. Kim, D., Subramanian, S. V., and Kawachi, I. Bonding versus bridging social capital and their associations with self-rated health: A multilevel analysis of 40 U.S. communities. *Journal of Epidemiology and Community Health,* 60, no. 2 (2006): 116–122.

18. Pridmore, P., Thomas, L., Havemann, K., Sapag, J., and Wood, L. Social capital and healthy urbanization in a globalized world. *Journal of Urban Health,* 84, no. 3, Suppl (2007): 130–143.

19. Stokols, D., Fuqua, J., Gress, J., Harvey, R., Phillips, K., Baezconde-Garbanati, L., Unger, J., Palmer, P., Clark, M. A., Colby, S. M., Morgan, G., and Trochim, W. Evaluating transdisciplinary science. *Nicotine and Tobacco Research,* Suppl 1 (December 5, 2003): S21–39.

20. Schulze, M. B., and Hu, F. B. Primary prevention of diabetes: What can be done and how much can be prevented? *Annual Review of Public Health,* 26 (2005): 445–467.

21. Finkelstein, E. A., Ruhm, C. J., and Kosa, K. M. Economic causes and consequences of obesity. *Annual Review of Public Health,* 26 (2005): 239–257.

22. French, S. A., Story, M., and Jeffery, R. W. Environmental influences on eating and physical activity. *Annual Review of Public Health,* 22 (2001): 309–335.

23. Berger, P. L., and Luckmann, T. *The Social Construction of Reality.* New York: Anchor Books, 1966.

24. Herek, G. M., Capitanio, J. P., and Widaman, K. F. Stigma, social risk, and health policy: Public attitudes toward HIV surveillance policies and the social construction of illness. *Health Psychology,* 22, no. 5 (2003): 533–540.

25. Shefer, T., Strebel, A., Wilson, T., Shabalala, N., Simbayi, L., Ratele, K., Potgieter, C., and Andipatin, M. The social construction of sexually transmitted infections (STIs) in South African communities. *Qualitative Health Research,* 12, no. 10 (2002): 1373–1390.

26. Mathema, B., Bifani, P. J., Driscoll, J., Steinlein, L., Kurepina, N., Moghazeh, S. L., Shashkina, E., Marras, S. A., Campbell, S., Mangura, B., Shilkret, K., Crawford, J. T., Frothingham, R., and Kreiswirth, B. N. Identification and evolution of an IS6110 low-copy-number *Mycobacterium tuberculosis* cluster. *Journal of Infectious Diseases,* 185, no. 5 (March 1, 2002): 641–649.

27. Minkler, M., and Wallerstein, N., eds. *Community-Based Participatory Research for Health.* San Francisco: Jossey-Bass, 2003.

28. Israel, B., Eng, E., Schulz, A. J., and Parker, E. A., eds. *Methods in Community-Based Participatory Research for Health.* San Francisco: Jossey-Bass, 2005.

29. Cook, W. K. Integrating research and action: A systematic review of community-based participatory research to address health disparities in environmental and occupational health in the USA. *Journal of Epidemiology and Community Health,* 62, no. 8 (2008): 668–676.

30. Lattuca, L. R. *Creating Interdisciplinarity.* Nashville, Tenn.: Vanderbilt University Press, 2001.

31. Hadorn, G. H., Hoffman-Reim, H., Biber-Klemm, S., Grossenbacher-Manusy, W., Joye, D., Pohl, C., Weisman, U., and Zemp, E., eds., *Handbook of Interdisciplinary Research.* New York: Springer, 2008.

32. UCLA. *2008–2009 Department of Community Health Sciences: Doctoral Program Handbook.* Available at http://www.ph.ucla.edu/chs/pdf/Doctoral_handbook.pdf. Accessed on January 23, 2009.

33. Freudenberg, N., and Klitzman, S. Teaching urban health. In S. Galea and D. Vlahov, eds., *Handbook of Urban Health* (pp. 521–538). New York: Springer Verlag, 2005.

34. Rosen, G. *A History of Public Health* (expanded ed.). Baltimore: Johns Hopkins University Press, 1993.

35. Gunnar, M., and Quevedo, K. The neurobiology of stress and development. *Annual Review of Psychology,* 58 (2007): 145–173.

36. Sapolsky, R. M. The influence of social hierarchy on primate health. *Science,* 308, no. 5722 (2005): 648–652.

37. Steffen, P. R., Smith, T. B., Larson, M., and Butler, L. Acculturation to Western society as a risk factor for high blood pressure: A meta-analytic review. *Psychosomatic Medicine,* 68, no. 3 (2006): 386–397.

38. Stewart, J. A. The detrimental effects of allostasis: Allostatic load as a measure of cumulative stress. *Journal of Physiological Anthropology,* 25, no. 1 (2006): 133–145.

39. Brondolo, E., Thompson, S., Brady, N., Appel, R., Cassells, A., Tobin, J. N., and Sweeney, M. The relationship of racism to appraisals and coping in a community sample. *Ethnicity and Disease,* 15, no. 4, Suppl 5 (2005): S5–14–9.

CHAPTER

2

ENVIRONMENTAL JUSTICE PRAXIS: IMPLICATIONS FOR INTERDISCIPLINARY URBAN PUBLIC HEALTH

TOM ANGOTTI, JULIE SZE

LEARNING OBJECTIVES

- Define environmental justice and explain its relevance to urban health.

- Describe the roles that social movements and activists can play in studying and reducing urban health problems.

- Compare the perspectives of health professionals and community activists in addressing urban health problems and analyze the strengths and weaknesses of each.

- Discuss the contributions the environmental justice movements bring to interdisciplinary research on health.

As public health professionals and academics seek to work across disciplines and sectors to solve complex public health problems, they often come into contact with two potential allies: (a) community activists who share the same objectives and who are unconcerned with disciplinary boundaries and (b) professionals from other fields who are similarly driven to cross disciplinary boundaries to achieve their goals. In this chapter, we tell the stories of professionals and activists who, without any training in public health, organized in their communities to successfully change public policies that had significant negative public health impacts in their own communities and far beyond. These activists are part of the environmental justice movement which, since it emerged in the 1980s, has addressed some of the most critical urban health crises that have disparate effects due to economic and racial inequalities, including high rates of asthma, obesity, and cancer. The stories suggest that public health practitioners need to take note of the field of environmental justice—both the social movements and the academic research on environmental justice—as an important source of lessons about how to analyze contemporary urban public health problems and find solutions to them.

We tell these stories from the perspective of two academics who have ourselves engaged with the environmental justice movements as practitioners and researchers. Although neither of us was trained in public health (Angotti has an advanced degree in urban planning, Sze in American studies), both of us became involved in urban public health problems through engagement with environmental justice issues and found ourselves crossing disciplines to address these issues. First, we were working in communities in which public health problems, as opposed to narrower concerns about environmental quality or the built environment per se, were the major focus of organizing. Second, although we were generally interested in the impact of the built environment on politically disenfranchised populations, environmental justice organizing questioned in a very dramatic way many public policies that partially shaped the built environment and had serious impacts on public health. Third, we were concerned with the complex relationship between academic institutions and local communities and the ways that educators engage with social justice issues, and our experiences with environmental justice helped shed light on these interactions.

Our own work encompasses an approach to research that emphasizes engagement in practical, problem-solving activity and shapes research in the pursuit of practical objectives through interaction with urban communities.[1] Julie Sze's early work for several environmental justice community-based organizations helped her develop an understanding of how environmental justice activism was linked to complex urban health epidemics,[2] work that she is continuing as director of the Environmental Justice Project at the University of California at Davis. Tom Angotti's work with community-based planning in New York City shows how environmental justice activists gravitated toward comprehensive community planning as a means to address complex urban health problems while at the same time forestalling displacement from neighborhoods in which economic and health conditions are improving.[3] This follows the tradition of advocacy planning,[4] which emerged when urban planners worked with low-income African American communities during the Civil Rights era to forestall displacement and develop strategies for community development and preservation, as we discuss later.

Although neither author was trained as a public health professional, we have learned to appreciate the importance of interdisciplinary knowledge and practice to solve the pressing urban public health problems in ways that go beyond traditional epidemiology and traditional urban planning. We attempt to use with flexibility the tools of applied social science research and exchange knowledge with community activists in a way that can lead to concrete solutions and policy changes. Our own experiences and engagement with other practitioners confirm that environmental justice can play a central role in the development of new approaches that combine an understanding of holistic and multi-level causation with complex multifaceted proposals for intervention.

In our own research and advocacy experience, we have identified what we call *environmental justice praxis*—a practice based on a holistic worldview that integrates environmental justice organizing, policy analysis, and research. Environmental justice praxis also opens up new roads to interdisciplinary practice. Our contention is that the environmental justice movement has been a major catalyst for holistic activism, research, and policy, and it has drawn on knowledge from a variety of fields. In this essay, we focus on the integration of urban planning and public health, but we do not doubt that important lessons can be learned from the relationships with other professional disciplines. We believe, therefore, that contemporary environmental justice praxis can help to reintegrate and reimagine the fields of public health and urban planning in bold and innovative ways. These two disciplines were founded over a century ago in response to urban epidemics, but over the years, they have divided for a variety of reasons.[2,5,6]

We draw on two case studies to illustrate what we mean by environmental justice praxis and give examples of how it can inform the theory and practice of interdisciplinary public health. The first is from New York City where, in response to the concentration of waste facilities in areas with high asthma rates, environmental justice activists played a central role in the development of a comprehensive citywide solid waste management plan informed by principles of community health and social justice. The second case study is in the San Francisco Bay Area where an innovative community-based organization, Asian Pacific Environmental Network (APEN), works to promote environmental justice, community development, and participatory democracy in low-income Asian immigrant and Asian American communities. Despite the significant differences between these cases—they revolve around distinct issues (waste and housing policies), involve different cultural and racial groups (African American, Latino, and Asian), and are on opposite sides of the country—in both cases, activists used environmental justice as their analytic framework to understand community health and environmental problems and to advocate for solutions through community organizing. In both cases, we found that disparate health and environmental effects triggered community organizing, but we also discovered that environmental justice advocates consistently defined health as more than reducing disease rates. They developed their own plans and strategies that reimagined urban development and the built environment and advanced public health policies in broad, holistic terms.

To present this argument, we first provide an overview of the environmental justice movement in U.S. cities and show the centrality of public health concerns in this movement. Second, we show how the built environment can exacerbate urban public health problems for racial minorities and how environmental justice organizing can suggest urban planning remedies. One of the major advances of the environmental justice movement has been its generation of strategies to reintegrate long-divided areas of knowledge and practice, particularly urban planning and public health, and reinject in these professions an explicitly social justice approach to health problems. Lastly, one of the key lessons that we hope to impart to students seeking to do the hard work of interdisciplinary, social justice oriented public health work is the importance of understanding the relationship between social justice movements and the politics of knowledge. By politics of knowledge, we mean how power relationships shape the production and use of knowledge. This requires us to highlight rather than obscure the occasionally fraught and contested relationships between communities and academic institutions.

ENVIRONMENTAL JUSTICE AND PUBLIC HEALTH

The U.S.-based environmental justice movement emerged in the 1980s as a result of a confluence of events and reports about the inequitable burden of toxic facilities and pollution on low-income communities and communities of color. This brought the terms *environmental racism* and *environmental justice* into the public sphere and policy discourse.[7] In response to pressures from social movements—and informed by academic research—government agencies also incorporated environmental justice as a basis for public policy at the federal, state, regional, and local levels. A landmark study in 1987 showed how toxic sites across the country were disproportionately located in and near communities of color.[8] In 1991, the first National People of Color Conference on Environmental Justice brought together groups from throughout the nation who were struggling with industries, utilities, and waste facilities that contaminated their communities and were suspected causes of major health problems such as cancer, asthma, and respiratory disease. One outcome of this gathering was the principles of environmental justice.[9] The environmental justice movement challenges public policies responsible for the disproportionate burden of pollution borne by people and communities of color, asserting that this is in fact a manifestation of racism.

The environmental justice movement broadly redefined the environment as the places where people of color live, work, play, pray, and learn, and not just phenomena measured by individual pollution indicators or exposure levels. The movement sought to show how environmental health risks are not uniform across social groups or geographically; for example, racial minority children, youth, and families in the United States disproportionately face risks associated with airborne pollution and exposure to lead paint. At the same time, the communities where they live and go to school have unequal access to environmental amenities such as parks and playgrounds. Thus, poor health and inadequate access to a healthy living environment are key features of the landscape of urban inequality, comparable to poor education, housing, income, and social mobility. In response to these conditions, communities of color have used the framework and language of the environmental justice movement and its focus on disproportionate pollution exposure to combat urban health problems in cities like San Diego, Boston, Detroit, Los Angeles, and New Orleans—in addition to our cases in Oakland and New York City.

Although environmental concerns are not always linked in theory or practice with public health issues, the environmental justice movement from the start established a strong link between environmental health and the built environment that led them to the public health and urban planning disciplines. In tackling complex urban environmental health problems, community-based activists gravitate toward engagement with the fields of public health and planning and many other specialized disciplines. Many activists learn how to "become" planners and health practitioners when they engage with highly specialized knowledge and practices, whether or not they are formally educated as such at any time in their careers.

Environmental justice practice that is broadly focused on community well-being as well as removing negative health impacts offers many opportunities for interdisciplinary professional and academic work. The intrinsically complex nature and unique characteristics of the problems activists face in large urban environments lead them to seek broad analyses and solutions. Because they have no particular stake in maintaining disciplinary boundaries, environmental justice activists are often natural partners for interdisciplinary researchers and professionals. Interdisciplinary and holistic approaches may help deal with complex, local problems where solutions are resistant to conventional discipline-based approaches. This is clearly one reason that many public health and urban planning practitioners have been naturally drawn to such approaches. Through our case studies, we show how environmental justice practitioners use technical knowledge that spans urban planning, public health, and other disciplines, and which incorporates professional expertise to achieve broad goals of social and environmental justice. We discuss the opportunities and barriers encountered by environmental justice advocates to illuminate these dynamics as the search for improved urban health continues in the twenty-first century.

THE BUILT ENVIRONMENT, URBAN PLANNING, AND URBAN PUBLIC HEALTH

Public health and urban planning arose in the early part of the twentieth century as related interdisciplinary fields that focused on urban public health problems and the conditions that caused them. As the nineteenth-century urban epidemics that gave rise to these professions subsided, the professions became more specialized and tended to work in separate local government administrative departments. The divergence between city planning and public health widened during the Progressive era in the early twentieth century due to a number of complex factors.[10] At the same time, the passion for social justice that had inspired the creation of these movements began to wane.[11]

The academic departments created at universities to train practitioners in these fields also expanded, developed specializations, and tended to reinforce divisions among the professions. As the presence of the professions in local governments grew, they developed complex regulatory systems and administrative institutions staffed by specialized professionals. In the long run, these have not been well equipped to engage complex, multifaceted health issues with multiple causes and enact policy changes to improve urban public health. This has been particularly noticeable in large, complex urban areas with significant social and health disparities.

All applied professions are subject to a tendency toward narrow determinism focused on quantifiable variables that are easily understood and interventions that produce immediate, local, quantifiable, and visible results that nevertheless fail to affect larger systemic problems. Within the field of urban planning in the United States, which was initially close to engineering and architecture, criticisms have long been raised against a prevailing tendency toward *physical determinism*. This refers to a tendency to propose changes to the built environment as solutions to social and political problems that require more comprehensive policy changes. Advocacy planners have criticized the efforts of some social reformers to address urban poverty by using "slum clearance" and urban renewal plans that displace poor people without necessarily attacking the conditions that result in poverty and social exclusion. Urban planning practice has come under fire for a narrow focus on solving problems of transportation mobility and access by simply building more highways or mass transit, dealing with inadequate recreational opportunities by simply building more parks, and fixing urban housing problems by simply building more housing for people with limited incomes. Jacobs[12] and Davidoff[4] have written the classic critiques of physical determinism in planning.

Urban planners commonly utilize the comprehensive master plan and zoning as tools to shape the physical environment. Although many master plans incorporate discussions of social equity and environmental health, for the most part they are focused narrowly on the physical environment and often serve only as advisory documents that are not implemented. They are most often prepared for municipal governments in metropolitan regions that are fragmented into many small municipalities. This fragmentation makes it difficult for municipal planning to address larger urban issues, including social, economic, and public health issues that affect entire metropolitan regions. Social and economic inequalities between municipalities are often significant. While regional planning could reduce fragmentation and inequalities, three-fourths of the nation's urban population live in large metropolitan regions with no comprehensive regional planning. As a result, market forces play a substantial role in land-use development, and the options of planning at the municipal level are limited. Zoning is urban planning's main regulatory tool that governs where and what kind of new development can occur. But while zoning originally separated land uses such as industry and housing to improve public health, it has come to be used as a mechanism for reinforcing social and racial separation.[13]

Since the 1980s, concurrent with the emergence of the environmental movements, urban planning began to branch into areas once exclusively occupied by public health and other professional disciplines. At a global level, the 1987 United Nations Conference on the Environment put forth the concept of *sustainability*—generally defined as addressing current needs without compromising the needs of future generations—which challenged all professions to engage in holistic analysis that moves beyond individual and easily defined measures. Planning for sustainability is a rapidly growing practice that includes environmental and public health concerns.[14, 15] In response to criticisms that urban planners contributed to the predominant pattern of suburban sprawl and the consequent problems of air pollution and auto dependence, energy waste, and the disappearance of farmland at urban peripheries, urban planners began to advocate for land-use policies that concentrated new development in already-developed areas. This "smart growth"[16] became a trademark of the American Planning Association. A group of architects and planners known as The New Urbanists emerged in recent decades and called for healthy, walkable communities and transit-oriented development that would reduce dependence on the private automobile and create healthier, more active cities.[17] To some extent, this has fed the growing intensity of real estate development in metropolitan regions, but it also spurred a renewal of interest in the public health consequences of urban growth, particularly the rise in the epidemics of asthma, obesity, and diabetes.

Often citing public health concerns, some urban planners have become advocates for better pedestrian, bicycle, and mass transit infrastructure.[18, 19] Others have begun to address problems of access to healthy food.[20–22] And in a link with the advocacy planning and the civil rights movements of the 1960s, many have focused on community-based planning as a tool for addressing the disparate impact of urban epidemics in a comprehensive, holistic fashion.[3] Still, the tendency toward physical determinism remains powerful. For example, researchers are now calling into question facile claims that building some new parks and bikeways will automatically induce greater physical activity and thus address epidemics such as obesity. In the area of housing, city planners have rejected the older myths that large-scale government-subsidized housing complexes would necessarily improve the lives of poor people, but many planners have also embraced the new myth that smaller scale, mixed-income housing would necessarily be better.[23] As a result, urban planners continue to give a lower priority to the preservation of housing in low-income communities and policies like rent control that help stabilize the lives of families and communities.

Because public health practitioners are increasingly looking at ways in which policies affecting the built environment can foster public health, it appears that there is now a greater appreciation in both professions for the historical roots that bound public health and planning together as interdisciplinary and related fields, both deeply concerned with social justice. This accompanies a growing understanding that they need to be brought together again to resolve today's new and complex urban issues. Environmental justice praxis can help foster this trend. It is not simply a matter of adding public health and urban planning tools to create a larger toolkit of practice but integrating the knowledge and experience from both fields. Although we have found that environmental justice activists often adopt the language and methods of urban planning, the scope of their practice transcends traditional urban planning, master plans, and zoning, as well as the new tools such as environmental impact statements that address narrow environmental concerns without necessarily looking at larger, cumulative impacts. Thus, while urban public health practitioners may learn from collaborations with urban planning practitioners, both face the challenge of moving beyond institutional borders and regulatory boundaries to solve broader problems and incorporate social justice as a fundamental principle.

For example, in arguing for innovative approaches to housing and health, Roderick Lawrence rejects the biomedical model and advocates a holistic approach that incorporates biological, cultural, economic, political, psychological, and social elements.[24] He proposes an ecological approach to health that looks at four components: (a) the individual, including genetic makeup; (b) agents and vectors (disease); (c) the physical and social environment; and (d) available resources. Ultimately, Lawrence defines health as not only freedom from disease but as the relationship of people to their social environment. Health allows people to achieve their potential in life. He defines housing as both a product and a process. Thus, planners and health professionals should not only focus on removing negative health impacts but also work to promote well-being through a careful focus on communities. This emphasis on urban community health, defined as more than removing pollution or the absence of disease, is also clear in housing-based environmental justice campaigns that link public health and urban planning, as shown in our second case study.

ENVIRONMENTAL AND SOCIAL JUSTICE, INTERDISCIPLINARITY, AND THE POLITICS OF KNOWLEDGE

We have defined environmental justice praxis as a holistic integration of organizing, policy analysis, and research. Environmental justice praxis also opens new roads to interdisciplinary practice. In this section, we discuss some key examples of research that we believe exemplify this integration of organizing, policy analysis, and research. These examples are particularly significant because they squarely focus on the social justice question: Why do so many racial minorities in urban and disenfranchised communities face such high rates of pollution exposure and the ensuing health risks?

Environmental justice activists are heavily invested in understanding why communities of color are disproportionately impacted by diseases that have an urban and environmental health component, such as asthma and lead poisoning. Health-disparities research and social epidemiology focus on "extrinsic" factors such as class, race, and power dynamics.[25] Environmental justice activists have also been a key factor in innovative public and environmental health research on complex urban problems such as disproportionately high minority childhood asthma rates.[26] Two recent studies, one in

New York and another in California, suggest new paths to knowledge emerging from environmental justice praxis.

The first study is Jason Corburn's *Street Science: Community Knowledge and Environmental Health Justice.*[27] In this book, Corburn discusses environmental justice activism and asthma research as one of his examples of "street science," which he defines as a framework that joins local insights with professional and scientific methods. The goal of street science is to improve scientific inquiry, environmental health policy, and decision making. At the heart of *Street Science* are four case studies from Greenpoint/Williamsburg in New York City, where diverse racial and ethnic, low-income populations practice what he calls "science on the streets of Brooklyn." The other case studies by Sze are on asthma, childhood lead poisoning, and small sources of air pollution.[2] Sze's study discusses asthma activism in West Harlem, another New York City neighborhood. Some of the larger issues addressed through these particular studies include the limits of traditional risk assessment and the politics of mapping health and environment risk.

Through these studies, Corburn provides a theoretical model for understanding key characteristics of what he calls "local knowledge," its paradoxes, and its contributions to environmental health policy. Street science, at its best, identifies health hazards and highlights research questions that professionals may otherwise ignore, provides hard-to-gather exposure data, involves difficult to reach populations, and expands possibilities for interventions, resulting in what he calls "improved science and democracy." Using a framework common among urban planners, Corburn explicitly calls for environmental and public health researchers, policymakers, and urban planners to become what Schön has called "reflective practitioners."[28] At the same time, he is careful to reject the idea of street science as a panacea. He states that it does not devalue but rather revalues science. He is not calling for a populism where the "community" replaces "experts" but for a better understanding of how knowledge that is "co-produced" by local and professional constituencies can lead to better health, science, and policy. This is consistent with other theoretical frameworks that emphasize the social production of knowledge. (See also Chapter One in this volume.)

Second, a series of major studies conducted in Los Angeles highlights how environmental and health inequalities are produced and reproduced. To highlight just one study, a 2004 analysis of ambient air toxics exposure and health risks among schoolchildren in Los Angeles found that African American and Latino youth bear the largest share of the burden of air pollution risks and that the respiratory hazards associated with air toxics appear to negatively affect indices of academic performance.[29] The research collaborative that conducted this study is notable for several reasons. First, the team is interdisciplinary in its composition: Pastor is an economist, Morello-Frosch is from public health, and Sadd is a geographer. Second, their interdisciplinary research was explicitly linked to environmental justice organizing. Third, the work addressed public policy.

The same collaborative team performed similar research in the San Francisco Bay Area. They completed a report, "Still Toxic After All These Years: Air Quality and

Environmental Justice in the San Francisco Bay Area"[30] for the Bay Area Environmental Health Collaborative, which includes some of the area's leading environmental justice and community health organizations. Their research is one of the few examples of team-based research in environmental justice, and each brings its own disciplinary methods to the larger collaboration. Team-based research is common in scientific disciplines and in public health but is far less common in urban planning and has rarely been used within an environmental justice framework.

In utilizing different disciplinary methods and frameworks, this research collaborative was able to ask better questions and provide better answers than existing research on air pollution in California. Their collaboration clearly "adds value" and opens up new ways of looking at phenomena beyond those favored in their disciplinary training. For example, Morello-Frosch, a trained public health specialist, in a critique that focuses on the political economy of place, thinks and writes in a disciplinary tradition distinct from the one she was trained in and partly draws from geography and ethnic studies.[31] By integrating relevant social and legal theories with a spatialized economic critique, she formulates a more supple theory of environmental discrimination that focuses on historical patterns of industrial development and racialized labor markets, suburbanization and segregation, and economic restructuring. Morello-Frosch et al.[29] discuss their collaboration, a multiyear project working with Communities for a Better Environment, a community-based organization in Los Angeles and the Bay Area.

This research collaborative has helped draw attention to the use of the *precautionary principle* in environmental justice praxis. This principle calls for preventing harm to the environment and human health by shifting the burden of proof from regulatory bodies and residents to polluters and producers, who must demonstrate the safety of a new product, process, or urban development proposal. Public health and cancer activists have advanced this notion with respect to asthma. Environmental justice activists are a major constituency among urban health advocates supporting the precautionary principle, particularly around asthma.[2,33]

This interdisciplinary research has also had a significant impact on policy, particularly at agencies like the California Air Resources Board where the researchers received a large grant for a study, "Integrating Indicators of Cumulative Impact and Socioeconomic Vulnerability into Regulatory Decision-making."[34] In addition to peer validation and respect from state agencies looking for guidance and research to direct policy, the research has enabled Morello-Frosch and her colleagues to continue to collaborate with community groups. For example, the group was contracted to write a report for the Bay Area Environmental Health Collaborative,[30] a coalition of groups concerned with air quality and its health impacts.

Corburn's *Street Science* and the interdisciplinary research of Pastor, Morello-Frosch, and Sadd show how engagement with social movements can drive innovative interdisciplinary research that asks better questions and informs urban public health policy. We now turn to our case studies to illustrate how the opportunities and challenges for environmental justice praxis can further advance urban public health.

ASTHMA AND THE ENVIRONMENTAL JUSTICE CAMPAIGN FOR A SOLID WASTE PLAN IN NEW YORK CITY

The environmental justice movement in New York City emerged in response to public health crises that had particularly significant impacts in low-income communities of color. The most important of these crises was asthma. The highest child hospitalization rates for asthma tend to be concentrated in low-income neighborhoods, among which the South Bronx, Harlem, and Central Brooklyn stand out, as shown in Figure 2.1.

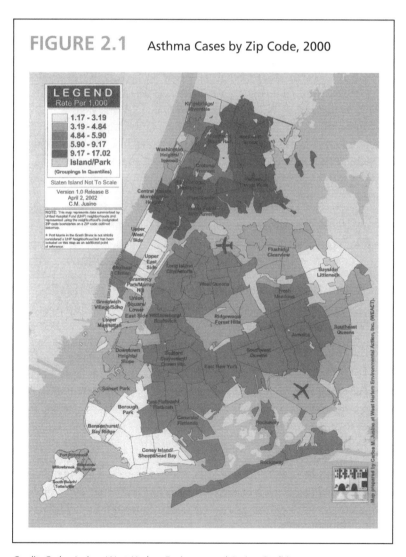

Credit: Carlos Jusino, West Harlem Environmental Action Coalition.

Neighborhood activists in these areas made the connection between high asthma rates (and other respiratory illnesses) and the concentration of noxious facilities, including waste transfer stations, bus depots, and dense highway networks. For those who live and work near such facilities, the operations at these facilities exacerbate asthma because of increased truck traffic, odors, noise, and vermin.[2] Given that most of the polluting activities involve functions that provide citywide and regional services, environmental justice activists found themselves confronting the need to understand not only their own neighborhoods but the larger city and region. In addition, activists focused not only on asthma but its relationship to broader issues of community well-being, to come up with effective solutions.

In July 2006, the New York City Council approved an updated Solid Waste Management Plan (SWMP) covering the city's five boroughs, which have a total population of about 8 million people. This complex, highly technical citywide plan was in large part an outgrowth of a plan put together years earlier by a coalition of neighborhood groups led by environmental justice activists in the Organization of Waterfront Neighborhoods (OWN). OWN formed in 1996 and, with the help of the Consumers Union, put forth a plan that attempted to provide a comprehensive, citywide solution to the waste problem. OWN's members, mostly neighborhood-based groups concerned about the health consequences of the concentration of privately owned waste transfer stations in their neighborhoods, developed a broad citywide strategy. The neighborhood activists, not the trained land-use or engineering professionals, were the catalyst for a more holistic, comprehensive city plan that cut across neighborhoods and disciplines. The urban planning and health departments were, for the most, absent from the official planning process, which was concentrated mostly in the Department of Sanitation, which contracted out the plan to engineering consultants.

Background and Genesis of the OWN Plan

In 1987, the city raised the fees it charged to private haulers to dump in the Fresh Kills landfill, the last of the city's landfills, the largest in the world, and an environmental hazard for the area in Staten Island where it is located. In 1998, Mayor Rudolph Giuliani announced the closing of the Fresh Kills landfill, in part to pay a political debt to the Borough of Staten Island, a largely European American borough that had given Giuliani the margin of votes he needed to win the election. In 2001, the last city sanitation truck made its delivery to Fresh Kills. Most of the city's waste is now exported under contract with the city.

Starting in 1987, however, the private waste haulers established some eighty-five waste transfer stations in the city where waste could be sorted and put on large tractor-trailers for shipment out of state. The waste companies went where land was cheapest and zoning permitted them. As a result, about 70 percent of all putrescible waste (all commercial waste, including food, except for construction waste and fill) went through transfer stations in north Brooklyn and the south Bronx, in and near low-income communities (the racially and geographically disproportionate problem of waste transfer station siting is not unique to New York City; see Pellow[35]). They brought with them heavy truck traffic, diesel fumes, noise, odors, vermin, and increased risks for asthma and other respiratory diseases. Despite legislation (Local Law 40) requiring the Department of Sanitation to issue siting regulations for these facilities, they had failed to do so. In 1993, regulations were proposed but never passed; in 1997, the city was ordered by a court to issue regulations; in 1998, they issued weak regulations that would have no effect on the concentration of sites; these were unsuccessfully contested in court by OWN, but Sanitation was forced by political pressure from community organizers to tighten up on enforcement.[36]

Although this was clearly a land-use issue, the Department of City Planning never addressed the location and concentration of waste facilities in the city. They could have proposed using the city's "fair share" rules, which were to ensure that no neighborhood had more than its fair share of certain facilities. Although these rules, established in the City's Charter, apply only to certain publicly owned facilities, the planners never evoked the principle or instituted efforts to apply them to all facilities serving a public function. Instead, they deferred to the Sanitation Department and missed an important opportunity to work across departments. The Department of Health instead recognized the critical importance of asthma and began an initiative that included research, education, and prevention; it targeted intervention in neighborhoods with high concentrations of childhood asthma cases. Three neighborhood-based health initiatives in affected areas went beyond traditional regulatory measures and promoted more comprehensive approaches that, in collaboration with community-based advocacy groups, identified elements in the built environment that tended to trigger asthma crises. However, the Department of Sanitation did not engage the health professionals, and they were not obligated to do so by the City. The City Planning Department was also not involved and did not make any changes to zoning regulations that would have restricted waste facilities, and they did not support community-based planning efforts that addressed unhealthy conditions in a comprehensive way.[3]

The OWN/Consumers Union solid waste management plan[37] is based on three principles that the Department of Sanitation had resisted adopting:

1. Retrofit the existing marine waste transfer stations, which are underutilized but relatively evenly spread throughout the city, to handle both domestic and commercial waste streams and substitute barges for polluting tractor-trailers

2. Fully support recycling

3. Enact measures to prevent and reduce waste

The marine-based transfer stations would export most garbage by barge; the city would take responsibility for the large portion of commercial waste (over half the total); and the impact would be distributed more equitably throughout the city. OWN's strategy was based on the understanding (which came out of their political organizing), that to resolve each individual neighborhood's problems there had to be a just plan for the citywide waste stream. This was a direct refutation of the charge often leveled against them by traditional city planners that community-based organizing and planning were necessarily based on the exclusionary Not in My Backyard (NIMBY) sentiments that would prevent any rational siting of public facilities (this argument failed to acknowledge that the city never had a comprehensive plan for siting such facilities). The charges of NIMBYism against OWN activists were also contradicted by the OWN plan itself, which required some neighborhoods with environmental justice claims to accept expanded and modernized marine transfer stations.

OWN activists demonstrated and lobbied elected officials and met with the mayor and his aides. In 2002, Mayor Michael Bloomberg announced that the city was planning to retrofit its existing marine waste transfer stations. The city essentially adopted the principles of OWN's solid waste plan. This decision was a historic moment for the environmental justice movement and the activist-led, community-based planning movement. The OWN plan made sense to the mayor's office because it would cut costs and remove a potential obstacle to gentrification in waterfront neighborhoods they were targeting for new housing development. It strengthened the hand of community groups angling for a greater say in land-use planning so that a better environment would not be accompanied by gentrification and displacement. City Hall followed the principles of growth and efficiency while OWN emphasized equity, but the two came together in a tactical compromise. According to environmental justice activist Eddie Bautista, the plan was resisted by the city's Department of Sanitation, whose job seemed to be defined as only "taking out the trash."[36]

Advocacy Planning and Environmental Justice

Eddie Bautista was OWN's lead organizer for most of its history and worked for the nonprofit New York Lawyers for the Public Interest. He became one of the city's leading experts on solid waste management and a central figure in the development and advancement of OWN's plan and then the city's SWMP. Bautista got involved as an advocate for the neighborhoods that were saturated with waste transfer stations and became a leader in the city's environmental justice movement. He had grown up in Red Hook, one of the Brooklyn neighborhoods affected by waste transfer stations. After the city adopted the principles of the OWN-backed solid waste plan, Bautista became an aide to Mayor Michael Bloomberg and went on to assist in development of the city's first long-term sustainability plan, PlaNYC2030.[38]

What led Bautista and OWN toward a comprehensive, citywide approach? First, according to Bautista, was the realization that the city's experts were always setting the agenda, and to get involved in the discussion, OWN had to have an alternative. OWN hired the Institute for Local Self Reliance, a Washington, D.C.–based nonprofit, to help find that alternative. However, according to Bautista, "one of the problems was that their experience was mostly in recycling, and that wasn't our priority. After a lot of discussion, we realized that what was missing in the traditional approach taken by the environmental movement, which emphasized recycling and waste reduction, was the infrastructure piece" (personal interview by Angotti, June 19, 2006). At a bidder's conference, an OWN member overheard a contractor propose that the city's existing marine-based transfer stations be retrofitted and in some cases expanded to handle the waste from the land-based transfer stations that were concentrated in residential and mixed use neighborhoods. This struck OWN's leadership as a possible citywide solution.

OWN's plan filled a vacuum left by the city's own technical experts in its various departments. But there was another impetus leading the activists to think more globally: solidarity. Bautista recounts how activists from different neighborhoods met at City Council hearings and other public events, developed ties, and supported each other: "There is a powerful emotional need for solidarity. . . . We were all in the same boat." (personal interview by Angotti, June 19, 2006). According to Bautista, it was a political necessity. The mayor and City Council govern on a citywide basis and are therefore more receptive to arguments about citywide policy. OWN activists also anticipated that the city would end up reshaping its solid waste policy, but based on their experiences at the grass roots, they had little confidence that their neighborhoods would be treated fairly. Bautista stated, "We knew that if the city was going to do a citywide strategy, some neighborhoods would get hit." In other words, principles of equity across the board would be sacrificed to keep waste out of the wealthier neighborhoods, a truly NIMBY outcome. (Even after the City Council passed the new SWMP, political leaders in Manhattan's Upper East Side, arguably the wealthiest neighborhood in the world, continued to oppose the plan.)

During the OWN campaign, Bautista entered the program in urban planning at Pratt Institute in Brooklyn and received a master's degree. Bautista said that he gravitated to planning because "so much of our urban life is connected." He says he learned from the battles fought by Jane Jacobs, and from advocacy planning, but also learned how Robert Moses, the city's master builder, "was able to get as much as he could." Throughout the campaign, he worked closely with urban planners, engineers, and public health professionals, including the coauthor of the OWN plan, Barbara Warren.

Tom Angotti first met Bautista when Angotti was a senior planner with the Department of City Planning in the early 1990s and worked on a community-generated plan for Red Hook, a low-income waterfront neighborhood that had successfully fought off two proposed sewage sludge treatment facilities and shut down several private waste transfer stations. After playing a critical role in the environmental justice campaign in Red Hook, Bautista collaborated in the development of the community plan. After Angotti left City Planning, he became professor and chair at the Pratt Institute Graduate Center for Planning and the Environment. He then joined OWN, representing Planners Network, a group of advocacy planners founded in 1975, and advised OWN in a court-endorsed mediation with the Department of Sanitation that was geared toward creating siting regulations for waste facilities (no agreement was reached). He also became Eddie Bautista's thesis advisor. Angotti's role followed closely that of the advocacy planner and is one illustration of how urban planners can step out of their assigned roles to support efforts that are aimed at improving environmental health. It is also an example of how learning and knowledge in academic, professional, and community arenas is a complicated process in which all teach and all learn from one another, as opposed to a top-down and hierarchial approach.[39]

ASIAN IMMIGRANT AND REFUGEE ORGANIZING FOR ENVIRONMENTAL HEALTH AND HOUSING IN THE BAY AREA

In Oakland, California, an environmental justice initiative illustrates how academic, social, and political forces interact to move practice toward new holistic and interdisciplinary approaches. This example is where a community-based organization, Asian Pacific Environmental Network (APEN), works to promote environmental justice, community development, and democracy in low-income Asian immigrant, refugee, and Asian American communities in the Bay Area. APEN was an important leader in the founding of the environmental justice movement, and their innovative programs and campaigns have been recognized nationally. Although the specific issues APEN focuses on are different from OWN, the holistic approach to urban public health and community development is similar. It emphasizes developing democracy (i.e., "speaking for ourselves," a key tenet of the environmental justice movement) and developing local leadership through the language and framework of environmental justice, specifically around issues of housing, displacement, gentrification, and tenants' rights.

Two ongoing campaigns in Oakland and Richmond demonstrate the complexity of APEN's approach to environmental justice in disenfranchised Asian immigrant and refugee communities. The first, called the Laotian Organizing Project (LOP), is based in Richmond, an extremely poor, primarily industrial city populated by African Americans and Laotians. The Laotian community in Contra Costa County lives in one of the most toxic regions in the nation. Surrounded by more than 350 industrial sites and toxic hazards, the people's home, school, and work environments are exposed to dangerous levels of lead, pesticides, and other chemicals on a daily basis. One of the LOP's early organizing successes was the implementation of a multilingual warning system when accidental toxic releases occurred. Before LOP began organizing on this issue, the warning system was only in English, which most of the Laotian community did not speak.[40]

The community's problems have multidimensional roots, and this has led APEN to multidimensional organizing. Because most families in the Laotian community are renters who tend to have less political power than homeowners, organizing on tenant issues was important. LOP's more than 300 active members have focused on the problem of weak housing standards, including endemic problems with mold and lead paint and weak health-based housing regulations and lack of enforcement. LOP launched a campaign to adopt a "just cause" ordinance similar to those in other Bay Area cities. The campaign argues that "everyone has a basic right to continue to live in their communities." LOP's newest front is fighting displacement and winning protections for tenants against unfair evictions. LOP's focus on housing justice strongly affirms a basic principle of environmental justice: "fighting for basic rights to protect our communities where we live, work and play."[41]

Vivian Chang, then-Executive Director of APEN, explained her view that the environment does not just mean pollution exposure (personal interview by Sze, August 5, 2006). For example, many Laotians grow their own food in their gardens (a practice they brought with them upon coming to the United States, journeys that were a result of U.S. interventions in Southeast Asia). Their view is that when tenants are evicted, these gardens and spaces that provide food as well as psychological connection to the land are also destroyed. Thus, environmental justice for Laotians also means community food security and access to environmental "goods" (e.g., gardens and open spaces). APEN also advocated for an enforcement board to deal with code violations and evictions in Richmond.

APEN's other organizing arm, Power in Asians Organizing (PAO), is focused on organizing Asian ethnic communities in the city of Oakland, including large numbers of Vietnamese, Chinese, Laotians, Cambodians, and Filipinos. Like LOP, PAO's core group of community resident/activists focused on safe and affordable housing through their Housing Justice Campaign. PAO, with two other organizations, worked for three years to secure affordable housing at Oak to Ninth, a large housing project of 3,100 residential units located in the heart of PAO's organizing area. The land, a sixty-four acre contaminated parcel on the waterfront, was originally proposed as 100 percent luxury condominiums (in a community where the average family is considered "very low income," i.e., under $35,000/year). Through their campaign, PAO also helped to negotiate 300 entry-level construction career-path placements for Oakland residents, with real penalties for noncompliance. Lastly, $1.65 million will be dedicated to training programs to support immigrants and those formerly incarcerated to get a start in the building trades.

What is perhaps as significant as the concrete goals achieved in both campaigns is that through their direct organizing APEN is taking steps to improve public participation and engagement with urban development and community health in historically and culturally disenfranchised immigrant and refugee populations in complex urban environments. LOP's organizing focuses simultaneously on health, environment, and housing rather than separating and narrowly defining these problems and solutions. LOP's ability to connect these domains, while increasing community engagement, can lead to more dynamic and effective solutions for the multidimensional community and health problems faced by urban low-income communities of color. The vision is dynamic and reflective of the environmental and public health conditions of real-world communities, individuals, and families. For example, as PAO suggested in their press release in response to the Oak to Ninth negotiations, "As a result of this and other community benefits campaigns, Oakland's elected officials are seriously grappling with policies like Inclusionary Zoning that can make sure that developers pay their fair share in Oakland." (Inclusionary zoning generally requires that a portion of new housing units be available to people with low and moderate incomes; some inclusionary zoning ordinances allow developers to develop more market-rate units if they include affordable units.) Like the OWN campaign, APEN focuses on how to use the language of fair share and environmental justice to develop more equitable housing, land use, health, and community economic development policies.

Does postgraduate education with an interdisciplinary focus matter, as it did to Eddie Bautista of OWN? It may in the case of Vivian Chang, who states that her personal experience with collaboration across the activist/academic divide shaped her political and practical vision. Chang previously worked as an organizer with Asian Immigrant Workers Advocates on their garment worker justice campaign, after which she worked briefly with the California Environmental Protection Agency (Cal/EPA) on their cumulative risk project. At Cal/EPA, she learned the importance of having an insider-outsider strategy to successfully implement positive policy change for environmental justice (as Angotti also learned). That is, to be effective, environmental justice activism and policy development needed to have both intermediaries and allies within public agencies and movement pressure from outside the agencies, specifically from community-based organizations. After those experiences, Chang attended the University of California at Los Angeles and received a masters in urban planning. For Chang, graduate education offered both a theoretical framework for interpreting regional economies and industries (e.g., the garment industry in Oakland) as well as pragmatic tools (GIS mapping and how to research particular industries and corporations). According to Chang, "graduate, academic, and professional training helped me develop smarter activist and organizing campaigns (such as living wage campaigns)," because this training helped her understand the dominant discourses and frameworks for policy development.

Chang believes that her personal work and academic experiences work synergistically, leading to innovative approaches to improving community development and public health in low-income Asian immigrant and refugee populations in Bay Area cities, specifically through the language and framework of the environmental justice movement. One of the key questions she grapples with in APEN's programmatic work is: "What does a public health approach to urban development look like?" In part, the answer depends on whether a particular development project or existing policy (whether land use, economic development, housing, environmental, or public health) promotes or negatively impacts community health and improves democracy, what environmental justice scholars call "participatory justice."

APEN strategically uses research as an organizing tool. To document environmental justice problems, APEN and four other environmental justice groups released "Building Healthy Communities from the Ground Up: Environmental Justice in California."[42] The 2003 report begins by outlining the "environmental justice crisis" in California (pollution, toxic waste, working conditions, environmental health risks, poor housing, and inequitable land uses). It then defines "environmental justice approaches to creating healthy communities" and the different strategies that environmental justice organizations have adopted to remediate the problems.

There are, however, notable gaps between the organizing-related research APEN has undertaken (as in the Health Impact Assessment Projects) and academic research in this development project. For instance, there was a health impact assessment (HIA) of the project performed by the University of California at Berkeley Health Impact Group (UCBHIG),[43] a nonpartisan, independent group of graduate students and faculty participating in a seminar on health impact assessment. The HIA differs from the traditional environmental impact assessment because it is voluntary but complements analysis required under law; evaluates environmental, social, and economic effects using the lens of human health; and estimates benefits as well as adverse consequences. On the issue of social equity (poverty, stereotypes, segregation, inequalities), the HIA reports no information. Although this report is quite extensive and is an example of graduate-level, applied training and education in public health related to a land-use and urban planning project, this lack of information on social equity is both disappointing and revealing of the limitations of much academic research, especially given the high profile of the activism by groups like APEN.

CONCLUSION

Opportunities for interdisciplinary urban research and education in academic institutions continue to be challenging and difficult. In the professions, specialization and not interdisciplinary collaboration continues to be of value to practitioners and employers. And government policy tends to focus on individual programs and agencies to solve specific issues and problems without necessarily looking at the whole picture. Holistic approaches are preached and promised by many, but they are often hard to come by in practice. Grand theories may promise efficient and equitable solutions to chronic urban health problems, but in practice, equitable solutions that address differences of race and class are often compromised.

Environmental justice praxis can help address these issues. Through environmental justice praxis, practitioners use technical knowledge that moves among urban planning, public health, and other disciplines, and they incorporate professional expertise to achieve broad goals of social and environmental justice in communities long disenfranchised by race and class. In doing so, environmental justice praxis embodies and represents the best possibilities for holistic urban health research and practice. In crossing disciplinary and organizational barriers, environmental justice practitioners are making both public health and urban policy better, particularly in helping to advance such concepts as cumulative impact and the precautionary principle. Although more orthodox approaches to comprehensive societywide problems often result in relatively greater health risks for low-income communities of color, environmental justice praxis can help ensure that "nobody's backyard" becomes a health risk.

This path is not without challenges, especially because existing divisions and categories are entrenched in both academic training and policy contexts. But environmental justice activists tend to understand that the problems faced by low-income and urban communities of color are relentless and that existing modes of practice are not working. This reality paradoxically creates better conditions for more dynamic and interdisciplinary urban health and environmental research and policy. Our real-world examples from New York and California, coming directly out of the environmental justice movement, show just how and why improved interdisciplinary approaches may help to remediate the worst examples of social injustice (and their health and environmental impacts) at community, city, and regional levels. Ultimately, interdisciplinary urban health is a framework that mirrors much of what is already happening "on the ground" as identified by environmental justice practitioners.

SUMMARY

In this chapter we have explored how interdisciplinary environmental justice praxis can help to reintegrate and reimagine the fields of public health and urban planning. We draw on two case studies of environmental activism: the development of a comprehensive citywide solid waste management plan in New York City and the promotion of environmental justice, community development and participatory democracy among low-income Asian immigrant and Asian American communities in the San Francisco Bay Area. In both cases, activists employed an environmental justice framework in seeking to understand community health and environmental problems and to advocate for solutions through community organizing. They adopted a broad a definition of community health and reimagined urban development, the built environment, and public health in broad, holistic terms. Lessons learned include the importance of understanding the relationship between social justice movements and the production of knowledge and understanding the occasionally fraught and contested relationships between communities and academic institutions.

DISCUSSION QUESTIONS

1. How did the Organization of Waterfront Neighborhoods (OWN) and the New York City government differ in how they viewed the problem of waste disposal in the city? How might these differences influence the questions researchers would ask?

2. How are the strategies used to achieve improved health and social outcomes and to promote environmental justice in New York City and the San Francisco Bay Area similar and how are they different?

3. What roles can social movements play in urban health research and practice? What are the limits of their role? How do they contribute to an interdisciplinary perspective?

4. What are the similarities and differences between the professions of public health and urban planning?

NOTES

1. Delemos, J. L. Community-based participatory research: Changing scientific practice from research on communities to research with and for communities. *Local Environment,* 11, no. 3 (2006): 329–338.

2. Sze, J. *Noxious New York: The Racial Politics of Urban Health and Environmental Justice.* Cambridge, Mass.: MIT Press, 2007.

3. Angotti, T. *New York for Sale: Community Planning Confronts Global Real Estate.* Cambridge, Mass.: MIT Press, 2008.

4. Davidoff, P. Advocacy and pluralism in planning. *Journal of the American Institute of Planners,* 31, no. 4 (1965): 186–197.

5. Corburn, J. Confronting the challenges in reconnecting urban planning and public health. *American Journal of Public Health,* 94, no. 4 (2004): 541–546.

6. Corburn, J. Urban planning and health disparities: Implications for research and practice. *Planning Practice and Research,* 20, no. 2 (2005): 111–126.

7. Cole, L., and Foster, S. *From the Ground Up: Environmental Racism and the Rise of the Environmental Justice Movement.* New York: NYU Press, 2000.

8. United Church of Christ Commission for Racial Justice. *Toxic Wastes and Race in the United States.* New York: Public Data Access, 1987.

9. Hofrichter, R., ed. *Toxic Struggles: The Theory and Practice of Environmental Justice.* Philadelphia: New Society, 1993.

10. Duffy, J. *The Sanitarians: A History of American Public Health.* Urbana: University of Illinois Press, 1990.

11. Schultz, S., and McShane, C. To engineer the metropolis: Sewers, sanitation and city planning in late nineteenth century America. *Journal of American History,* 65, no. 2 (1978): 389–411.

12. Jacobs, J. *The Death and Life of the Great American City.* New York: Vintage Books, 1961.

13. Angotti, T., and Hanhardt, E. Problems and prospects for healthy mixed-use communities in New York City. *Planning Practice and Research,* 16, no. 2 (2001): 145–154.

14. Beatley, T., and Manning, K. *The Ecology of Place: Planning for Environment, Economy, and Community.* Washington, D.C.: Island Press, 1997.

15. Portney, K. E. *Taking Sustainable Cities Seriously: Economic Development, the Environment, and Quality of Life in American Cities.* Cambridge, Mass.: MIT Press, 2003.

16. American Planning Association. *Knowledge exchange: A smart growth reader.* Available at http://myapa.planning.org/sgreader. Accessed February 2, 2009.

17. Duany, A., Plater-Zyberk, E., and Speck, J. *Suburban Nation: The Rise of Sprawl and the Decline of the American Dream.* New York: North Point Press, 2000.

18. Vuchic, V. R. *Transportation for Livable Cities.* New Brunswick, N.J.: Rutgers Center for Urban Policy Research, 1999.

19. Tolley, R. *The Greening of Urban Transport.* London: Belhaven, 1990.

20. Crewe, K., Ed. Special issue: Food and planning. *Progressive Planning Magazine,* 158 (Winter 2004).

21. Kaufman, J., Ed. Special issue: Planning for community food systems. *Journal of Planning Education and Research* (2004).

22. Gottlieb, R. *Environmentalism Unbound.* Cambridge, Mass.: MIT Press, 2002.

23. Angotti, T. It's not the housing, it's the people. *Planners Network,* 126 (November/December 1997): 7–9.

24. Lawrence, R. J. Housing and health: From interdisciplinary principles to trans-disciplinary research and practice. *Futures,* 36 (2004): 417–502.

25. Berkman, L., and Kawachi, I., eds. *Social Epidemiology.* New York: Oxford University Press, 2000.

26. Vasquez, V., Minkler, M., and Shepard, P. Promoting environmental health policy through community based participatory research: A case study from Harlem, New York. *Journal of Urban Health,* 83, no. 1 (2006): 101–110.

27. Corburn, J. *Street Science: Community Knowledge and Environmental Health Justice.* Cambridge, Mass.: MIT Press, 2005.

28. Schön, D. A. *The Reflective Practitioner: How Professionals Think in Action.* New York: Basic Books, 1983.

29. Morello-Frosch, R., Pastor, M., Jr., Sadd, J., Porras, C., and Prichard, M. Citizens, science, and data judo: Leveraging secondary data analysis to build a community-academic collaborative for environmental justice in southern California. In B. A. Israel, E. Eng, A. J. Schulz, and E. A. Parker, Eds., *Methods for Conducting Community-Based Participatory Research for Health,* pp. 371–392. San Francisco: Jossey-Bass, 2005.

30. Pastor, M., Jr., Sadd, J., and Morello-Frosch, R. *Still Toxic After All These Years: Air Quality and Environmental Justice in the San Francisco Bay Area.* Prepared for the Bay Area Environmental Health Collaborative by the Center for Justice, Tolerance & Community, University of California, Santa Cruz. Available at http://ucsc.edu/docs/bay_final.pdf. Published February 2007. Accessed June 26, 2008.

31. Morello-Frosch, R. A. Discrimination and the political economy of environmental inequality. *Environment and Planning C: Government and Policy,* 20 (2002): 477–496.

32. Whiteside, K. *Precautionary Politics: Principle and Practice in Confronting Environmental Risk.* Cambridge, Mass.: MIT Press, 2006.

33. Morello-Frosch, R., Pastor, M., Jr., and Sadd, J. Integrating environmental justice and the precautionary principle in research and policy making: The case of ambient air toxics exposures and health risks among schoolchildren in Los Angeles. *Annals of the American Academy of Political and Social Science,* 584 (2002): 47–68.

34. California Environmental Protection Agency Air Resources Board. *Integrating indicators of cumulative impact and socioeconomic vulnerability into regulatory decision-making.* Dr. Manuel Pastor, University of California, Santa Cruz. Available at www.arb.ca.gov/research/apr/archive/oct04/oct04–1.htm. Accessed June 26, 2008.

35. Pellow, D. N. *Garbage Wars: The Struggle for Environmental Justice in Chicago.* Cambridge, Mass.: MIT Press, 2002.

36. Bautista, E. *Taking Out the Garbage.* New York: n.d.

37. OWN/Consumers Union. *Taking Out the Trash.* New York: n.d.

38. The City of New York. *PlaNYC2030.* Available at www.nyc.gov/html/planyc2030. Published April 22, 2007. Accessed June 26, 2008.

39. Freire, P. *Pedagogy of the Oppressed.* New York: Continuum, 2002.

40. Tai, S. Environmental hazards and the Richmond Laotian American community: A case study in environmental justice. *Asian Law Journal,* 6, no. 1 (1999): 189–207.

41. Asian Pacific Environmental Network (APEN). Available at www.apen4ej.org. Accessed June 26, 2008.

42. Asian Pacific Environmental Network, Communities for a Better Environment, Environmental Health Coalition, People Organizing to Demand Environmental & Economic Rights, Silicon Valley Toxics Coalition/Health and Environmental Justice Project. *Building healthy communities from the ground up: Environmental justice in California.* Available at www.rachel.org/files/document/Building_Healthy_Communities_from_the_Ground_Up.pdf. Accessed February 2, 2009.

43. University of California at Berkeley Health Impact Group (UCBHIG). *Health impact assessment projects: Oak to Ninth Avenue health impact assessment.* Available at http://ehs.sph.berkeley.edu/hia/O2N.HIA.ExecSum.pdf (Executive Summary). Accessed February 2, 2009.

INTERDISCIPLINARY APPROACHES TO STUDYING CAUSES OF URBAN HEALTH PROBLEMS

CHAPTER

3

INTERDISCIPLINARY, PARTICIPATORY RESEARCH ON URBAN FOOD ENVIRONMENTS AND DIETARY BEHAVIORS

SHANNON N. ZENK, AMY J. SCHULZ,
ANGELA M. ODOMS-YOUNG, MURLISA LOCKETT

LEARNING OBJECTIVES

- Describe how differences in neighborhood food environments can contribute to differences in the health of populations in different neighborhoods.

- Analyze the different ways that individual-level and neighborhood-level factors influence diet, nutrition, and obesity.

- Present a rationale for using community-based participatory research methods to study neighborhood food environments.

■ Discuss the challenges that interdisciplinary researchers working with communities face and some of the strategies they can use to overcome these challenges.

INTRODUCTION

Poor diet is a major risk factor for several diseases, including diabetes, cardiovascular disease, and certain cancers, from which African Americans experience excess morbidity and mortality when compared with whites. Until recently, research had mainly focused on the role of individual and familial factors in dietary practices and disparities. However, over the past few years, an explosion of research has documented inequalities in the accessibility of retail food outlets (e.g., supermarkets, fast-food restaurants) and in the food supply (e.g., food availability, selection, quality, price) across neighborhoods, with low-income and racial/ethnic minority neighborhoods often having fewer nutritional resources (e.g., supermarkets) and more nutritional hazards (e.g., low-quality fresh produce).[1-10] There is growing interest in understanding whether and how neighborhood "food environments" affect dietary behaviors and contribute to racial/ethnic disparities in diet and related health outcomes. From the early work of Cheadle and colleagues to more contemporary studies,[11-18] accumulating evidence suggests that people who have food options closer to home that support healthy eating have better dietary quality or healthier body weights. Given that 81 percent of African Americans live in urbanized areas (densely populated areas with at least 50,000 residents) and 60 percent live in urban centers (generally incorporated places or census-designated places with the most population within urbanized areas),[19] understanding whether and how neighborhood food environments affect residents' dietary intake and health is especially important in urban settings to eliminate black-white disparities in health.

In this chapter, we draw on research conducted in Detroit, Michigan, between 1996 and 2008 as a case study of one approach for understanding how the neighborhood retail food environment affects dietary behaviors and the health of urban populations. This research engaged academic researchers and representatives of health service and community-based organizations. It employed theoretical perspectives and research methodologies (i.e., spatial mapping, community surveys, in-person observations) of several academic disciplines: health behavior and health education, sociology, community nutrition, nursing, epidemiology, and geography. We first consider distinctive determinants of contemporary retail food environments in cities, highlighting circumstances in Detroit. We then describe efforts of, and lessons learned by, community-based participatory research (CBPR) partnerships working to understand the health implications of retail food environments in Detroit. We conclude by discussing next steps for research that examines the contributions of retail food environments to dietary behaviors and the health of urban populations.

DETERMINANTS OF RETAIL FOOD ENVIRONMENTS IN CITIES

Detroit, like many other cities, has experienced dramatic shifts in the retail food landscape over the past few decades. The spatial distribution of grocery stores is one aspect of the retail food environment that has changed. Factors contributing to grocery store closures and rare store openings within cities are multifaceted.[20-25] However, many of the factors that have shaped the contemporary retail food environment in Detroit and other midwestern and northeastern cities in the United States stem from at least three interrelated historical forces: racial residential segregation, economic restructuring, and restructuring in the retail food industry.

Racial Residential Segregation

A major factor shaping the retail food environment in metropolitan Detroit since 1950 has been racial residential segregation. Following World War II, fears of racial integration prompted white residents to flee the city for the suburbs, as increasing numbers of African Americans moved into previously all-white neighborhoods. Between 1950 and 2000, Detroit lost over half of its population and transitioned from 16 percent to 81 percent African American.[19, 26] In contrast, by 2000, more than 80 percent of residents in metropolitan Detroit were non-Hispanic white.[19] Metropolitan Detroit is currently one of the most racially segregated urban areas in the United States.[27]

The closing of white-owned grocery stores and opening of Middle Eastern–owned food stores were two outcomes of white flight in Detroit.[28] According to informal estimates from trade associations, people of Middle Eastern descent now own 80 to 90 percent of Detroit's grocery and liquor stores.[28] Some African American residents view the fact that most food store owners and employees are of a different racial/ethnic background as a symbol of economic inequalities in Detroit.[29, 30] Moreover, many Detroit residents report being discriminated against—watched, followed, treated with disrespect—when frequenting local food stores.[28, 31] Strained race relations between many residents and store owners and employees may negatively influence residents' perceptions of foods available to them, their food shopping behaviors, and their mental well-being.[32-34]

Economic Restructuring

The contemporary retail food environment in Detroit has also been profoundly shaped by economic restructuring. Fueled by the rise in the automotive industry, Detroit was growing and prosperous in the early to mid-twentieth century.[30, 35, 36] However, economic restructuring after World War II, particularly relocation of industries from the city to the suburbs and deindustrialization, led to the loss of over 250,000 manufacturing jobs between 1947 and 1992.[36] Further job loss and economic divestment followed the loss of manufacturing jobs. Between 1960 and 1990, the city of Detroit lost about 350,000 jobs, whereas the surrounding metropolitan area gained more than twice that number.[36] Stemming in part from the disappearance of good-paying, blue-collar employment opportunities, the percentage of residents living below the federal poverty line in Detroit was over four times greater than in the rest of metropolitan Detroit in 2000 (26 percent vs. 6 percent).[24, 37, 38] Although research documents untapped purchasing power in urban neighborhoods, including Detroit,[21, 24, 38] food retailers cite lack of profitability as a reason they pulled out and continue to avoid investing in Detroit and other cities.

Restructuring in the Retail Food Industry

A third historical factor shaping Detroit's current retail food environment is restructuring of the retail food industry. Consolidation in the retail food industry beginning in the 1950s is one aspect of restructuring, including movement from independently owned stores to corporately owned chains, as well as mergers and leveraged buyouts that created even larger corporations.[21, 22] By the 1970s, many independent grocery stores could not compete with the prices offered at chain stores, which could exploit economies of scale; thus, many independent grocers were forced to close.[22] Unfortunately, as Detroit's white population shifted from the city to the suburbs after World War II, grocery stores began closing in the city, and many chains avoided locating new stores in Detroit due in part to racial stereotypes and associated fears of crime in an increasingly African American city.[21–23] Instead, grocery chains took advantage of abundant and inexpensive land in the suburbs, which allowed them to build large store formats at a lower cost. Scarcity of land to accommodate large store formats (e.g., supercenters, superstores), high prices to develop sites, or both also contributed to the loss of supermarkets from cities.[24] Supermarkets' abandonment of the city, with accompanying loss of jobs and tax revenues, exacerbated already deteriorating economic conditions in Detroit.

In sum, racial residential segregation, economic restructuring, and restructuring in the retail food industry have had negative repercussions for the current retail food landscape in Detroit. As one Detroit resident, participating in a focus group on facilitators and barriers to healthy eating and physical activity, observed: "You've got to go out into the suburbs now to get some decent food. And therefore, it's not available to us in this community. By the time you get to that store and get some fresh fruits and vegetables, you're going to pass about 30 fast food joints and about 100 liquor stores."[31]

USING CBPR TO UNDERSTAND THE HEALTH IMPLICATIONS OF DETROIT'S FOOD ENVIRONMENT

As highlighted by the preceding quotation, Detroit residents do not view the local retail food environment as supportive of healthy eating. In this section, we describe how the retail food environment in Detroit became a focus of the work of two community-based participatory research (CBPR) partnerships: the East Side Village Health Worker Partnership (ESVHWP) and the Healthy Environments Partnership (HEP). We also describe how expansion of the research teams to include scholars with a wider range of disciplinary perspectives facilitated work of these partnerships between 1996 and 2008 as we began and have proceeded with work aimed at understanding the role of the retail food environment in health variations among Detroit residents. We will then discuss lessons learned in using an interdisciplinary, participatory approach to study the urban retail food environment.

Concern about the retail food environment emerged initially in the context of the ESVHWP. Initiated in 1996, the goal of the ESVHWP was to identify and address, using a lay health advisor approach, social determinants of women's health in eastside Detroit.[39] Lay health advisors (known as "village health workers") and community representatives (including coauthor Murlisa Lockett) involved in the ESVHWP identified diabetes as a priority in 1999. Facilitated by disciplinary training in health behavior, health education, and sociology of the initial academic researchers (including coauthor Amy J. Schultz), as well as by the engagement of a postdoctoral fellow with a community nutrition background (coauthor Angela M. Odoms-Young) and other individuals and community organizations with expertise in diabetes, the ESVHWP in 2000–2001 developed a pilot project to prevent diabetes, Healthy Eating and Exercising to Reduce Diabetes (HEED).[40] In conversations among those involved in HEED, residents in eastside Detroit described the scarcity of fresh fruits and vegetables at local stores and difficulties securing rides from family and friends to reach suburban supermarkets to obtain fresh produce. They also described how the dearth of supermarkets and high-quality, reasonably priced nutritious foods made it difficult for residents to maintain a healthful diet. In response, the ESVHWP initiated healthy soul food cooking demonstrations to provide skills in healthy food preparation and monthly fruit and vegetable "minimarkets," which were later expanded to bimonthly due to high demand.[40] Designed to increase the availability of a wide variety of high-quality fresh produce at low prices in eastside Detroit, the minimarkets sold a variety of produce items at wholesale prices at readily accessible community sites, including community centers and churches. In addition, as described below, members of the ESVHWP began new data collection efforts to understand the retail food environment, which required knowledge and research methodologies from other disciplines (e.g., geography, urban planning).

Documenting Locations of Food Resources

A public health doctoral student working with the ESVHWP (Shannon N. Zenk) had general interests in nutrition and the role of neighborhood environments in health disparities. She initiated new data collection to systematically document the distribution of food resources across Detroit area neighborhoods. Training was offered through other disciplines (e.g., a semester-long geographic information system [GIS] course offered through the University's Department of Natural Resources), and it was distinctly interdisciplinary (e.g., a five-day workshop on accessibility measurement sponsored by the Center for Spatially Integrated Social Science [CSISS]). There were also interactions with geographers at the university's map library and statistical consulting center and an economist with expertise in spatial statistics. All provided opportunities to learn new research methodologies for data collection (e.g., GIS) and data analysis (e.g., spatial econometrics).

To examine the spatial accessibility of supermarkets, we used GIS to map the locations of supermarkets in metropolitan Detroit. We found that the city of Detroit had only nine supermarkets for 950,000 residents in late 2002, whereas supermarkets were abundant in the surrounding metropolitan area. The results also showed inequities in the distance to the nearest supermarket by neighborhood racial composition and poverty level, with the longest distances to supermarkets found for the most economically disadvantaged neighborhoods where African Americans lived.[41] At the same time, we also conducted in-person audits of food stores in four Detroit area communities to explore whether a good selection of affordable, high-quality fresh fruits and vegetables was less available in an economically disadvantaged African American community than in more advantaged communities. This project entailed developing an instrument to measure fresh fruit and vegetable availability, selection, quality, and price; mapping food stores located in each community using GIS; training data collectors; and visiting the food stores to conduct the audits. We found differences in the types of food stores present and in the quality of fresh produce for sale, but not fresh produce selection or prices, among the four communities.[34]

Examining Health Implications of the Food Environment

The ESVHWP, and later HEP, also initiated new data collection to examine implications of inequalities in the neighborhood retail food environment for the health of Detroit residents. The ESVHWP added items to a 2001 second-wave survey of African American women living in eastside Detroit. The questions included the name and location (street intersection) of the primary store where they shopped for food; perceptions of the selection, quality, and affordability of fresh produce at that store; and frequency of fruit and vegetable intake. Results of analyses using those data showed that women with higher incomes were more likely to shop at suburban supermarkets and suggested that the type of food store to which women had access (using stores where they shopped as proxies) and the selection and quality of fresh produce for sale may have influenced women's fruit and vegetable consumption.[42] Conversations about the results of this analysis in 2002 among members of the ESVHWP encouraged efforts to document the demand for fresh fruits and vegetables in the community, increase the visibility and frequency of the fruit and vegetable minimarkets, expand the minimarkets to other areas of the city, and work with local store owners to increase the availability of healthy foods.

The Healthy Environments Partnership (HEP) expanded efforts to understand the role of the retail food environment in dietary behaviors and health outcomes among Detroit residents. As part of the National Institute of Environmental Health Sciences Health Disparities Strategic Plan, HEP began in 2000 to examine relationships between neighborhood social and physical environments and cardiovascular disease risk among adults in three Detroit communities (eastside, southwest, and northwest) using a CBPR approach.[43] HEP engaged scholars from a variety of academic disciplines, including health behavior and health education, sociology, epidemiology, human nutrition, and environmental health sciences, as well as a wider range of community partners, including organizations working on issues of environmental justice.

These new interdisciplinary collaborations enabled the collection of a number of nutrition-related measures as part of the survey of residents: a semiquantitative food frequency questionnaire; anthropometric measures of height, weight, and waist circumference; and a variety of biomarkers (e.g., cholesterol).[43] The survey also included measures of participants' perceptions of the neighborhood food environment. Community partners provided space where survey participants could come to have their blood drawn and helped to ensure that data collection procedures were culturally appropriate and had suitable safeguards for participants' confidentiality. Using these data, HEP has begun a series of analyses examining relationships among independently observed and perceived measures of the retail food environment (e.g., proximity of different types of retail food outlets; food availability, quality, and price), dietary behaviors, and related health outcomes (e.g., obesity, serum cholesterol) in residents of eastside, southwest, and northwest Detroit. Among the initial findings of these analyses are that residents' perceptions of the neighborhood food environment are associated with factors at multiple levels, including their individual educational attainment, neighborhood racial composition, and store availability.[44] Another analysis revealed that availability of a large neighborhood grocery store was positively associated with fruit and vegetable intake and that the neighborhood food environment had stronger effects on consumption in Latinos compared with African Americans.[45]

In 2005, HEP brought in new colleagues from urban planning and received additional financial support to examine associations between aspects of the built environment and obesity risk and to evaluate multilevel interventions centered on the introduction of greenways in Detroit. In fall 2008 through winter 2009, HEP conducted a second-wave community survey and reassessed the retail food environment, including mapping food store and restaurant locations and assessing the availability, quality, and price of a range of healthy food options (e.g., produce, low-fat foods, whole-grain foods) at stores. This new data collection will allow HEP to examine the effects of changes in the retail food environment on residents' dietary behaviors and health indicators over a six-year period. HEP anticipates that the new disciplinary collaborations will allow for a better understanding of the role of the retail food environment in obesity and related health outcomes by allowing simultaneous examination of the retail food environment and aspects of the built environment relevant for physical activity (e.g., land use, street connectivity). It will also assist in identifying relevant community change strategies.

With the addition of supplemental pilot funding and the engagement of a geographer, HEP will also invite a subsample of survey participants to participate in additional data collection that uses portable global positioning system (GPS) units to measure the environment to which they are exposed during daily activities ("activity-space" environments). This will allow HEP to characterize environmental exposures and resources, including the food environment, in a broader area beyond the residential neighborhood and to examine relationships among aspects of activity-space environments, health behaviors including dietary intake, and health outcomes.

Challenges and Lessons Learned

The ESVHWP and HEP both used an interdisciplinary, participatory approach to study the retail food environment in Detroit. Involvement of community partners and expansion of the research teams to include investigators from a wider range of disciplines enriched the work of the partnerships by providing content and methodological expertise, offering multiple interpretive lenses, and identifying implications for community change efforts. Based on our experience studying the retail food environment using an interdisciplinary, participatory approach in an urban context, we suggest several lessons.

Competing Priorities   Interdisciplinary, participatory research projects that are interested in issues of social justice in urban communities often have ambitious goals and multiple components. One reason is that economically vulnerable urban communities face numerous challenges that warrant attention.[40] Another contributing factor is the wide range of interests of individual members, which reflect not only diverse disciplinary backgrounds but also organizational priorities. Although the ESVHWP's and HEP's concentration on the retail food environment arose from community concerns, nutrition, and more specifically the retail food environment, was only one of the foci of these projects. Limited resources often force partnerships to choose to address a small number of urban communities' many needs. Community planning processes that engage not only members of the partnership but also community residents and other stakeholders can help to prioritize community change efforts as well as identify connections to other concerns faced by the community. HEP has recently completed such a community planning process that prioritized interventions addressing the local food environment as well as other aspects of the built and social environment that may influence obesity and cardiovascular risk.

Communicating Across Disciplines   As we have described, as the need for additional content and methodological expertise became apparent, members of the partnerships sought researchers and professionals with a broader range of disciplinary backgrounds: human nutrition, social and spatial epidemiology, economics, and geography. Some joined the research teams; others provided critical input into the projects. This array of disciplinary perspectives introduced disciplinary language and challenges to communication. The need to communicate with community partners added another layer of complexity. Reaching common conceptual and methodological understandings required willingness across partnership members to ask questions when terminology (e.g., social structure, food security, spatial autocorrelation, land use) or methodologies (e.g., GPS, accelerometer, spatial regression) were unclear and to provide more detailed explanations. The fact that many members of the partnerships had training and/or worked in public health, regardless of disciplinary homes, provided some common language and experiences that facilitated communication.

Incorporating Diverse Cultural Food Preferences Racial and ethnic diversity is a distinct characteristic of most U.S. cities. One lesson learned regarding studying the retail food environment in a multiethnic urban context is the importance of incorporating cultural food preferences and norms of multiple racial/ethnic groups. Although more than 80 percent of Detroit residents are African American, communities involved in the HEP have substantial Latino and white populations, too. Thus, in designing instruments we used to audit food stores, we attempted to include items that were popular among all three racial/ethnic groups. We learned that our efforts were partially successful and have identified area for improvement (e.g., adding more fruits and vegetables popular among Mexican Americans in Detroit) in future work. Working closely with community members can help to ensure that data collection tools are appropriate for the populations under study.

Understanding the Relationship Between Race and Economics Racial residential segregation, a defining characteristic of metropolitan Detroit and other U.S. metropolitan areas, adversely impacts socioeconomic circumstances of many people of color and the urban neighborhoods in which they live.[46] As a result, race and socioeconomic status (SES) are highly correlated at not only the individual level but also the neighborhood level, which makes it difficult to tease apart whether spatial access to nutritional resources and hazards differs by neighborhood racial composition, SES, or both.[6, 41] Yet, because solutions will differ, understanding the role race plays in decisions regarding the placement of retail food outlets, above and beyond the role of SES, is important. Although more difficult to achieve in some urban contexts than in others, study designs that incorporate neighborhoods in both the city and surrounding suburbs can introduce sufficient variation in economic conditions within neighborhoods of the same racial composition and help to answer questions regarding the role of race in the distribution of food resources and risks.

Time-Intensive Nature of Research As referenced earlier, considerable time passed from when residents brought problems of inadequate availability of healthy foods in Detroit to the forefront of these CBPR initiatives to subsequent stages in the research: documentation of inequalities in neighborhood retail food environments and examination of the associations with health behaviors and outcomes. Indeed, HEP's research examining the role of retail food environment in dietary behaviors and related health outcomes among Detroit residents is still in its early stages. The time-intensive realities of forming interdisciplinary, participatory research collaborations; securing funding; and collecting and analyzing data presented two challenges.

A first challenge was balancing research to understand contributions of the retail food environment to Detroit residents' dietary intakes and health with action. Community-based participatory research calls for a balance between research and action.[47] Indeed, Detroit residents described pressing challenges of inadequate availability of healthy food options in their neighborhoods and limited transportation options to reach suburban food sources. These needs conflicted with the timeline required to develop data to inform evidence-based community change strategies that would lead to improvements in the health of Detroit residents. Ultimately, the ESVHWP pursued short-term strategies to increase the availability of healthy food options (e.g., development of fruit and vegetable minimarkets) at the same time that research continued, which allowed the partnership to respond to a community-identified need. Yet, while both partnerships would have liked large-scale policy and program development to proceed more quickly, these interim strategies were critical to address community concerns in the short term.

Another challenge posed by the time-intensive nature of the research process is that investigators who offered valuable disciplinary perspectives related to nutrition and who provided GIS skills have since left the area, which was due to the structure of academia (postdoctoral and doctoral training) and individual career trajectories. Still, the initial interdisciplinary relationships that were developed, sustained involvement of many of the original research team members, engagement of new investigators with requisite knowledge and skills, and long-distance participation of some team members using technology (e.g., teleconference, e-mail) have enabled the interdisciplinary work to continue.

DIRECTIONS FOR FUTURE RESEARCH

Our experiences highlight the importance of engaging communities and casting a wide disciplinary net in efforts to understand and address the retail food environment in cities. Because issues may not be the same across cities, community residents and representatives can play a critical role in defining problems and resources related to the retail food environment, interpreting findings, and prioritizing and designing change strategies. In addition to public health, sociology, and nutritional science, theoretical perspectives and methodologies from disciplines such as geography, economics, anthropology, and urban planning can greatly enrich research and the understandings gained from that research. Extant research aimed at understanding and addressing contributions of the retail food environment to the health of urban populations has implications for future observational and intervention research.

First, an underlying assumption of most extant epidemiologic research is that residents, especially in economically disadvantaged urban neighborhoods, rely on foods available within their residential neighborhood. As a result, most studies have methodologically equated food availability in residential neighborhoods with food access or as a set of available options with respect to food sources (e.g., grocery stores, restaurants) and the food supply. In fact, an individual's or household's food access likely depends on their physical (e.g., physical mobility, transportation), economic (e.g., income, food assistance receipt), and social (e.g., social networks, time-budget) resources and constraints. These resources and constraints may, for example, shape individuals' activity spaces and consequently the food environments to which they are exposed beyond the residential neighborhood. Yet, the interplay of individual/household resources and constraints and the local and regional food environment in shaping food access, both in the residential neighborhood and broader activity space, in shaping food access and consequently the use of the retail food environment is poorly understood[48] and thus is an important direction for future research.

Second, studies examining the potential influence of the retail food environment on the health of city populations have generally focused on retail outlet availability and characteristics of the food supply (e.g., availability, quality, price). Yet, the retail food environment may impact city residents' health through pathways beyond the type of retail food outlets present and the food supply. For example, utilizing the retail food environment in economically disadvantaged urban neighborhoods often involves encountering crime and harassment when entering and leaving stores, deteriorated conditions inside and surrounding stores, and unfair treatment from store employees and owners. Stress stemming from these conditions and experiences may negatively impact urban residents' mental well-being and have indirect negative repercussions for dietary behaviors, weight status, and physical health.[49] Thus, research that examines health implications of these and other aspects of the retail food environment, above and beyond food outlet locations and the food supply, will be critical in understanding the retail food environment and its implications for health. Community members can inform the identification and investigation of these other pathways.

Third, understanding the role of the retail food environment in the health of city populations necessitates reliable and valid measures of multiple dimensions of the retail food environment. Although measures are increasing, they are currently scarce, particularly perceptual measures of the retail food environment. Moreover, few studies have demonstrated the reliability and validity of existing perceived or observational measures.[50] Interdisciplinary teams, which include community members, can work together to create and test the properties of these food environment measures.

With respect to intervention research, studies are needed to evaluate the impact of natural and planned changes in the retail food environment on health status. Additional studies that evaluate the opening and closing of retail food outlets (e.g., supermarkets, fast-food restaurants) and changes in food availability, quality, pricing, or product mix would be informative. Relatively little research has been conducted to date in the United States, with most research in this area taking place in the United Kingdom.[51–53] Moreover, multilevel interventions that combine environmental changes with individual behavioral change strategies may be an even more promising approach. Still, researchers should address other aspects of the food environment (e.g., safety, customer service, cleanliness), beyond increasing the availability of high-quality, reasonably priced healthy foods, that affect urban residents' comfort and willingness to shop at a store. Furthermore, it is important that researchers pay particular attention to how change efforts directed at the retail food environment affect the most vulnerable populations in cities. For example, opening a supermarket in an economically disadvantaged urban neighborhood may not benefit economically vulnerable residents if they cannot afford to shop there. Assuring that all residents have economic as well as spatial access to healthy foods is essential if we are to address racial and socioeconomic disparities in health.

In conclusion, we found that use of an interdisciplinary, participatory approach enhanced our research on the retail food environment in Detroit in several ways. Community participation and priorities motivated this research. They shaped the research trajectory, framed the research questions, and helped to ensure the work was grounded in Detroit's historical and contemporary context. Engagement of multiple disciplines provided substantive and methodological expertise to conduct the research. By combining perspectives from disciplines that have traditionally focused on individuals (such as nursing and nutrition) with those that have focused on societies (such as sociology and public health), we have moved toward research questions that recognize multiple levels of influence on dietary intake reflecting both structure and individual agency. New theoretical and methodological ideas have continued to emerge as we have expanded our literature reviews and research partners to include other disciplines such as time geography and economics. Ultimately, drawing on the epidemiologic research we have conducted, we anticipate that use of an interdisciplinary, participatory approach will facilitate our change efforts directed at the urban retail food environment in the future.

SUMMARY

In this chapter, we presented a case study of a research project designed to understand how the neighborhood retail food environment affects the dietary behaviors and health of urban populations. In this project, academic researchers and representatives of health service and community-based organizations used theoretical perspectives and research methodologies (spatial mapping, community surveys, and in-person observations) from several academic disciplines: health behavior and health education, sociology, community nutrition, nursing, epidemiology, and geography. We considered the determinants of contemporary retail food environments in cities, illustrating them with examples from Detroit. We found that community participation and priorities motivated this research and helped to ensure the work was grounded in Detroit's historical and contemporary context. Ultimately, we anticipate that our findings and the use of an interdisciplinary, participatory approach will facilitate broader efforts directed at improving the urban retail food environment.

DISCUSSION QUESTIONS

1. Why was the research team interested in understanding how the food environment in Detroit influenced diet and health?

2. What were the unique contributions that community residents made to this study?

3. How did the research collaborative overcome the challenges they faced?

4. What were the specific contributions that each discipline made to this study?

ACKNOWLEDGMENTS

We wish to acknowledge the contributions of the East Side Village Health Worker Partnership and Healthy Environments Partnership in Detroit, Michigan, to this research. The East Side Village Health Worker Partnership involved representatives from Butzel Family Center, Detroit Department of Health and Wellness Promotion, Friends of Parkside, Henry Ford Health System, Kettering/Butzel Health Initiative, University of Michigan, and Warren Conner Development Corporation and was funded by the Centers for Disease Control (U48/CCU515775). The Healthy Environments Partnership (www.sph.umich.edu/hep) includes representatives from Boulevard Harambee, Brightmoor Community Center, Detroit Department of Health and Wellness Promotion, Detroit Hispanic Development Corporation, Friends of Parkside, Henry Ford Health System, Southwest Detroit Environmental Vision, Southwest Solutions, University of Detroit Mercy, and University of Michigan and is funded by National Institute of Environmental Health Sciences (R01 ES10936–05, R01 ES014234–01) and National Center on Minority Health and Health Disparities (R24 MD001619–01). The research described here was also funded in part by the National Institute of Nursing Research (K01 NR010540).

NOTES

1. Baker, E. A., Schootman, M., Barnidge, E., and Kelly, C. The role of race and poverty in access to foods that enable individuals to adhere to dietary guidelines. *Preventing Chronic Disease,* 3 (2006): A76.

2. Block, J. P., Scribner, R. A., and DeSalvo, K. B. Fast food, race/ethnicity, and income: A geographic analysis. *American Journal of Preventive Medicine,* 27 (2004): 211–217.

3. Cummins, S., and Macintyre, S. Food environments and obesity—neighbourhood or nation? *International Journal of Epidemiology,* 35 (2006): 100–104.

4. Helling, A., and Sawicki, D. Race and residential accessibility to shopping and services. *Housing Policy Debate,* 14 (2003): 69–101.

5. Horowitz, C. R., Colson, K. A., Hebert, P. L., and Lancaster, K. Barriers to buying healthy foods for people with diabetes: Evidence of environmental disparities. *American Journal of Public Health,* 94 (2004): 1549–1554.

6. Moore, L. V., and Diez Roux, A. V. Associations of neighborhood characteristics with the location and type of food stores. *American Journal of Public Health,* 96 (2006): 325–331.

7. Morland, K., Wing, S., Diez Roux, A., and Poole, C. Neighborhood characteristics associated with the location of food stores and food service places. *American Journal of Preventive Medicine,* 22 (2002): 23–29.

8. Powell, L. M., Chaloupka, F. J., and Bao, Y. The availability of fast-food and full-service restaurants in the United States: Associations with neighborhood characteristics. *American Journal of Preventive Medicine,* 33 (2007): S240–5.

9. Powell, L. M., Slater, S., Mirtcheva, D., Bao, Y., and Chaloupka, F. J. Food store availability and neighborhood characteristics in the United States. *Preventive Medicine,* 44 (2007): 189–195.

10. Sloane, D. C., Diamant, A. L., Lewis, L.V.B., et al. Improving the nutritional resource environment for healthy living through community-based participatory research. *Journal of General Internal Medicine,* 18 (2003): 568–575.

11. Auchincloss, A. H., Diez Roux, A. V., Brown, D. G., Erdmann, C. A., and Bertoni, A. G. Neighborhood resources for physical activity and healthy foods and their association with insulin resistance. *Epidemiology,* 19 (2008): 146–157.

12. Laraia, B. A., Siega-Riz, A. M., Kaufman, J. S., and Jones, S. J. Proximity of supermarkets is positively associated with diet quality index for pregnancy. *Preventive Medicine,* 39 (2004): 869–875.

13. Mehta, N., K., and Chang, V. W. Weight status and restaurant availability: A multi-level analysis. *American Journal of Preventive Medicine,* 34 (2008): 127–133.

14. Moore, L. V., Diez Roux, A. V., Nettleton, J. A., and Jacobs, D. R., Jr. Associations of the local food environment with diet quality—a comparison of assessments based on surveys and geographic information systems: The multi-ethnic study of atherosclerosis. *American Journal of Epidemiology,* 167 (2008): 917–924.

15. Morland, K., Wing, S., and Diez Roux, A. The contextual effect of the local food environment on residents' diets: The atherosclerosis risk in communities study. *American Journal of Public Health,* 92 (2002): 1761–1767.

16. Morland, K., Diez Roux, A. V., and Wing, S. Supermarkets, other food stores, and obesity: The atherosclerosis risk in communities study. *American Journal of Preventive Medicine,* 30 (2006): 333–339.

17. Powell, L. M., Auld, M. C., Chaloupka, F. J., O'Malley, P. M., and Johnston, L. D. Associations between access to food stores and adolescent body mass index. *American Journal of Preventive Medicine,* 33 (2007): S301–7.

18. Rose, D., and Richards, R. Food store access and household fruit and vegetable use among participants in the U.S. food stamp program. *Public Health Nutrition,* 7 (2004): 1081–1088.

19. U.S. Census Bureau. *Summary File 1: Census 2000* [electronic data]. Available at www.census.gov/Press-Release/www/2001/sumfile1.html. Accessed March 2006.

20. Bolen, E., and Hecht, K. Neighborhood groceries: New access to healthy food in low-income communities. *Report prepared for the California Food Policy Advocates* (January 2003).

21. Donohue, R. M. *Abandonment and revitalization of central city retailing: The case of grocery stores.* Doctoral dissertation. Ann Arbor: University of Michigan, 1997.

22. Eisenhauer, E. In poor health: Supermarket redlining and urban nutrition. *GeoJournal,* 53 (2001): 125–133.

23. Policylink. *Healthy Food, Healthy Communities: Improving Access and Opportunities Through Food Retailing.* Oakland, Cal.: Policylink, 2005.

24. Pothukuchi, K. Attracting supermarkets to inner-city neighborhoods: Economic development outside the box. *Economic Development Quarterly,* 19 (2005): 232–244.

25. Smoyer-Tomic, K. E., Spence, J. C., and Amrhein, C. Food deserts in the prairies? Supermarket accessibility and neighborhood need in Edmonton, Canada. *The Professional Geographer,* 58 (2006): 307–326.

26. Schulz, A. J., Williams, D. R., Israel, B. A., and Lempert, L. B. Racial and spatial relations as fundamental determinants of health in Detroit. *Milbank Quarterly,* 80 (2002): 677–707.

27. Iceland, J., Weinberg, D. H., and Steinmetz, E. *Racial and Ethnic Residential Segregation in the United States, 1980–2000.* Washington, D.C.: U.S. Census Bureau, 2002.

28. David, G. C. Behind the bulletproof glass: Iraqi Chaldean store ownership in metropolitan Detroit. In N. Abraham and A. Shryock, eds., *Arab Detroit: From Margin to Mainstream,* pp. 151–178. Detroit, Mich.: Wayne State University Press, 2000.

29. Israel, B. A., Schulz, A. J., Estrada-Martinez, L., et al. Engaging urban residents in assessing neighborhood environments and their implications for health. *Journal of Urban Health,* 83 (2006): 523–539.

30. Sugrue, T. J. *The Origins of the Urban Crisis: Race and Inequality in Postwar Detroit.* Princeton, N.J.: Princeton University Press, 1996.

31. Kieffer, E. C., Willis, S. K., Odoms-Young, A. M., et al. Reducing disparities in diabetes among African-American and Latino residents of Detroit: The essential role of community planning focus groups. *Ethnicity and Disease,* 14 (2004): S27–37.

32. Essed, P. *Understanding Everyday Racism: An Interdisciplinary Theory.* Newbury Park, Cal.: Sage, 1991.

33. Siegelman, P. Racial discrimination in "everyday" commercial transactions: What do we know, what do we need to know, and how can we find out. In M. Fix and M. A. Turner, eds., *A National Report Card on Discrimination in America: The Role of Testing,* pp. 69–98. Washington, D.C.: Urban Institute, 1999.

34. Zenk, S. N., Schulz, A. J., Israel, B. A., James, S. A., Bao, S., and Wilson, M. L. Fruit and vegetable access differs by community racial composition and socio-economic position in Detroit, Michigan. *Ethnicity and Disease,* 16 (2006): 275–280.

35. Darden, J. T., Hill, R. C., Thomas, J., and Thomas, R. *Detroit: Race and Uneven Development.* Philadelphia: Temple University Press, 1987.

36. Farley, R., Danziger, S., and Holzer, H. J. *Detroit Divided.* New York: Russell Sage Foundation, 2000.

37. U.S. Census Bureau. Summary File 3: Census 2000 [electronic data]. Washington, D.C.: 2001. Available at www.census.gov.

38. Initiative for a Competitive Inner City. *The Business Case for Pursuing Retail Opportunities in the Inner City.* Boston: Initiative for a Competitive Inner City, 1998.

39. Schulz, A. J., Israel, B. A., Parker, E. A., Lockett, M., Hill, Y., and Wills, R. The East Side Village Health Worker Partnership: Integrating research with action to reduce health disparities. *Public Health Reports,* 116 (2001): 548–558.

40. Schulz, A. J., Zenk, S., Odoms-Young, A., et al. Healthy eating and exercising to reduce diabetes: Exploring the potential of social determinants of health frameworks within the context of community-based participatory diabetes prevention. *American Journal of Public Health,* 95 (2005): 645–651.

41. Zenk, S. N., Schulz, A. J., Israel, B. A., James, S. A., Bao, S., and Wilson, M. L. Neighborhood racial composition, neighborhood poverty, and the spatial accessibility of supermarkets in metropolitan Detroit. *American Journal of Public Health,* 95 (2005): 660–667.

42. Zenk, S. N., Schulz, A. J., Hollis-Neely, T., et al. Fruit and vegetable intake in African Americans: Income and store characteristics. *American Journal of Preventive Medicine,* 29 (2005): 1–9.

43. Schulz, A. J., Kannan, S., Dvonch, J. T., et al. Social and physical environments and disparities in risk for cardiovascular disease: The healthy environments partnership conceptual model. *Environmental Health Perspectives,* 113 (2005): 1817–1825.

44. Zenk, S. N., Schulz, A. J., Lachance, L. L., et al. Multilevel correlates of satisfaction with neighborhood availability of fruits and vegetables. *Annals of Behavioral Medicine*. (in press).

45. Zenk, S. N., Lachance, L. L., Schulz, A. J., Mentz, G., Kannan, S., and Ridella, W. Neighborhood retail food environment and fruit and vegetable intake in a multiethnic urban population. *American Journal of Health Promotion,* 23 (2009): 255–264.

46. Williams, D. R., and Collins, C. Racial residential segregation: A fundamental cause of racial disparities in health. *Public Health Reports,* 116 (2001): 404–416.

47. Israel, B. A., Schulz, A. J., Parker, E. A., and Becker, A. B. Review of community-based research: Assessing partnership approaches to improve public health. *Annual Review of Public Health,* 19 (1998): 173–202.

48. Barnes, S. L. *The Cost of Being Poor: A Comparative Study of Life in Poor Urban Neighborhoods in Gary, Indiana.* Albany: State University of New York Press, 2005.

49. Aylott, R., and Mitchell, V. An exploratory study of grocery shopping stressors. *British Food Journal,* 101 (1999): 683–700.

50. Glanz, K., Sallis, J. F., Saelens. B. E., and Frank, L. D. Nutrition environment measures survey in stores (NEMS-S): Development and evaluation. *American Journal of Preventive Medicine,* 32 (2007): 282–289.

51. Glanz, K., and Yaroch, A. L. Strategies for increasing fruit and vegetable intake in grocery stores and communities: Policy, pricing, and environmental change. *Preventive Medicine,* 39, Suppl 2 (2004): S75–80.

52. Cummins, S., Petticrew, M., Higgins, C., Findlay, A., and Sparks L. Large scale food retailing as an intervention for diet and health: Quasi-experimental evaluation of a natural experiment. *Journal of Epidemiology and Community Health,* 59 (2005): 1035–1040.

53. Wrigley, N., Warm, D., and Margetts, B. Deprivation, diet and food retail access: Findings from the Leeds "food deserts" study. *Environment and Planning A,* 35 (2003): 151–188.

CHAPTER

4

AN ECOLOGICAL MODEL OF URBAN CHILD HEALTH

KIM T. FERGUSON, PILYOUNG KIM,
JAMES R. DUNN, GARY W. EVANS

LEARNING OBJECTIVES

- Define the term *ecological model* and explain its utility in interdisciplinary research in urban health.

- Describe key influences on the health of urban children at various levels of social organization (e.g., individual, family, community, policy).

- Describe some of the ways that researchers have studied these influences on child health across multiple levels.

- Identify questions on the health of urban children that require ecological research approaches to answer.

INTRODUCTION

Approximately 10 million children under the age of five, including 4 million infants under the age of one month, die every year from causes that are largely preventable,[1-3] including preventable and/or treatable diseases such as diarrheal dehydration, acute respiratory infection, measles, malaria, and HIV.[1,2] In fact, three of the five most significant contributors to the global burden of disease are primarily or exclusively childhood diseases—namely, perinatal conditions, lower respiratory infections, and diarrheal diseases.[1,2] In addition, malnutrition contributes to over a third of all child deaths worldwide.[2,4] Although children living in rural areas are almost twice as likely to be malnourished as children living in urban areas,[2] and child mortality rates are typically higher in rural areas,[1] high morbidity, mortality, and malnutrition rates are nevertheless serious concerns for urban children worldwide, especially in the developing world. Furthermore, there is some evidence that, with increasing rates of rural-urban migration and the resulting growth of the urban poor, this urban advantage is decreasing and may not exist when socioeconomic status is controlled for.[5-7]

Urbanization has been on the incline since the Industrial Revolution, with 46 percent of the world's population living in cities in 2000 as opposed to just 5 percent at the beginning of the nineteenth century.[8,9] This trend is expected to continue, and in fact, global population growth in the next thirty years will be primarily in cities, with approximately two-thirds of the world's population living in cities by 2040.[9,10]

Children may be disproportionately affected by the environmental challenges inherent in poor urban neighborhoods.[11-13] Child illnesses and malnutrition influence various aspects of child development, including cognitive development and intellectual performance.[14-24] Further, child mental and physical health predict later health during adolescence and adulthood.[22,23] Thus, healthy children grow up to be healthy adults.[22] It is therefore critical that public health researchers and practitioners consider the specific factors affecting the health of urban children in developing intervention strategies for improving global health and development. In this chapter, we suggest a conceptual framework wherein the complex interrelations among biological, psychosocial, and physical factors influencing child health in urban environments can be studied.

AN ECOLOGICAL MODEL

Ecological contexts have long been recognized as influential in determining population health. For example, in a discussion on housing conditions and health, Saegert and Evans[25] described the powerful influence of housing location and its determinants in shaping the multiple social and physical risks low-income and minority urban families face.

Although some research on urban public health has adopted an ecological perspective, individual studies tend to assess the influences of very specific ecological contexts at only one level (e.g., housing and health, neighborhood poverty and crime).

By contrast, in its World Health Report for 2005, the World Health Organization suggests taking an integrated rather than an isolated approach in developing both assessments of and interventions to improve child health.[26] Indeed, considerable research indicates that health interventions are most effective when implemented at multiple levels.[27-33] Thus, this chapter calls for an integrated ecological approach to the study of urban public health, employing Bronfenbrenner's bioecological model to assess the influences of the ecological context at multiple levels over time on child health. We use this theoretical framework as a heuristic to examine what is known and what needs to be looked at further among the multiple, intersecting ecological niches cities provide for children and their families, with a specific focus on how such complex urban contexts influence children's health. We then lay out an agenda for future work in light of the Bronfenbrenner bioecological model.

BRONFENBRENNER'S BIOECOLOGICAL MODEL

Bronfenbrenner originally conceptualized his bioecological model as a framework for studying development within the actual environments in which people live.[34-40] Therefore, this framework lends itself well to the study of urban health within an ecological framework, which necessarily emphasizes the interaction between characteristics of the person and characteristics of the environment in determining specific health outcomes.[29] Further, in contrast to other ecological models employed in urban health research, in the formulation of their bioecological framework, Bronfenbrenner and colleagues have specifically identified some of the characteristics of the person and the environment that have an impact on development. They have further specified mechanisms through which interactions between person and environment characteristics may influence development and health.

Process-Person-Context-Time

Within Bronfenbrenner's bioecological model are four interacting dimensions that should be considered when studying development in context—namely, *process, person, context,* and *time* (PPCT; see Figure 4.1).[40] The first of these, *process,* is at the core of the model, and it encompasses exchanges of energy between an organism and the environment that operate over time.[37, 39, 40] These enduring forms of progressively more complex reciprocal interactions between active and evolving human organisms and the persons, objects, and symbols in their immediate external environments, termed *proximal processes,* are critically important in driving development.[39, 40] For the purposes of this chapter, proximal processes can be thought of as two-way interactions between the child and the objects and people in his or her immediate environment that may influence health (see Figure 4.1). A simple example would be the ways a child learns to communicate to her parent whether she is ill and needs medical treatment, while at the same time the parent learns to identify the child's need for medical treatment from her behavior.

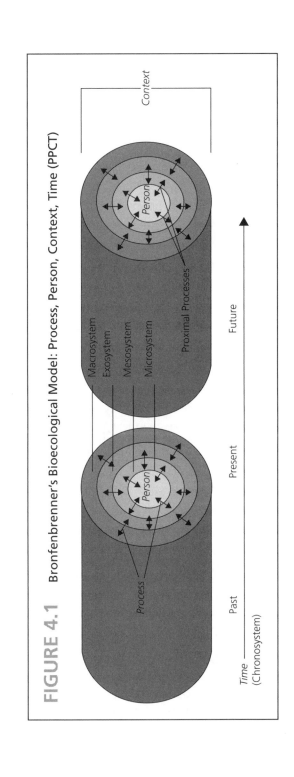

FIGURE 4.1 Bronfenbrenner's Bioecological Model: Process, Person, Context, Time (PPCT)

The power of proximal processes in directing development is posited to vary as a function of various characteristics of the developing *person,* including behavioral dispositions, resources, and demand characteristics.[40] The distinction between these different types of person characteristics as conceptualized in Bronfenbrenner's model is not essential for our present purposes. What *is* important to note is that much research evidence indicates that various characteristics of the developing person do indeed shape both mental and physical health. For example, self-motivation, self-efficacy, and self-esteem all positively influence health and well-being.[41, 42] Some evidence suggests that the aggressiveness of physicians' treatments for persons suffering from heart attacks varies by gender, whereby physicians treat males more aggressively than females.[43]

Another defining property of Bronfenbrenner's bioecological model is *time,* which is characterized at three different levels—namely, microtime (continuity vs. discontinuity within episodes of proximal processes), mesotime (the periodicity of these episodes of proximal processes across longer time intervals such as days or weeks), and macrotime (changing expectations and events in the larger society that may influence individual development).[40] As with the specific aspects of the person as conceptualized in the Bronfenbrenner model, the different levels of time are not a critical consideration for our present purposes. However, given the importance of enduring reciprocal interactions between persons and their environment in directing development, we can see that the regularity and predictability of events across time directly influences children's development, including their health. For example, children living in families with greater turmoil (e.g., frequent arguments between parents and parental divorce or separation) have elevated cardiovascular activity.[44, 45] Further, the regularity of events and levels of unpredictability and confusion in the home are related to children's mental health, independent of socioeconomic status (SES).[46–48]

Finally, in terms of the ecological *context,* Bronfenbrenner and colleagues have argued that development occurs within four nested and interacting systems—namely the microsystem, the mesosystem, the exosystem, and the macrosystem (see Figure 4.2).[40] All four systems are important for understanding children's health in urban environments. The microsystem consists of the settings directly experienced by the child (e.g., the family, the peer group, the school, and the immediate neighborhood). The mesosystem consists of connections between these microsystems (e.g., the interaction between parents' expectations of the child in terms of nonrisky health behavior and the expectations of the child's peers). The exosystem is comprised of linkages and processes between settings that do not contain but directly influence the child (e.g., parental work settings, the larger neighborhood). The macrosystem is the overarching pattern of micro-, meso-, and exosystems that is characteristic of a given culture or subculture. Thus, the ecological context influences the critical proximal processes that underlie human development at multiple levels. In the present chapter, we focus on how both physical and social environmental factors at these different levels influence child health.

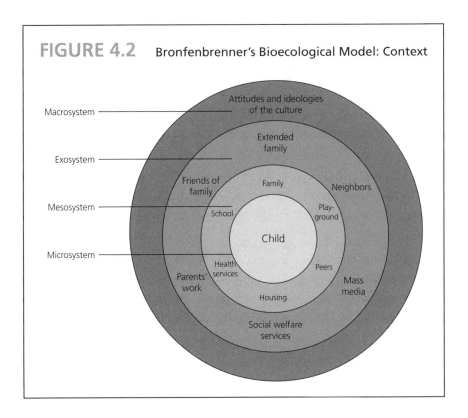

FIGURE 4.2 Bronfenbrenner's Bioecological Model: Context

INFLUENCES ON CHILDREN'S HEALTH IN THE URBAN CONTEXT

We turn now to a brief discussion of some of the key factors having an impact on urban children's health. It should be emphasized that our purpose here is not to provide a comprehensive overview of the current literature on urban children's health but instead to consider some ways this literature could be understood, and future research could be conducted, within an ecological framework. Thus, we have identified key factors of the physical and social environment that have demonstrated impacts on children's health at each level of the child's environment, from her immediate surroundings to the larger culture in which she is embedded. Some of these factors have been identified by public health researchers as "leverage points"—individual and environmental factors that have the most significant impact on a given health outcome.[29, 31] Understanding the impact of such critical factors on child health is an essential first step in developing appropriate intervention strategies at multiple levels.

Macrosystem

Physical and Social Environment: Urban Environments The macrosystem is the overarching pattern of micro-, meso-, and exosystem factors characteristic of a given culture or subculture.[40] Urban environments can be seen as a macrosystem that leads to specific micro-, meso-, and exosystem characteristics, as well as to certain proximal processes acting over time. For example, three hallmark characteristics of urban environments—namely, complexity, diversity, and density—were introduced in the introductory chapter of this volume. These characteristics operate at multiple levels of the urban environment (including at the immediate level of the family and at the more external level of parents' work environments) and influence practices and beliefs of parents and their children, thus affecting child health in a unique way (Figure 4.3). These characteristics are briefly considered here in light of their possible role in the health of urban children. We also discuss how these factors fit within Bronfenbrenner's ecological model.

Complexity is one of the defining characteristics of an urban environment.[49] Two dimensions of complexity in cities are the heterogeneity of urban populations (microsystem) and neighborhoods (microsystem and exosystem),[33, 49–51] both encompassed within the overall characteristic of diversity, and the heterogeneity of both housing (microsystem) and neighborhood (exosystem) density.[52] This heterogeneity is partly a result of the high immigration rates that are typical of cities. Further, cities change over time, a characteristic important to consider in assessing the most critical factors influencing urban child health, which may well change as cities evolve.[49] Some of this high rate of change over time is partly due to the high mobility and residential turnover that

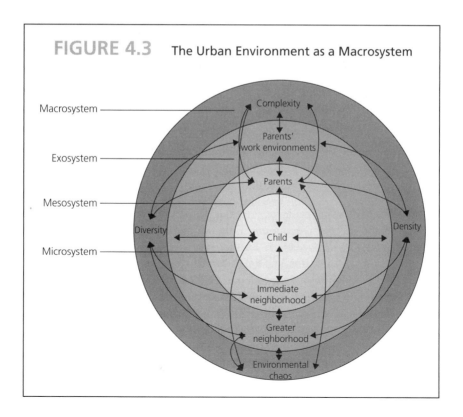

FIGURE 4.3   The Urban Environment as a Macrosystem

are typical of urban environments, which result in disruptions in the child's immediate environment (microsystem) as well as in environments not immediately affecting the child, such as parents' work environments (exosystem).

These dimensions of complexity render urban environments particularly challenging to study in terms of identifying the various factors influencing health. The development and application of multilevel, multidimensional models in studying urban health is thus of critical importance.[27–33, 49]

Diversity exists both between and within cities. Between different cities in different parts of the world, different characteristics of the physical and social environment may be more or less salient and may influence health in different ways.[49] For example, the lack of safe water and poor sanitation critically influence urban child health in the developing world,[11, 13] factors that may be less critically important influences in the developed world. These can be conceptualized as factors operating at the level of the macrosystem, as they differ between large, complex environments. By contrast, overcrowding and other factors characteristic of poor quality housing in urban areas have a direct impact on child mental and physical health in both developing and developed cities.[11, 25, 46, 50, 53, 54] They can thus be considered components of the child's microsystem. These differences require researchers to be cautious in making generalizations about the critical influences of urban living on health in urban environments. It is also essential that differences between different children's experiences be considered at the level at which they operate.

Within cities, diversity encompasses the heterogeneity of both urban populations and neighborhoods and housing quality and type.[33, 49–51] Urban populations are heterogeneous along the dimensions of ethnicity, income, and socioprofessional status, among other factors.[33, 49] As we will discuss in some detail later, characteristics such as SES critically influence child health and operate both in the microsystem (e.g., within families, schools, and immediate neighborhoods) and the exosystem (e.g., the larger neighborhood).[55–56] Differing neighborhood characteristics are similarly correlated with differential child mental and physical health outcomes, again as detailed later in this chapter.[11, 46, 50, 51, 53, 54]

Yet another level of complication in assessing the influences of various ecological factors on child health in urban environments is the fact that person and neighborhood characteristics are often interrelated; for example, neighborhood segregation tends to occur along ethnic and socioeconomic lines.[25,50] We thus discuss SES as operating across levels in the following section. Further, both housing and neighborhood density are heterogeneous within cities such that low-income, minority families are more likely to live in homes and neighborhoods characterized by residential crowding.[52] Thus, poor, ethnic minority urban children are exposed to considerably more environmental and psychosocial stressors related to poverty than are suburban white children; these stressors in turn influence child health at multiple levels.[15, 52, 55, 56]

In many urban areas, inequality is pervasive; low-income residents, including children, lack access to adequate health and social services, which typically operate at the level of the mesosystem and/or exosystem (see Figure 4.2) in both developing and developed world cities.[6–8, 57–59] As a result, large numbers of children under the age of five die from causes that would have been preventable given adequate care.[1–4] In fact, in the forty-two countries that in 2000 accounted for 90 percent of all deaths of children under age five, 63 percent of those deaths could have been prevented if these children had adequate access to basic health services.[60] In the U.S. context, persons of lower SES often lack critical health insurance coverage.[61, 62]

A third defining characteristic of cities is *density*.[49] This density may influence such physical environmental factors affecting child health within the microsystem as the availability of green space and other play or recreational space for children,[63] the urban climate, traffic, noise and air pollution,[46, 64, 65] exposure to lead and other environmental toxins and hazardous waste,[46, 66–68] and water scarcity, pollution, and sanitation.[11, 26] In addition, density contributes to diversity; in urban areas, social environmental factors result in the physical proximity of rich and poor neighborhoods.[56, 69] The physical proximity of these different neighborhoods usually influences children at the level of the exosystem.

One salient aspect of urban as opposed to rural contexts that affects child health is traffic congestion.[46] This typically operates at the level of the microsystem. Street traffic raises the risk of pediatric injuries[70] and is also related to restrictions in outdoor play for five-year-old children and to poorer social and motor skills.[71] Further, children and families have smaller social networks and interact less with their neighbors on congested streets.[71, 72] Additionally, traffic congestion is related to higher levels of pollutants and noise pollution, which both adversely affect child health.[46]

Another distinguishing feature of the urban environment is the built environment, which again typically operates at the level of the microsystem. The quality of the built environment, as assessed by housing quality or crowding, has demonstrated effects on mental and physical health for both children and adults, including asthma and other respiratory conditions, lead poisoning, accidents and injuries, and psychological distress.[11, 46, 52, 73–79] Exposure to noise, particularly chronic airport noise, similarly influences children's physical and mental health.[46]

Another salient aspect of urban as opposed to rural environments is children's lack of access to nature. Children prefer to play in natural, outdoor settings and engage in more complex play in such settings as opposed to built play spaces, perhaps because they afford a greater variety of motoric and social play opportunities as well as more independent play.[46] Such settings also enhance positive affect and may buffer some of the negative effects of exposure to chronic stressors in children.[46, 63] Given the adverse impact of chronic stress on children's physical and mental health,[15, 52, 55, 56] it is likely that access to green space contributes to children's health.

Two other related characteristics of urban environments are *social disorganization* and *environmental chaos*. Interestingly, the third proposition of Bronfenbrenner's bioecological model posits that chaos, which is likely more common in urban than in rural environments, can interfere with proximal processes and/or directly lead to proximal processes that foreshadow dysfunctional social development.[39] The regularity of events and levels of unpredictability and confusion in the home[47, 48] are related to children's socioemotional functioning[46] and mental and physical health.[50, 80, 81]

Chaos typically influences the proximal processes at the level of the microsystem. Many of the defining characteristics of urban environments (i.e., *complexity, diversity,* and *density*) contribute to chaos. Some urban characteristics that contribute to chaos are noise, traffic, high mobility, residential turnover, and the high rate of migration into cities, particularly in the developing world.[82] Thus, chaos can influence children's mental and physical health at multiple levels.

Social support and connectedness,[22, 50, 83–85] spatial segregation along racial/ethnic and socioeconomic lines,[86–90] and inequality[53, 87, 89, 91–93] also have demonstrated effects on child health in urban areas. These factors influence child health most noticeably at the family (microsystem) and neighborhood (microsystem and exosystem) levels,[22, 50, 51, 87–89, 94] as will be discussed later.

Exosystem

Physical Environment: Neighborhood and Parents' Work Environments   The exosystem includes linkages and processes between settings that do not contain but directly influence the child.[40] Children's interactions with their immediate neighbors and immediate neighborhood play areas may be classified as part of the microsystem directly affecting proximal processes. However, larger neighborhood contexts may be conceptualized as part of the exosystem (i.e., environmental contexts that children are not a part of but nevertheless influence their development).[50]

The neighborhood may affect children's mental and physical health in a number of ways. For example, living in a poor neighborhood is associated with poorer individual health, even after controlling for SES.[95] In an evaluation of the New York City Moving to Opportunity program, researchers demonstrated that male children who moved to low-poverty areas from poor neighborhoods showed improvements in mental health.[96] Similarly, the concentration of neighborhood poverty is a strong predictor of child maltreatment.[97, 98] Thus, it can be seen that various neighborhood characteristics, and most important, poverty, may significantly influence urban children's mental and physical health.

Parents' work contexts, which typically represent settings not directly experienced by children, influence children's health as part of both the social and physical environment. A good example of the way parents' physical work environments have an impact on their children's health is the transfer of pesticides from farm workers' worksites to their homes.[99, 100] These pesticides, which are accumulated on farm workers' skin and clothing, contribute to cancer risk, neurobehavioral deficits, and other health risks for children.[100]

Social Environment: Parents' Work Environments   Parents' work contexts can also influence children's health by affecting the social environment parents provide for their children. For example, extensive research by Menaghan and Parcel[101] documents the negative effect of poor quality, low-status, and low-complexity maternal work conditions on the home environment, which then contributes to children's behavioral problems and general mental health. Similarly, Crouter and colleagues have found that parents' experiences of high work pressure (work stress) may make them more likely to engage in conflict with their adolescent children.[102] Conflict is, in turn, linked to lower feelings of psychological well-being (i.e., poorer mental health) in adolescents. Likewise, parents' working conditions and the family's economic stress have been demonstrated to affect their parenting behaviors.[103] More specifically, low-SES parents and parents with stressful working conditions tend to discourage self-directedness and are more restrictive than are other parents.[103, 104] Such parenting trends, in turn, lead to lower self-efficacy among adolescents[103] and may also influence general mental and physical health.[22]

Mesosystem

Physical and Social Environment: Crowding and Parent-Child Relationships   The mesosystem consists of connections between microsystems (settings directly experienced by the child).[40] Thus, mesosystem influences on child health assess the ways that various aspects of the microsystems children inhabit interrelate across settings to affect health. There is little direct evidence for these cross-microsystem impacts.

Evans and Saegert[52] found that family turmoil (e.g., frequent arguments between parents and parental divorce or separation) was associated with residential density. Physiological stress for children living in low-turmoil households was largely unaffected by residential density, whereas crowding elevated stress in high-turmoil families.

Other researchers have found that the effects of density on children's health may be moderated by other factors. For example, Evans et al.[105] found that residence in larger, multifamily structures exacerbated the negative effects of crowded housing on third- and fourth-graders' psychological distress. By contrast, low-density housing has been linked with resilience in terms of low birthweight babies' socioemotional development at age three.[106] Similarly, Maxwell[107] found that the adverse impacts of day care crowding on preschoolers' social development (including mental health) were amplified by living in more crowded homes.

Microsystem

Physical Environment: Housing Quality and Crowding   The microsystem consists of the settings directly experienced by the child.[40] We have already briefly mentioned the effects of housing quality and crowding on child mental and physical health.[25, 46, 52–54, 76, 108, 109] Considering children specifically, Evans et al.[54] found that high-rise, multiple-family dwellings have a negative impact on children's mental health, especially among preschoolers. Similarly, their review indicated that housing quality may influence child health by contributing to parental and child stress.[15, 52, 55, 56] Housing quality can also directly influence child physical health. For example, cold and damp housing causes respiratory problems in children.[108] Dust mites, cockroaches, and other allergens are known asthma triggers and one component of the epidemic of asthma in low-income urban centers in the United States.[76, 109] Asthma is a growing problem disproportionately affecting children in low-income and/or minority households. Mold, dampness, dust, and smoking are all significant—and preventable—indoor asthma triggers.

Turning to crowding, residential density has been shown to predict children's psychological distress,[52, 110] which may influence both mental and physical health[15, 52, 55, 56] and physical development.[111, 112] Further, crowding is associated with higher rates of respiratory and infectious diseases, especially in the developing world.[11, 73, 113]

Social Environment: Family   As we have seen, the family is a critical component of the social environment and thus has a significant impact on child mental and physical health.[22, 26]

The family influences child mental and physical health in a number of ways. For example, parental worldviews in the form of beliefs, attitudes, and behaviors influence both children's health and well-being and children's own beliefs, attitudes, and behaviors, which may themselves later influence child health.[114–117]

Children's health is also directly and powerfully influenced by parental care through parental provision of care, adequate nutrition, access to external health care services, and parent-child interactions.[22, 26, 118–122] For example, Richter and Griesel[120] demonstrated that the absence of sensitive, responsive parental care is related to both malnutrition and a failure to thrive in young children. Similarly, Repetti et al.[22] review substantial evidence that negative family interactions such as cold, unsupportive, and neglectful relationships significantly affect both the present and future health of children growing up in such environments. For example, maternal-infant conflict is associated with lower infant weight gain, even after controlling for infant birthweight, maternal height, and maternal eating disorders.[123] Numerous other research studies assessing the impacts of various family interaction characteristics on different child mental and physical health outcomes show similar results.[22]

Factors Operating Across Systems

Physical and Social Environment: Socioeconomic Status   Socioeconomic status (SES) is often conceptualized as a component of the macrosystem. The spatial segregation along socioeconomic lines that is characteristic of urban environments creates low-income, predominantly minority neighborhoods as specific subcultures within the broader urban environment.[50, 86, 88, 89] However, it should be noted that SES can also operate more directly and specifically within individual families and small neighborhoods (i.e., at the level of the microsystem) and at the level of the mesosystem as well, as has been discussed. For example, urban children in low-income households typically attend predominantly low-income schools. This is in contrast, at least in the United

States, to rural, low-income children, who typically attend schools largely populated by middle-income students. Finally, SES can also operate at the level of the exosystem; for example, parents' workplaces influence their children's health. The larger neighborhood within which a child lives can also be considered part of the exosystem, as has already been discussed. It is thus important in evaluating the effects of SES on child health to evaluate at which level or levels SES affects the child.

A considerable body of research has documented the inverse relationship between SES and health for both children and adults.[125–128] This inverse relationship has been described as a gradient, whereby health differences have been observed between adjacent SES levels.

Socioeconomic status has been shown to affect various aspects of child mental and physical health.[89, 125–128] Numerous studies that assess the impacts of various family interaction characteristics on child mental and physical health show similar results.[22, 124] The overall consensus is that SES significantly influences multiple aspects of child health at multiple levels. Although low SES does not directly cause poor health, it is most often its indicator. The relationship between SES and poor health is usually mediated by other factors in the environment, such as decreased social support to assist single mothers to cope with their children's demands and a decrease in social support networks that provide good mentoring for adolescents. In this way, SES is operating at a higher level (macrosystem) than at the level of the immediate family alone (microsystem).

Evans[56] provides an overview of the environment of childhood poverty, specifically, and documents the higher incidence of multiple psychosocial and physical risk factors accompanying child poverty. There is also evidence that higher levels of cumulative risk exposure help to account for poverty's ill effects on children.[121, 129, 130] In addition, not only are low-income children more likely to be exposed to a plethora of suboptimal environmental conditions, but personal and social resources for coping with these poor conditions are often wanting. Low-income parents may themselves be contending with these same stressors and hence be less able to provide support for their children. Parents in crowded and noisy homes, for example, are less responsive to their children.[131] Here, SES influences the child at the level of the microsystem.

Residential segregation along racial/ethnic and socioeconomic lines,[50, 86–90] which is typical of urban areas, perpetuates racial disparities in poverty and perpetuates both racial and socioeconomic inequities in education and economic opportunities for children and their parents, which in turn contribute to health inequalities.[87] Further, substandard housing, residential crowding, and environmental hazards are concentrated in such areas, which further contributes to racial and socioeconomic disparities in health. All of these aspects of the environment affect child health. Such disparities are present at both the individual (microsystem) and neighborhood (microsystem and exosystem) levels; we have already discussed how neighborhood characteristics, including poverty, may influence children's mental and physical health.

Low-income urban neighborhoods tend to be the site for greater risks, fewer resources, including fewer recreational resources,[63, 132] and less positive social environments, all of which contribute to child health and development. For example, the usually positive impact of social capital (conceptualized as trusting and reciprocal relationships between neighbors) for children and youth can actually negatively affect children's mental health in neighborhoods of concentrated poverty.[133] In general, high levels of social capital are positively associated with good population health.[133–135] However, in an investigation of the influence of social capital on African American children's behavioral problems, a recent study indicated that, in poor urban neighborhoods, children whose parents knew few of the neighbors had lower levels of internalizing problems such as anxiety and depression (i.e., better mental health).[133] In contrast, in wealthier urban neighborhoods, children whose parents knew few of the neighbors had higher levels of internalizing problems.[133] This research highlights the importance of studying child health in context, as well as the importance of conceptualizing the effects of SES on children's health at the level of the macrosystem. Given the complex, multilevel relationship between SES and health, a critical assessment of the various factors mediating this SES-health correlation will provide urban health practitioners with specific avenues for possible intervention in urban children's mental and physical health outcomes.

In conclusion, we can see the complexity of urban environments and the existence of multiple interacting factors influencing child health at multiple levels. Disentangling these effects, and thus understanding both the individual and cumulative effects of various aspects of the ecological context on urban children's mental and physical health, is a critical precursor to the development of effective assessments and interventions.

RESEARCH ACROSS MULTIPLE LEVELS

Although recent research on urban public health has adopted an ecological perspective, individual studies tend to assess the influences of very specific ecological contexts at only one level (e.g., housing and health, neighborhood poverty and crime). There is thus a critical need for multilevel analyses of the various interacting factors of the physical and social environment, as well as individual characteristics, that influence child health within the complexity and diversity of urban environments. We turn now to three specific examples of research assessing the influence of the ecological context on child health across multiple levels.

Health, Family, and Residential Crowding

Evans and Saegert[52] propose an ecological model of the effects of the interactive relations between residential density and inner-city stressors on children's mental health and the mediation of these effects by parent-child proximal processes (enduring two-way interactions). This model was tested through an assessment of forty minority children ($M = 9.8$ years) living in a low-income, inner-city, predominantly minority neighborhood of New York City. Their results indicated that, for low-income children living in inner-city neighborhoods, family turmoil compounded the negative effects of residential crowding on child health. Moreover, some of the impact appeared to be accounted for by less responsive parenting. Thus, their results highlight the importance of studying the influences of environmental stressors such as residential crowding on child health within the broader, ecological context so as to better understand the multiple interacting factors influencing child health.

Health, Family, and Neighborhood

Oliver, Dunn, Kohen, and Hertzman[136] investigated the influence of six neighborhood characteristics (percentage speaking English as a first language; median family income; percentage with a high school certificate; unemployment rate; percentage of lone parent families; percentage who haven't moved in the last five years) on urban kindergarten children's physical health and well-being. They also studied children's social knowledge and competence, emotional health and maturity, language and cognitive development, and communication skills and general knowledge. They statistically controlled for individual characteristics such as family income and whether English is the primary language spoken at home. Thus, the impact of various aspects of the microsystem (family and immediate neighborhood) as well as various aspects of the exosystem (larger neighborhood) on child outcomes was investigated. Further, they employed hierarchical linear modeling to investigate the influence of neighborhood factors on children's health and other outcomes, and thus developed a two-level model with individuals nested in neighborhoods, similar to Bronfenbrenner's ecological model. The primary goal was to investigate whether neighborhood characteristics were independently associated with any of the five child outcomes assessed (including physical health and well-being) after adjusting for family characteristics that might contribute to these outcomes.

Family-level characteristics generally influenced children's outcomes more than did neighborhood-level characteristics.[136] However, some neighborhood-level factors were independently associated with some outcomes, including physical health and well-being. Their results thus suggest that interventions to improve children's physical health and well-being might be more effective if implemented at the family level rather than at the neighborhood level, but that some specific interventions at the neighborhood level may also be effective. Thus, again we can see the additional information garnered in developing a multilevel, nested model to assess the independent influences of various aspects of the ecological context at different levels on children's health.

Health, Family, School, and Neighborhood

Previous research on the relationship between stress and children's adjustment, including their mental health, has shown that specific types of stressors in specific contexts can predict a variety of adjustment problems in children. However, little previous research had examined the influence of different types of stressors across multiple contexts on multiple indicators of poor mental health. Morales and Guerra[137] investigated the effects of a number of stressful experiences within three different contexts (family, school, and neighborhood), as well as cumulative stress and stress across multiple contexts, on three different indices of adjustment, including depression (a mental health measure), in a large sample of urban elementary schoolchildren from economically disadvantaged communities over a two-year period. Children were initially assessed when they were in Grades 1–4 and then again two years later, when they were in Grades 3–6. Thus, the impact of different stressors within various aspects of the microsystem (family, school, and immediate neighborhood) on various child outcomes (including depression) was longitudinally investigated within a specific macrocontext (low-income urban communities). The majority of the children assessed were ethnic minorities.

Stressful experiences in each of the three measured contexts (family, school, and neighborhood) were related to negative outcomes across each of the three adjustment measures assessed, including depression, both at the time of the measured stress and longitudinally.[137] Morales and Guerra further found that cumulative stress was related to increases in depression. Stress across multiple contexts, however, did not contribute uniquely to increases in depression independent of cumulative stress. These findings are an important contribution to our understanding of the impact of multiple stressful events across multiple ecological contexts on disadvantaged urban children's health.

AGENDA FOR FUTURE RESEARCH AND PRACTICE

As we have described, much is known about some of the specific factors influencing child health, especially at the level of the individual. However, despite recent arguments for an ecological approach to urban public health, relatively few studies, particularly in the realm of child health, have adopted such a comprehensive approach. Instead, the majority of studies tend to assess the influences of very specific ecological contexts at only one level. One of the reasons for this is, perhaps, that such comprehensive research projects are beyond the resources and capacities of individual researchers. We thus offer some suggestions for practical steps to take in applying Bronfenbrenner's model to research and practice in urban public health.

Agenda for Research

First, critical reviews of the literature should identify those individual factors that have demonstrated effects on specific health outcomes, such as asthma, depression, or substance abuse. We have begun to do this in the present chapter, identifying some key factors that influence child health at each level of Bronfenbrenner's model (microsystem, mesosystem, exosystem, macrosystem; see also Figure 4.2). The magnitudes of such effects should be noted, and some key "leverage points" (individual and environmental factors that have the most significant impact on a given health outcome) should be identified.

Next, a comprehensive model detailing the effects known to have an impact on a given health outcome should be developed based on Bronfenbrenner's bioecological framework or another systems model. Using this framework, researchers should identify other factors that may be hypothesized to influence this given health outcome at each level. Hypothesized and known interactions between various factors should also be identified. Thus, a comprehensive model of the various factors and their interactions as they influence a specified health outcome should be developed. Earlier, we described three studies that have begun to do this in the broad area of urban child health—Evans and Saegert;[52] Oliver et al.;[136] Morales and Guerra.[137] We have also provided a basic outline of key aspects of the urban environment that may operate on child health at multiple levels in Figure 4.3.

In studying child health, it is also important to consider how different factors may vary in their impact on a given child health outcome across time,[138, 139] as is outlined in Bronfenbrenner's bioecological framework (see Figure 4.1).[40] This perspective helps to clarify whether the same factors influence child health in infancy and adolescence, and the cumulative effects of a particular environment on child outcomes. For example, Morales and Guerra found that stressful experiences affected child mental health (depression) both at the time of the measured stress and longitudinally.[137] Further, cumulative stress was related to increases in depression. Without a consideration of time, this more nuanced understanding of the effects of stress on child mental health would have been missed.

The next step, of course, is to test these models. To do this effectively, large-scale studies involving teams of researchers from multiple disciplines will be needed to identify the relative influences of each physical and social factor at multiple levels on the health outcome of interest, as well as the interactions between these various influences. The use of advanced statistical analyses, such as multiple regression models and hierarchical linear modeling (HLM), is also warranted, as in Oliver et al.[136]

Agenda for Practice

Once we have a better understanding of the multiple factors influencing a given child health outcome at multiple levels across time, we can link this knowledge with practice. We should emphasize that we believe the most effective child health interventions will be clearly based on research conducted within an ecological-contextual framework that also takes developmental time into account, as described earlier and elsewhere.[138, 139] This will provide researchers with a clear understanding of all the interacting factors influencing the health outcome of interest, both at the time that each factor operates and longitudinally.

In an ideal world, once we have a clear understanding of the interacting, multi-level factors that influence a particular child health outcome across time, we would implement interventions to positively alter the influence of each factor. However, this is not always practically possible. Thus, it is important to identify key leverage points that have the most significant impact on a given health outcome[29, 31] so as to identify the factors that are most malleable to change.[138, 139]

Finally, once key intervention strategies have been implemented, investigators must evaluate their effectiveness in positively altering the specified child health outcome.[138, 139] This evaluation process will also help to evaluate the accuracy of the model developed during the research process. Alterations can be made to this model based on the results of this evaluation. Thus, researchers will develop a more comprehensive

SUMMARY

In this chapter, we have argued that improving the health of urban children is critical to improving the future health of individuals and communities worldwide. Such improvements must rest on an understanding of the various factors contributing to child health, as well as the ways in which different factors interact at multiple levels in determining overall mental and physical health outcomes. To assist in this daunting task, we have suggested a conceptual framework based on Bronfenbrenner's bioecological model. We use this framework to assess the influences of multiple environmental factors operating at multiple levels over time as they influence critical two-way interactions between children and the objects and people in their immediate environments that may influence health. Applications of this model can assist urban health researchers become more effective in assessing and improving the health of children growing up in cities, both locally and globally.

understanding of the multiple factors influencing this aspect of child health at multiple levels across time.

DISCUSSION QUESTIONS

1. Why are ecological models useful in studying the health of urban children?

2. What does Bronfenbrenner mean by microsystem, mesosystem, exosystem, and macrosystem influences? Give some examples of factors that influence child health at each of these levels.

3. What are some ways that exposure to stress influences child health? What are examples of urban stressors at each of Bronfenbrenner's levels?

4. If you were to apply an ecological approach to study food availability for low-income urban children (see Chapter Three), what might be key influences of availability at individual, family, neighborhood, and municipal levels?

ACKNOWLEDGMENTS

This work was partially supported by a fellowship from the College of Human Ecology, Cornell University, the W. T. Grant Foundation, and the John D. and Catherine T. MacArthur Foundation Network on Socioeconomic Status and Health. Many thanks to Dr. Marianella Casasola, Dr. Barbara Lust, Dr. N'Dri Assie-Lumumba, and an anonymous reviewer for helpful comments on earlier versions of this manuscript.

NOTES

1. UNICEF. *Child mortality.* Available at www.childinfo.org/mortality.html. Updated November 2007. Accessed April 25, 2008.

2. World Health Organization. What are the key health dangers for children? Available at www.who.int/features/qa/13/en/index.html. Updated December 2008. Accessed February 1, 2009.

3. World Health Organization. 10 facts on child health. Available at www.who.int/features/factfiles/child_health2/en. Updated October 02007. Accessed April 25, 2008.

4. UNICEF. *Malnutrition.* Available at www.childinfo.org/undernutrition.html. Updated January 2009. Accessed February 1, 2009.

5. Fotso, J-C. Urban-rural differentials in child malnutrition: Trends and socioeconomic correlates in sub-Saharan Africa. *Health and Place,* 13 (2007): 205–223.

6. Brockerhoff, M., and Brennan, E. The poverty of cities in developing regions. *Population and Development Review,* 24 (1998): 75–114.

7. Panel on Urban Population Dynamics, Montgomery, M. R., Stren, R., Bohen, B., and Reed, H. E. *Cities Transformed: Demographic Change and Its Implications in the Developing World.* Washington, D.C.: National Academies Press, 2003.

8. Brockerhoff, M. P. An urbanizing world. *Population Bulletin,* 55 (2000): 3–4.

9. Guidotti, T. L., de Kok, T., Kjellstrom, T., and Yassi, A. *Basic Environmental Health.* New York: Oxford University Press, 2001.

10. Satterthwaite, D. Will most people live in cities? *British Medical Journal,* 321 (2000): 1143–1145.

11. Bartlett, S. Children's experience of the physical environment in poor urban settlements and the implications for policy, planning and practice. *Environment and Urbanization,* 11 (1999): 63–73.

12. Stephens, C. Healthy cities of unhealthy islands? The health and social implications of urban inequality. *Environment and Urbanization,* 8 (1996): 9–30.

13. World Health Organization. *World Health Report 1995: Bridging the Gaps.* Geneva: World Health Organization, 1995.

14. Boivin, M. J. Effects of early cerebral malaria on cognitive ability in Senegalese children. *Journal of Developmental and Behavioral Pediatrics,* 23, no. 5 (2002): 353–364.

15. Brooks-Gunn, J., Duncan, G. J., and Britto, P. R. Are socioeconomic gradients for children similar to those for adults? Achievement and health of children in the United States. In D. P. Keating and C. Hertzman, eds., *Developmental Health and the Wealth of Nations: Social, Biological, and Educational Dynamics,* pp. 94–124. New York: Guilford Press, 1999.

16. Carter, J. A., Murira, G. M., Ross, A., Mung'ala-Odera, V., and Newton, C. R. J. C. Speech and language sequelae of severe malaria in Kenyan children. *Brain Injury,* 17 (2002): 217–224.

17. Carter, J. A., Munga'ala-Odera, V., Neville, B. G. R., Murira, G. M., Mturi, N., Musumba, C., and Newton, C. R. J. C. Persistent neurocognitive impairments associated with severe falciparum malaria in Kenyan children. *Journal of Neurology, Neurosurgery, and Psychiatry,* 76 (2004): 476–481.

18. Dougbartey, A. T., Spellacy, F. J., and Dougbartey, M. T. Somatosensory discrimination deficits following pediatric cerebral malaria. *American Journal of Tropical Medicine and Hygiene,* 59 (1998): 393–396.

19. Glewwe, P., Jacoby, H. G., and King, E. M. Early childhood nutrition and academic achievement: A longitudinal analysis. *Journal of Public Economics,* 81 (2001): 345–368.

20. Holding, P. A., Stevenson, J., Peshu, N., and Marsh, K. Cognitive sequelae of severe malaria with impaired consciousness. *Royal Society of Tropical Medicine and Hygiene,* 93 (1999): 529–534.

21. Molteno, C., Woods, D., and Hollingshead, J. A 5-year follow-up study of full term small for gestational age infants in Cape Town. *Developmental Brain Dysfunction,* 8 (1995): 119–126.

22. Repetti, R. L., Taylor, S. E., and Seeman, T. E. Risky families: Family social environments and the mental and physical health of offspring. *Psychological Bulletin,* 128 (2002): 330–366.

23. Sameroff, A. J. Environmental risk factors in infancy. *Pediatrics,* 102 (1998): 1287–1292.

24. Scrimshaw, N. S. Malnutrition, brain development, learning, and behavior. *Nutrition Research,* 18 (1998): 351–379.

25. Saegert, S., and Evans, G. W. Poverty, housing niches, and health in the United States. *Journal of Social Issues,* 59 (2003): 569–589.

26. World Health Organization. *World Health Report 2005: Make Every Mother and Child Count.* Geneva: World Health Organization, 2005.

27. Ansari, Z., Carson, N. J., Ackland, M. J., Vaughan, L., and Serraglio, A. A public health model of the social determinants of health. *Sozial- und Präventivmedizin,* 48 (2003): 242–251.

28. Green, L. W., and Krueter, M. W. *Health Promotion Planning: An Education and Ecological Approach,* 3rd ed. Mountain View, Cal.: Mayfield, 1999.

29. Grzywacz, J. G., and Fuqua, J. The social ecology of health: Leverage points and linkages. *Behavioral Medicine,* 26 (2000): 101–115.

30. Parker, E. A., Baldwin, G. T., Israel, B., and Salinas, M. Application of health promotion theories and models for environmental health. *Health Education and Behavior,* 31 (2004): 491–509.

31. Stokols, D. Social ecology and behavioral medicine: Implications for training, practice, and policy. *Behavioral Medicine,* 26 (2000): 129–138.

32. Lawrence, R. J. Urban health: An ecological perspective. *Reviews on Environmental Health,* 14 (1999): 1–10.

33. Lawrence, R. J. Inequalities in urban areas: Innovative approaches to complex issues. *Scandinavian Journal of Public Health,* 30 (2002): 34–40.

34. Bronfenbrenner, U. Developmental research, public policy, and the ecology of childhood. *Child Development,* 45 (1974): 1–5.

35. Bronfenbrenner, U. Toward an experimental ecology of human development. *American Psychologist,* 32 (1977): 513–531.

36. Bronfenbrenner, U. *The Ecology of Human Development: Experiments by Nature and by Design.* Cambridge, Mass.: Harvard University Press, 1979.

37. Bronfenbrenner, U., and Ceci, S. J. Nature-nurture reconceptualized in developmental perspective: A bioecological model. *Psychological Review,* 101 (1994): 568–586.

38. Bronfenbrenner, U., and Crouter, A. C. The evolution of environmental models in developmental research. In W. Kessen, series ed., and P. H. Mussen, vol. ed., *Handbook of Child Psychology: Vol. 1. History, Theory, and Methods,* 4th ed., pp. 357–414. New York: John Wiley, 1983.

39. Bronfenbrenner, U., and Evans, G. W. Developmental science in the 21st century: Emerging questions, theoretical models, research designs and empirical findings. *Social Development,* 9 (2000): 115–125.

40. Bronfenbrenner, U., and Morris, P. A. The ecology of developmental processes. In W. Kessen, series ed., and P. H. Mussen, vol. ed., *Handbook of Child Psychology: Vol. 1. Theoretical Models of Human Development,* 5th ed., pp. 993–1028. New York: John Wiley, 1998.

41. Bandura, A. Self-efficacy: Toward a unifying theory of behavioral change. *Psychological Review,* 84 (1977): 191–215.

42. World Health Organization. *Social Determinants of Health: The Solid Facts.* Copenhagen: World Health Organization, 1998.

43. Iezzoni, L. I., Ash, A. S., Shwartz, M., and Mackiernan, Y. D. Differences in procedure use, in-hospital mortality, and illness severity by gender for acute myocardial infarction patients. *Medical Care,* 35 (1997): 158–171.

44. El-Sheikh, M., Cummings, E., and Goetsch, V. Coping with adults' angry behavior: Behavioral, physiological, and verbal responses in preschoolers. *Developmental Psychology,* 25 (1989): 490–498.

45. Matthews, K, A., Gump, B., Block, D., and Allen, M. Does background stress heighten or dampen children's responses to acute stress? *Psychological Medicine,* 59 (1997): 488–496.

46. Evans, G. W. Child development and the physical environment. *Annual Review of Psychology,* 57 (2006): 1–28.

47. Wachs, T. D., and Corapci, F. Environmental chaos, development and parenting across cultures. In C. Raeff and J. Benson, eds., *Social and Cognitive Development in the Context of Individual, Social, and Cultural Processes,* pp. 54–83. New York: Routledge, 2003.

48. Fiese, B. H., Tomcho, T. J., Douglas, M., Josephs, K., Poltrock, S., and Baker, T. A review of 50 years of research on naturally occurring family routines and rituals: Cause for celebration? *Journal of Family Psychology,* 16 (2002): 381–390.

49. Galea, D., and Vlahov, D. Urban health: Evidence, challenges, and directions. *Annual Review of Public Health,* 26 (2005): 341–365.

50. Leventhal, T., and Brooks-Gunn, J. The neighborhoods they live in: The effects of neighborhood residence on child and adolescent outcomes. *Psychological Bulletin,* 126 (2000): 309–337.

51. Wandersman, A., and Nation, M. Urban neighborhoods and mental health: Psychological contributions to understanding toxicity, resilience, and interventions. *American Psychologist,* 53 (1998): 647–656.

52. Evans, G. W., and Saegert, S. Residential crowding in the context of inner city poverty. In D. Wapner, J. Demick, T. Yamamoto, and H. Minami, eds., *Theoretical Perspectives in Environment-Behavior Research,* pp. 247–267. New York: Kluwer Academic/Plenum Press, 2000.

53. Dunn, J. R., and Hayes, M. V. Social inequality, population health, and housing: A study of two Vancouver neighborhoods. *Social Science & Medicine,* 51 (2000): 563–587.

54. Evans, G. W., Wells, N. M., and Moch, A. Housing and mental health: A review of the evidence and a methodological and conceptual critique. *Journal of Social Issues,* 59 (2003): 475–500.

55. Bradley, R. H., and Corwyn, R. F. Socioeconomic status and child development. *Annual Review of Psychology,* 53 (2002): 371–399.

56. Evans, G. W. The environment of childhood poverty. *American Psychologist,* 59 (2004): 77–92.

57. Agnew, R. Foundation for a general strain theory of crime and delinquency. *Criminology,* 30 (1992): 47–87.

58. Hoffman, M., Pick, W. M., Cooper, D., and Myers, J. E. Women's health status and use of health services in a rapidly growing peri-urban area of South Africa. *Social Science & Medicine,* 45 (1997): 149–157.

59. Wan, T. T. H., and Gray, L. C. Differential access to preventive services for young children in low-income urban areas. *Journal of Health and Social Behavior,* 19 (1978): 312–324.

60. Jones, G., Steketee, R. W., Black, R., Bhutta, Z. A., and Morris, S. Bellagion Child Survival Study Group. How many child deaths can we prevent this year? *Lancet,* 362 (2003): 65–71.

61. Grumbach, K., Vranizan, K., and Bindman, A. B. Physician supply and access to care in urban communities. *Health Affairs,* 16 (1997): 71–86.

62. Williams, D. R., and Rucker, T. D. Understanding and addressing racial disparities in health care. *Health Care Financing Review,* 21 (2000): 75–90.

63. Wells, N. M., and Evans, G. W. Nearby nature: A buffer of life stress among rural children. *Environment and Behavior,* 35 (2003): 311–330.

64. Dockery, D. W., Pope, C. A., 3rd, Xu, X., et al. An association between air pollution and mortality in six U.S. cities. *New England Journal of Medicine,* 329 (1993): 1753–1759.

65. Samet, J. M., Dominici, F., Curreriro, F. C., Coursac, I., and Zeger, S. L. Fine particulate air pollution and mortality in 20 U.S. cities, 1987–1994. *New England Journal of Medicine,* 343 (2000): 1742–1749.

66. Dietrich, K., Ris, M. D., Succop, P., Berger, O., and Bornschein, R. Early exposure to lead and juvenile delinquency. *Neurotoxicology Teratology,* 23 (2001): 511–518.

67. Mendelsohn, A. L., Dreyer, B. P., Fierman, A. H., et al. Low-level lead exposure and behavior in early childhood. *Pediatrics,* 101, no. e10 (1998): 1–7.

68. Vrijheid, M. Health effects of residence near hazardous waste landfill sites: A review of the epidemiologic literature. *Environmental Health Perspectives,* 108, Suppl 1 (2000): 101–112.

69. Evans, G. W. Environmental stress and health. In A.B.T. Revenson, ed., *Handbook of Health Psychology,* pp. 365–385. Hillsdale, N.J.: Erlbaum, 2001.

70. Macpherson, A., Roberts, I., and Pless, I. B. Children's exposure to traffic and pedestrian injuries. *Journal of Public Health,* 88 (1998): 1840–1843.

71. Huttenmoser, M. Children and their living surroundings: Empirical investigations into the significance of living surroundings for the everyday life and development of children. *Children's Environments,* 12 (1995): 403–413.

72. Appleyard, D., and Lintell, M. The environmental quality of city streets. *Journal of the American Institute of Planners,* 38 (1972): 84–101.

73. Awasthi, S., Glick, H. A., and Fletcher, R. H. Effect of cooking fuels on respiratory diseases in school children in Lucknow, India. *American Journal of Tropical Medicine and Hygiene,* 55 (1996): 48–51.

74. Evans, G. W., and Kantrowitz, E. Socioeconomic status and health: The potential role of environmental risk exposure. *Annual Review of Public Health,* 23 (2002): 203–231.

75. Evans, G. W., Wells, N. M., Chan, E., and Saltzman, H. Housing and mental health. *Journal of Consulting and Clinical Psychology,* 68 (2000): 526–530.

76. Matte, T. D., and Jacobs, D. E. Housing and health: Current issues and implications for research programs. *Journal of Urban Health,* 77 (2000): 7–25.

77. Northridge, M. E., Sclar, E. D., and Biswas, P. Sorting out the connections between the built environment and health: A conceptual framework for navigating pathways and planning healthy cities. *Journal of Urban Health,* 80 (2003): 556–568.

78. Oie, L., Nafstad, P., Botten, G., Magnus, P., and Jaakkola, J. K. Ventilation in homes and bronchial obstruction in young children. *Epidemiology,* 10 (1999): 294–299.

79. Warner, M., Barnes, P. M., and Fingerhut, L. A. Injury and poisoning episodes and conditions: National Health Interview Survey, 1997. *Vital Health Statistics,* 10 (2000): 202.

80. Ackerman, B. P., Kogos, J., Youngstream, E., Schoff, K., and Izzard, C. Family instability and problem behaviors of children from economically disadvantaged families. *Developmental Psychology,* 35 (1999): 258–268.

81. Evans, G. W., Gonnella, C., Marcynyszyn, L. A., Gentile, L., and Salpekar, N. The role of chaos in poverty and children's socioemotional adjustment. *Psychological Science,* 16 (2005): 560–565.

82. Satterthwaite, D., Hart, R., Levy, C., et al. *The Environment for Children.* London: Earthscan, 1996.

83. Kawachi, I., and Berkman, L. F. Social ties and mental health. *Journal of Urban Health,* 78 (2001): 458–467.

84. Kawachi, I., Kennedy, B. P., and Glass, R. Social capital and self-rated health: A contextual analysis. *American Journal of Public Health,* 89 (1999): 1187–1193.

85. McLeod, L., and Kessler, R. Socioeconomic status differences in vulnerability to undesirable life events. *Journal of Health and Social Behavior,* 31 (1990): 162–172.

86. Acevedo-Garcia, D. Residential segregation and the epidemiology of infectious diseases. *Social Science & Medicine,* 51 (2000): 1143–1161.

87. Fiscella, K., and Williams, D. R. Health disparities based on socioeconomic inequities: Implications for urban health care. *Academic Medicine,* 79 (2004): 1139–1147.

88. Leventhal, T., and Brooks-Gunn, J. Poverty and child development. *International Encyclopedia of the Social and Behavioral Sciences,* 3, Article 78 (2002): 11889–11893.

89. McLoyd, V. C. Socioeconomic disadvantage and child development. *American Psychologist,* 53 (1998): 185–204.

90. Williams, D. R., and Collins, C. Racial residential segregation: A fundamental cause of racial disparities in health. *Public Health Reports,* 116 (2001): 404–416.

91. Kaplan, G. A., Pamuk, E. R., Lynch, J. W., Cohen, R. D., and Balfour J. L. Inequality in income and mortality in the United States: Analysis of mortality and potential pathways. *British Medical Journal,* 312 (1996): 999–1003.

92. Lynch, J., Smith, G. D., Hillemeier, M., Shaw, M., Raghunathan, T., and Kaplan, G. A. Income inequality, the psychosocial environment and health: Comparisons of wealthy nations. *Lancet,* 358 (2001): 1285–1287.

93. Ross, N. A., Wolfson, M. W., Dunn, J. R., Berthelot, J. M., Kaplan, G., and Lynch, G. W. Income inequality and mortality in Canada and the United States. *British Medical Journal,* 320 (2000): 898–902.

94. Henderson, C., Diez Roux, A. V., Jacobs, D. R., Kiefe, C. I., West, D., and Williams, D. R. Neighborhood characteristics, individual level socioeconomic factors, and depressive symptoms in young adults: The CARDIA study. *Journal of Epidemiology and Community Health,* 59 (2005): 322–328.

95. Haan, M., Kaplan, G. A., and Camacho, T. Poverty and health: Prospective evidence from the Alameda County Study. *American Journal of Epidemiology,* 125 (1987): 989–998.

96. Leventhal, T., and Brooks-Gunn, J. Moving to Opportunity: An experimental study of neighborhood effects on mental health. *American Journal of Public Health,* 93 (2003): 1576–1582.

97. Garbarino, J., and Crouter, A. Defining the community context for parent-child relations: The correlates of child maltreatment. *Child Development,* 49 (1978): 604–616.

98. Garbarino, J., and Sherman, D. High-risk neighborhoods and high-risk families: The human ecology of child maltreatment. *Child Development,* 51 (1980): 188–198.

99. Eskenazi, B., Bradman, A., and Castorina, R. Exposures of children to organophosphate pesticides and their potential adverse health effects. *Environmental Health Perspectives,* 107, Suppl 3 (1999): 409–419.

100. Thompson, B., Coronado, G. D., Grossman, J. E., Puschel, K., Solomon, C. C., Islas, I., et al. Pesticide take-home pathway among children of agricultural workers: Study design, methods, and baseline findings. *Journal of Occupational Environmental Medicine,* 45 (2003): 42–53.

101. Parcel, T. L., and Menaghan, E. G. *Parents' Jobs and Children's Lives.* Edison, N.J.: Aldine Transaction, 1994.

102. Crouter, A. C., Bumpus, M. F., Maguire, M. C., and McHale, S. M. Linking parents' work pressure and adolescents' well-being: Insights into dynamics in dual-earner families. *Developmental Psychology,* 35 (1999): 1453–1461.

103. Whitbeck, L. B., Simons, R. L., Conger, R. D., Wickrama, K. A. S., Ackley, K. A., and Elder, G. H., Jr. The effects of parents' working conditions and family economic hardship on parenting behaviors and children's self-efficacy. *Social Psychology Quarterly,* 60 (1997): 291–303.

104. Kohn, M. L. *Social Class and Conformity.* Chicago: University of Chicago Press, 1977.

105. Evans, G. W., Lercher, P., and Kofler, W. W. Crowding and children's mental health: The role of house type. *Journal of Environmental Psychology,* 22 (2002): 221–231.

106. Bradley, R. H., Whiteside, L., Mundfrom, D. J., Casey, P. H., Kelleher, K., et al. Early indications of resilience and their relation to experiences in the home environments of low birth weight, premature children living in poverty. *Child Development,* 65 (1994): 346–360.

107. Maxwell, L. Multiple effects of home and day care crowding. *Environment and Behavior,* 28 (1996): 494–511.

108. Shaw, M. Housing and public health. *Annual Review of Public Health,* 25 (2004): 397–418.

109. Kreiger, J., and Higgins, D. L. Housing and health: Time again for public health action. *American Journal of Public Health,* 92 (2002): 758–768.

110. Saegert, S. Environment and children's mental health: Residential density and low-income children. In E. Baum and J. E. Singer, eds., *Handbook of Psychology and Health, Vol. II, Issues in Child Health and Adolescent Health,* pp. 247–271. Hillsdale, N.J.: Erlbaum, 1982.

111. Goduka, I. N., Poole, D. A., and Aotaki-Phenice, L. A comparative study of black South African children from three different contexts. *Child Development,* 63 (1992): 509–525.

112. Widmayer, S., Peterson, L., Larner, M., Carnahan, S., Calderon, A., Wingerd, J., and Marshall, R. Predictors of Haitian-American infant development at twelve months. *Child Development,* 61 (1990): 410–415.

113. Evans, G. W. Environmental stress and health. In A.B.T. Revenson, ed., *Handbook of Health Psychology,* pp. 365–385. Hillsdale, N.J.: Erlbaum, 2001.

114. Campbell, T. L. Family's impact on health: A critical review. *Family Systems Medicine,* 4 (1986): 135–200.

115. Denham, S. A. Family routines: A construct for considering family health. *Holistic Nursing Practice,* 9 (1995): 11–23.

116. Doherty, W. J., and McCubbin, H. I. Families and health care: An emerging arena of theory, research, and clinical intervention. *Family Relations,* 34 (1985): 5–11.

117. Litman, T. J. The family as a basic unit in health and medical care: A social behavior overview. *Social Science & Medicine,* 8 (1974): 495–519.

118. Pollitt, E., Golub, M., Gorman, K., et al. A reconceptualization of the effects of undernutrition on children's biological, psychosocial, and behavioral development. *SRCD Social Policy Report No. X5.* Ann Arbor, Mich.: Society for Research in Child Development, 1996.

119. Richter, L. *The Importance of Caregiver-Child Interactions for the Survival and Healthy Development of Young Children: A Review.* Geneva: World Health Organization, 1994.

120. Richter, L., and Griesel, D. Malnutrition, low birthweight and related influences on psychological development. In A. Dawes and D. Donald, eds., *Childhood and*

Adversity: Psychological Perspectives from South African Research, pp. 66–91. Cape Town, South Africa: David Philips, 1994.

121. Rutter, M., Yule, B., Quinton, D., Rowlands, O., Yule, W., and Berger, M. Attainment and adjustment in two geographic areas: III—Some factors accounting for area differences. *British Journal of Psychiatry,* 125 (1974): 520–533.

122. Taylor, S. E., Repetti, R. L., and Seeman, T. Health psychology: What is an unhealthy environment and how does it get under your skin? *Annual Review of Psychology,* 48 (1997): 411–447.

123. Stein, A., Wooley, H., Cooper, S. D., and Fairburn, C. G. An observational study of mothers with eating disorders and their infants. *Journal of Child Psychology and Psychiatry,* 35 (1994): 733–748.

124. Cohen, S., Evans, G. W., Stokols, D., and Krantz, D. S. *Behavior, Health, and Environmental Stress.* New York: Plenum Press, 1986.

125. Aber, J. L., Bennett, N. G., Conley, D. C., and Li, J. The effects of poverty on child health and development. *Annual Review of Public Health,* 18 (1997): 463–483.

126. Adler, N. E., Boyce, T., Chesney, M. A., et al. Socioeconomic status and health: The challenge of the gradient. *American Psychologist,* 49 (1994): 15–24.

127. Chen, E., Matthews, K. A., and Boyce, T. W. Socioeconomic differences in children's health: How and why do these relationships change with age? *Psychological Bulletin,* 128 (2002): 295–329.

128. Grant, K. E., Compas, B. E., Stuhlmacher, A. F., Thurm, A. E., McMahon, S. D., and Halpert, J. A. Stressors and child and adolescent psychopathology: Moving from markers to mechanisms of risk. *Psychological Bulletin,* 129 (2003): 447–466.

129. Evans, G. W., and English, K. The environment of poverty: Multiple stressor exposure, psychophysiological stress, and socioemotional adjustment. *Child Development,* 73 (2002): 1238–1248.

130. Felner, R. D., Brand, S., DuBois, D. L., Adan, A. M., Mulhall, P. F., and Evans, E. G. Socioeconomic disadvantage, proximal environmental experiences, and socioemotional and academic adjustment in early adolescence: Investigation of a mediated effects model. *Child Development,* 66 (1995): 774–792.

131. Evans, G. W., Maxwell, L. R., and Hart, B. Parental language and verbal responsiveness to children in crowded homes. *Developmental Psychology,* 35 (1999): 1020–1023.

132. Cummins, S., and Macintyre, S. The price and availability of food in Glasgow: A systematic study of an urban foodscape. *Urban Studies,* 39, no. 11 (2002): 2115–2130.

133. Caughy, M. O., O'Campo, P. J., and Muntane, C. When being alone might be better: Neighborhood poverty, social capital, and child mental health. *Social Science & Medicine,* 57 (2003): 227–237.

134. Lochner, K. A., Kawachi, I., Brennan, R. T., and Buka, S. L. Social capital and neighborhood mortality rates in Chicago. *Social Science & Medicine,* 56, no. 8 (2003): 1791–1805.

135. Sampson, R. J., Raudenbush, S. W., and Earls, F. Neighborhoods and violent crime: A multilevel study of collective efficacy. *Science,* 277, no. 5328 (1997): 918–924.

136. Oliver, L. N., Dunn, J. R., Kohen, D. E., and Hertzman, C. Do neighborhoods influence the readiness to learn of kindergarten children in Vancouver? A multi-level analysis of neighbourhood effects. *Environment and Planning A,* 39, no. 4 (2007): 848–868.

137. Morales, J. R., and Guerra, N. G. Effects of multiple context and cumulative stress on urban children's adjustment in elementary school. *Child Development,* 77 (2006): 907–923.

138. Louw, J., Donald, D., and Dawes, A. Intervening in adversity: Towards a theory of practice. In D. Donald, A. Dawes, and J. Louw, eds., *Addressing Childhood Adversity,* pp. 244–260. Cape Town, South Africa: David Philip, 2000.

139. Dawes, A., and Donald, D. Improving children's chances: Developmental theory and effective interventions in community contexts. In D. Donald, A. Dawes, and J. Louw, eds., *Addressing Childhood Adversity,* pp. 1–25. Cape Town, South Africa: David Philip, 2000.

CHAPTER

5

GEOGRAPHIC INFORMATION SYSTEMS, ENVIRONMENTAL JUSTICE, AND HEALTH DISPARITIES

JULIANA MAANTAY, ANDREW R. MAROKO,
CARLOS ALICEA, A. H. STRELNICK

LEARNING OBJECTIVES

- Describe some of the benefits and challenges of integrating biomedical and geographic perspectives for the study of childhood asthma.
- Assess the role of differing exposure to urban environmental pollutants in creating or maintaining health disparities.
- Identify specific roles that community organizations, medical centers, and academic institutions can play in the study of urban health conditions such as childhood asthma.

◼ Assess different strategies for collecting data on the urban environment and analyze their strengths and limitations.

INTRODUCTION

In scientific research, the most interesting questions are very often at the interstitial zones and boundaries of disciplines, neither firmly within one or another. These are frequently the questions that go unasked or unanswered. They may also provide evidence that stimulates reconceptualization (e.g., physicians considering environmental aspects of asthma). One of the challenges of interdisciplinary research is to leverage input from many different disciplines. Embracing this challenge enables thinking about and solving problems in ways not possible using the methods and techniques of just a single discipline. In this chapter, we apply this approach to the study of asthma and air pollution in the Bronx, New York City. Our organizing framework for this chapter is based on two important themes: the *process* of interdisciplinary research (i.e., the benefits and challenges of an academic-medical-community partnership, which brought together expertise in geographic information science, clinical epidemiology, and street science), and the *outcomes* of interdisciplinary research (i.e., the enhanced understanding of the association between environmental conditions and asthma hospitalizations).

Environmental conditions are believed to contribute to producing and maintaining minority health disparities.[1] In the past four decades, numerous studies have demonstrated the existence of environmental injustices in the United States,[2,3] and there have been efforts by communities and governmental agencies to define and advance environmental justice (EJ). The objectives of environmental justice include overcoming and rectifying past and present inequities—the now commonplace recognition that disadvantaged communities suffer a disproportionate share of toxic burdens and hazards.[4] Environmental justice refers to the conditions necessary to assure the right to a safe, healthy, productive, and sustainable environment for all, including biological, ecological, physical (both natural and human-made), social, political, aesthetic, and economic environments. The National Institute of Environmental Health Sciences (NIEHS) Health Disparities Strategic Plan for eliminating such disparities and injustices notes:

> *Both social and environmental exposures represent an important area of investigation for understanding and ameliorating the health disparities suffered by the disadvantaged of this nation . . . Recent results suggest that factors such as access to quality health care and individual lifestyle choices, e.g., smoking or alcohol consumption, are not the primary causative agents underlying disparate health outcomes for those of low SES [socioeconomic status]. Indeed, these findings act to shift research emphasis toward examination of mechanisms by which social and physical environments interact with SES to produce health disparities.[5]*

In the next sections, we set the stage for our study by providing a brief overview of three key foundations for our study: community-based participatory research, multilevel models of causation, and geographic information systems.

COMMUNITY-BASED PARTICIPATORY RESEARCH

Since the 1990s, there has been growing and convergent interest in minority health disparities and community-based participatory research (CBPR). Historically, research conducted in low-income areas and communities of color has rarely benefited and often harmed the communities involved. Because these communities were not included in the development of the research question and design, interventions often proved ineffective because they were not tailored to the concerns and cultures of those being recruited to participate.

In a study commissioned by the Agency for Healthcare Research and Quality, CBPR was defined as "a collaborative research approach that is designed to ensure and establish structures for participation by communities affected by the issue being studied, representatives of organizations, and researchers in all aspects of the research process to improve health and well-being through taking action, including social change."[6] CBPR also involved (a) "co-learning and reciprocal transfer of expertise by all research partners; (b) shared decision-making power; and (c) mutual ownership of the processes and products of the research enterprise." The study found that using CBPR improved research quality and enhanced community involvement and research capacity.

Israel and her colleagues at the Detroit Community-Academic Urban Research Center have outlined the following CBPR principles: (a) recognizes the community as a unit of identity; (b) builds on the strengths and resources within the community; (c) facilitates collaborative, equitable partnership in all phases of the research and is an empowering process; (d) promotes co-learning and capacity-building among all partners that attends to social inequalities; (e) integrates knowledge generation and intervention for the mutual benefit of all partners; (f) emphasizes the local relevance of public health problems and the multiple determinants of health and disease, including biomedical, social, economic, and physical environmental factors; (g) is cyclical, iterative, and long term with research goals not always known at the beginning of work with a community; (h) disseminates findings and knowledge gained to all partners and involves them in dissemination; (i) addresses health from both positive and ecological perspectives; and (j) continues after the funding ends.[7, 8]

The advantages and rationale for CBPR include (a) enhanced relevance and usefulness of the research findings to all partners involved; (b) improved quality and validity of research by engaging local knowledge and theory based on the experience of those involved; (c) strengthened research and program development capacity of all partners; (d) convened the diverse skills, knowledge, expertise, and sensitivities needed to address complex problems; (e) reduced community mistrust of research; (f) bridged gaps in culture; (g) reduced fragmentation and increased contextualization of research; (h) provided employment for community partners; (i) reduced marginalization; and (j) improved health directly from interventions and indirectly from increased power and control over the research process.[9] From the community's perspective, an empowering CBPR must also include questioning of the political and economic underpinnings of the scientific research proposed, the methodology selected to conduct that research, and the decision-making process to determine where and how the research project is going to be conducted.

MULTILEVEL MODELS OF CAUSATION

Social characteristics vary systematically across communities along a number of dimensions, including socioeconomic status (e.g., poverty, wealth, education, occupation), family structure and life cycle (e.g., female-headed households, child density), residential stability (e.g., home ownership and tenure), and racial and ethnic composition (e.g., residential segregation).[10, 11] Evidence shows that the ecological concentration of poverty and inequality has increased in American neighborhoods during the 1980s and 1990s.[12, 13]

A growing body of multilevel research has examined community characteristics and individual-level health and has found mixed, often modest, but consistent evidence that links health outcomes to neighborhood context even when controlling for individual attributes and behaviors. Outcomes examined have included cardiovascular risk factors and mortality, low birthweight, smoking, all-cause mortality, and self-reported health status.[14, 15] Although ecological and observational study designs limit causal inferences, recent experimental studies, such as the Moving to Opportunity program, have confirmed that improving community environment leads to better health outcomes.[16] In summary, social and behavioral science research has found broad agreement (with causality and magnitude still at issue) that (a) much inequality persists between neighborhoods and local communities along multiple dimensions of socioeconomic status; (b) health problems tend to cluster together geographically in ecological units such as neighborhoods; (c) individual- and community-level predictors themselves interact in relation to health outcomes; and (g) the association of community context and health outcomes, especially all-cause mortality, depression, and violence, persists even when controlled for individual-level risk factors.[11]

ROLE OF GEOGRAPHIC INFORMATION SYSTEMS

We used geographic information systems (GIS) as the primary analytic tool in this study. GIS refers to a structured system of computer hardware, specialized spatial analysis and mapping software, spatial and nonspatial attribute data, and an informed analyst. Geographic information science (GISc) is a discipline grounded in geographic spatial analytic theory, requiring a myriad of spatial decisions and constant use of expert judgment, knowledge, training, and experience. GIS have been extensively used in public health research in recent years, including disease mapping for epidemiological studies, as well as mapping for planning and analyzing health services provision, health care administration, environmental health justice, health disparities, hazard and risk assessment, exposure analyses, and research on many other types of public health issues.[3, 17–32]

GIS can help the health researcher discover and analyze the spatial relationships among populations and their sociodemographic characteristics, health outcomes, patterns of diseases, and access to health care, as well as a host of other variables that may be spatially linked to health and specific locations and populations. Although GIS is becoming more common among health researchers, it is still not widely used due to lack of awareness of the potential analytic power of GIS and the steep learning curve required to use GIS in a meaningful way. Knowledge of the geographic aspects of health issues is very often crucial to fully understanding them, and the spatial perspective gives unique insights that cannot be obtained in any other way. Additionally, being a visual medium as well as an analytic tool, GIS is a means of incorporating, integrating, and enhancing the participatory research process with disparate groups. However, the extensive time and effort necessary for novice GIS users to become proficient was our reason for undertaking interdisciplinary research among geographers, medical professionals, and community advocates. Interdisciplinary research eliminates the need for everyone to be an expert in everything and makes it possible for everyone to have a sufficiently deep understanding of the basics to participate in a meaningful way in the research design and interpretation of results.

In the project described in this chapter, GIS was used to examine the spatial correspondence between the residence of people hospitalized for asthma and major sources of air pollution. The following section outlines some of the issues that must be resolved when using GIS for health research and the specific methodology used for this project to address and optimize these issues.

There are a number of limitations in using GIS for health research, such as spatial and attribute data deficiencies, the limits of ecological research designs, and methodological problems, especially those related to geographic considerations.[3,33,34] Geographic considerations include the delineation of the boundaries of the optimal study area, determining the level of resolution and the unit of spatial data aggregation, and estimating the areal extent of exposure, as well as the various problems encountered in trying to statistically analyze and summarize spatial data. Due to the principle of spatial autocorrelation, which states that data from locations near one another in space are more likely to be similar than data from locations remote from one another, spatial data are by their very nature not randomly distributed, as traditional statistical approaches require.[35] Spatial autocorrelation, which is a given in geography, becomes an impediment to the application of conventional statistical tests.

ENVIRONMENTAL JUSTICE AND HEALTH IN THE BRONX

The Bronx is the nation's poorest urban county and home to more than 1.3 million people.[36] Of New York City's five boroughs, the Bronx is the poorest and contains the highest percentage of black and Latino populations (85.5 percent) and the least well educated—37.7 percent of adults have not graduated from high school. The Sixteenth Congressional District in the South Bronx had the highest poverty rate (40.2 percent), lowest median income, and highest proportion of children living below poverty (50.1 percent) in the United States.

In addition to these economic disadvantages, residents of the Bronx bear severe environmental burdens. In New York City, as in many urban areas, minorities and poor people are more likely to be concentrated in or near industrial zones that typically carry higher environmental burdens than residentially zoned areas.

In the Bronx, many of the industries occupying these areas are waste related or pollute land in other ways. From the 1970s to the 1990s, other areas of New York City were gentrifying, and city planners were changing industrial zones into areas zoned for residential and commercial uses; however, during that same time period, the Bronx had many acres of residential land rezoned for industrial uses, and existing light industrial land was rezoned for heavier industrial uses.[37, 38] By decreasing the extent of industrial zones in the rest of the city and increasing those in the Bronx, the historical zoning changes virtually assured that industrial areas in the Bronx became home of many new noxious facilities such as waste transfer stations and hazardous materials storage centers. Although these rezoning actions may not be malicious or racist in intent, the effect of disproportionate environmental burdens remains, with the highest exposures to pollutants in neighborhoods that are poorer and have higher proportions of blacks and Latinos. Our study seeks to ascertain whether or not proximity to these disproportionate environmental burdens corresponds to an increased risk for asthma hospitalization.

Geographic Scale and Context of the Project

The geographic extent (scale) of this study is Bronx County. The Bronx is the only borough of New York City located on the mainland, and therefore, it serves the important purpose of providing surface accessibility and connectivity with the city's four boroughs, the counties of Long Island, and the rest of the United States. As a result, the Bronx has one of the highest volumes of vehicular traffic in the nation.[39] The Bronx is approximately forty-two square miles, and it was selected as a study area primarily due to its high rates of asthma hospitalizations (approximately 7 hospitalizations per 1,000 people annually), high quantities of noxious land uses, and the availability of relatively complete and accurate asthma hospitalization data sets for this area.

Role of Asthma and Air Pollution in Health Disparities in the Bronx

Since 1980, asthma has become epidemic in low-income urban areas and is now the leading cause for hospitalization of children over one year of age. The precise causes of asthma are not known, and there may be a multiplicity of triggers. These include indoor and outdoor air pollution, pollen, allergies, and smoking or exposure to second-hand smoke.[40] Previous research has linked high concentrations of known air pollutants with morbidity (including hospitalization) and mortality from respiratory diseases, including asthma.[41, 42] Many researchers have investigated the link between outdoor air pollution and asthma in other cities and have demonstrated that exposure to major

air pollutants, including ozone, sulfur dioxide, nitrogen dioxide, and suspended particulate matter, is related to asthma prevalence or hospitalizations.[42–48] Many of these
studies focused on exposure based on proximity to roadways.[40–44, 46–49]

Asthma is the leading cause of preventable hospitalizations in New York City for
both children and adults, and the Bronx has the city's highest rates of asthma hospitalizations and deaths.[50] Residents of the Bronx, especially children under the age of
fifteen years, suffer from rates of asthma hospitalization that are among the highest in
the nation.[50] In 1999, the asthma hospitalization rate for children was 70 percent higher
in the Bronx than in New York City as a whole and 700 percent higher in the Bronx
than for the rest of New York State (excluding New York City).[50] The asthma hospitalization rate for children in the Mott Haven/Hunts Point sections of the South Bronx is
23.2 per 1,000 children, which is more than double New York City's rate of 9.9 per
1,000 children.

On average, approximately 9,000 Bronx residents per year, nearly half of them
children, were hospitalized for asthma for each of the five years studied, 1995–1999.[51]
Asthma hospitalization rates for children in the Bronx doubled between 1988 and
1997, peaking in 1993. Although reductions in asthma hospitalization rates have been
seen in children and young adults, there have been no changes in the past fifteen years
in the asthma hospitalization rate of adults over thirty-five years of age.

General air quality, however, has improved during the same time period. The Bronx
also has many facilities that are known stationary sources of air pollution such as waste
transfer stations and power plants as well as high quantities of pollution from mobile
sources. Figure 5.1 shows that in the Bronx, pollution sources are concentrated in areas
with high proportions of minority populations. We tested the hypothesis that there is a
significant increase in asthma hospitalization rates in *microenvironments* for those
residing near major sources of both mobile and stationary air pollution.

Research Partnership

Given the multiplicity of causes and consequences, solving the myriad environmental
health issues facing the Bronx requires a partnership that includes community, academia,
health professionals, and government. The South Bronx Environmental Justice Partnership (SBEJP) was developed in 2001 as a consortium of organizations, funded by NIEHS
and led by a community organization, For a Better Bronx; a large clinical system,
Montefiore Medical Center; a minority-serving educational institution, Lehman College;
and a research-oriented medical school, Albert Einstein College of Medicine. The partnership's goal has been to improve the health and well-being of the people who live and
work in the South Bronx by building capacity for and delivering community-driven environmental health research, education, and clinical and public health programs.

Community Partners   For a Better Bronx (FABB) was founded in August 2004,
evolving from the South Bronx Clean Air Coalition (SBCAC), which was founded in
1991 when several dozen community-based organizations, including churches and tenant, neighborhood, health, and civil rights groups, joined together to stop the operation

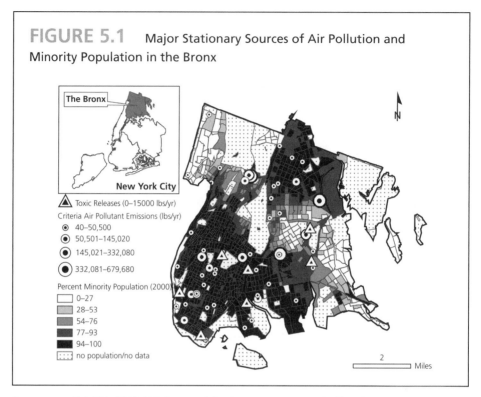

FIGURE 5.1   Major Stationary Sources of Air Pollution and Minority Population in the Bronx

Data sources: U.S. EPA, 2002; U.S. Bureau of the Census, 2000. Compiled by Juliana Maantay.

of a hospital-sponsored medical waste incinerator. SBCAC finally succeeded in closing it in June 1997. FABB now campaigns against large solid waste handlers, sludge processors, and fossil-fuel power plants and for sustainable community development initiatives, such as community-sponsored agriculture, community and rooftop gardens, "green" buildings, solar energy, and an environmental youth corps. FABB brings first-hand experience to the partnership with local traffic and air pollution point sources.

Medical Partners   Albert Einstein College of Medicine (AECOM) is the only medical school in the Bronx and the largest private medical school in New York State. AECOM is a premier basic science research institution with clinical affiliations not only in the Bronx but extending to Manhattan, Queens, and Long Island with a total enrollment of more than 800 medical and PhD students and a full-time and voluntary faculty of more than 3,000 physicians and researchers.

Montefiore Medical Center (MMC) is AECOM's university teaching hospital and provides more than 60 percent of the clinical training for all AECOM medical students. MMC is the largest hospital and health system in the Bronx. AECOM and MMC jointly sponsor the Institute for Community and Collaborative Health, which contributes administrative and clinical expertise and access to our study's hospitalization database.

Academic Partners   Lehman College, City University of New York (CUNY) became CUNY's only four-year liberal arts college in the Bronx in 1968. Lehman's Department of Environmental, Geographic, and Geological Sciences sponsors a certificate program in GISc and brings technical expertise in GIS to the partnership. Research based in geographic information science (GISc) and environmental and health spatial analyses is conducted in the Urban GISc Lab.

Partnership Organization

The South Bronx Environmental Justice Partnership (SBEJP) has operated with funding from the NIEHS since 2001 with Montefiore Medical Center (MMC) serving as the grantee and For a Better Bronx (FABB) and Lehman College receiving subcontracts. Although this structure represents the organizational and administrative resources of the partners, it does not reflect the relative commitment to environmental justice or environmental health expertise of the partners. In fact, only FABB has a mission focused on promoting environmental justice, whereas AECOM, MMC, and Lehman have a variety of clinical, educational, and research goals. SBEJP has operated generally by consensus and has aims that include organizational development. Currently, meetings rotate between each partner's offices with a member of the host organization developing the agenda and chairing the meeting.

To better understand health disparities in the Bronx, we set out to explore whether environmental factors, such as poor outdoor air quality, could be shown to have a spatial association with the increased rates of asthma hospitalization in the Bronx. To conduct this multifaceted study, we needed to develop a team of experts in several fields as well as community-based scientists.

For the asthma and air pollution study, the academic, medical, and community-based organizations have joined together, and all three partners have been instrumental in crafting the methods for the analyses. The process of our collaboration and contribution of each partner is summarized in Table 5.1. In this project, geographic information systems were instrumental in the research design, and one of the strengths behind GIS is that it can take large amounts of data and examine complex interactions, making the complex visible and intelligible. GIS also provides an excellent foundation for meaningful community participation in research design, development of methodology, data needs assessment, data acquisition, and the actual analytic portions of the work. In other words, it permits the integration of local knowledge bases and "street science" into the more traditional health and environmental assessments.

METHODS

Community-Scale Assessment Techniques and Units of Analysis

Within Bronx County, not all areas are equally affected by high asthma hospitalization rates. Smaller geographic units may show contradictory trends regarding concentrations, hot spots, or prevalence. Therefore, we must look at the subcounty level to discern important differences and potential spatial correlations with air pollution sources. The unit of

TABLE 5.1. Phases of South Bronx Environmental Justice Partnership's Geographical Information Systems and Asthma Study and Partners' Contributions

Phase of asthma and GIS study	Role of collaborating partners	Description of analysis	Results
I: Proximity Analysis[a] I A—Use of census tract data as areal unit of analysis I B—Use of individual hospitalization and census block group as units of analysis	Community focused on influence of outdoor air pollution in asthma; Lehman conducted GIS analysis; Montefiore provided SPARCS data; funding from Einstein	Original creation of circular and linear "buffers" or "impact" zones and calculation of odds ratios inside vs. outside impact zones	Statistically significant increases in odds ratios for most exposures except major truck routes (MTRs) for children and limited access highways (LAHs) for both adults and children
II: Regression Analysis[b]	Einstein and Montefiore statisticians performed analysis to control for influence of poverty and racial/ethnic minority of original findings	Multiple regression analysis to determine contribution of minority and poverty status in relation to buffer zone exposure	Most hospitalization variance explained by minority and poverty status with 1 percent residual contribution from air pollution exposure
III: Multiple Exposure Analysis[c]	In response to FABB's concern about excess burden of multiple exposures, Lehman restructured data and analyzed for zones affected by two or more sources of air pollution	Creation of "multiple exposure" buffer zones and calculation of odds ratios	Multiple exposure zones have higher odds ratios for hospitalizations than single exposure zones

IV: Dasymetric Population Mapping: Development of CEDS[d]	Analysis developed by Lehman in response to all partners' skepticism of original findings that proximity to LAHs were "protective" against asthma hospitalizations	Dasymetric analysis: Application of cadastral (tax assessment) database to calculating population distribution within block groups and calculation of odds ratios	Odds ratios for LAHs now show statistical significance; odds Ratios increase for all individual, combined, and multiple exposure impact buffers
V: Loose-Coupling an Air Dispersion Model and the GIS[e]	Analysis developed by Lehman in response to concerns that circular "impact zones" were unrealistic and did not reflect local geography, prevailing winds, height of apartment buildings, etc.	Air dispersion modeling: Loose coupling air dispersion modeling estimates more accurate exposure plumes and, therefore, different "buffers"	Odds ratios increased for stationary point sources impact buffers

[a] Maantay, J. A. Asthma and Air Pollution in the Bronx: Methodological and Data Considerations in Using GIS for Environmental Justice and Health Research Health & Place. Special issue: Linking Environmental Justice, Population Health, and Geographical Information Science, 13 (2007): 32–56.

[b] Fletcher, J. Report on the Regression Analysis of Asthma Hospitalization Rates and Proximity to Major Air Pollution Sources. Bronx, NY: Albert Einstein College of Medicine, 2006.

[c] Maantay, J. A., Maroko, A. R., Porter-Morgan, H. A New Method for Population Mapping and Understanding the Spatiality of Disease in Urban Areas. Urban Geography, 29, no. 7 (2008); 724–738.

[d] Maantay, J. A., Maroko, A. R., and Herrmann, C. Mapping Population Distribution in the Urban Environment: The Cadastral-Based Expert Dasymetric System (CEDS). Cartography 2007: Reflections, Status, and Prediction. Special issue: Cartography and Geographic Information Science. Special issue: Cartography 2007: Reflections, Status, and Prediction. 34 no. 2 (2007): 77–102.

[e] Maantay, J. A., Tu, J., and Maroko, A. R. Loose-Coupling an Air Dispersion Model and a Geographic Information System (GIS) for Studying Air Pollution and Asthma in the Bronx, New York City. International Journal of Environmental Health Research, 2008.

analysis for demographic and socioeconomic data is the *census block group,* the smallest census enumeration unit for which demographic and socioeconomic data are consistently available. The Bronx has 957 block groups, each containing an average of about 1,400 people.

The unit of analysis for the asthma hospitalization cases is the *individual patient record* for each admission, and this level of resolution was crucial in developing accurate rates of asthma hospitalization inside and outside buffered areas around polluting land uses, as described later. These individual hospital discharge records were drawn from the publicly available Statewide Planning and Research Consortium System (SPARCS) database of the New York State Department of Health. The home address of each individual hospitalized with a primary discharge diagnosis of asthma was geocoded to exact longitude and latitude with protections put into place to assure confidentiality and prevent back-coding. Rates were developed by dividing the number of asthma cases by the block group populations. Prior studies have used *census tract* data (a larger geographic unit than the block group) for both. The units of analysis for the environmental data are the individual polluting land uses and impact zones constructed around each. Figure 5.2 shows the spatial distribution of asthma hospitalization rates for various age groups.

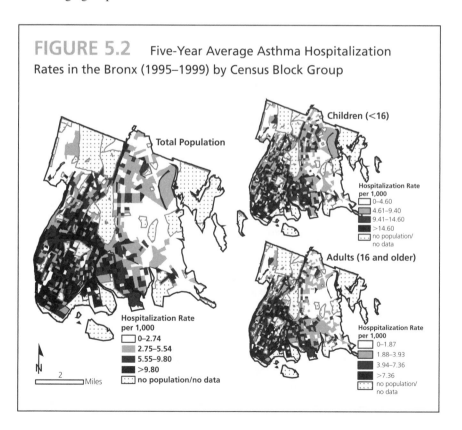

FIGURE 5.2   Five-Year Average Asthma Hospitalization Rates in the Bronx (1995–1999) by Census Block Group

Environmental Hazards and Pollutants Investigated

The locations of known sources of air pollution were used to derive approximations of the areas with poor air quality in the Bronx. In ascertaining which land uses are most likely associated with the suspected pollutants of concern for asthma, we decided to focus on major stationary point sources of air pollutants and the Toxic Release Inventories (TRIs) as well as mobile sources from major highways and truck routes as proxies for local areas of poor air quality.

Our GIS analysis used the publicly available TRI, maintained by the U.S. Environmental Protection Agency (EPA), which is a fairly consistent database and covers the entire United States. Facilities within certain Standard Industrial Classification (SIC) codes (e.g., chemical, printing, electronic, plastics, refining, metal, paper industries, etc.) must report their emissions and waste to the EPA if they meet certain conditions, such as manufacturing more than 25,000 pounds per year or using more than 10,000 pounds per year of one or more of the 650 listed toxic chemicals.[52] Because of the high thresholds in the reporting regulations, TRI includes only the largest users and emitters of toxic substances.

In many communities, TRI facilities and other listed major stationary point sources represent just one component of the total environmental burden, and many other facilities (which individually are below the reporting thresholds for quantities of emissions, use, or production of toxic chemicals and, thus, are not required to report to the EPA) may contribute as much or more on a cumulative basis to the overall air emissions. Unfortunately, it is difficult to obtain reliable data about these facilities because they are not listed in a publicly accessible format and often do not receive any governmental oversight. Many smaller facilities, such as auto body painting and repair shops, electroplating firms, waste transfer stations, and factories, also emit contaminants to the air, but these emissions for the most part remain undocumented and, thus, are difficult to incorporate into the analysis.

Another major contributor to air pollution, especially fine particulate matter, is the high level of truck traffic in the Bronx, which is especially prevalent in the industrial zones. It is not uncommon for 1,000 trucks to enter one solid waste transfer station each day, and there are more than a dozen such transfer stations in the Bronx.[53] Also of note, FABB has observed significant truck traffic on streets other than the truck routes designated by the Department of Transportation.

Although other vehicular traffic is a significant source of air pollution in the Bronx, it is more difficult than the major truck routes to isolate and quantify. Limited access highways, which carry in excess of 50,000 vehicles per day (average annual daily count), were selected to represent the most significant pollution sources from vehicular traffic in addition to trucks. The Hunts Point Terminal and Fulton Fish Markets, the major fish, meat and produce wholesale exchange in the metropolitan area are also located in the South Bronx, resulting in more than 15,000 trucks entering the area per day.

Most researchers now consider air pollutants to be a risk factor for asthma, although the roles that specific air pollutants play in various respiratory illnesses remain unclear.[54, 55] However, if we examine the general effects of air pollution, rather than the effects of specific pollutants, we find there is a large body of literature demonstrating their relationship to adverse respiratory events, suggesting that air pollutants are best treated as a whole. Therefore, air pollution in this article refers to the substances that constitute the pollutant mixture from traffic and industrial-related sources that has been associated with respiratory effects and typically includes particulate matter (e.g., PM_{10}, $PM_{2.5}$), volatile organic compounds (e.g., VOCs, benzene, acetaldehyde, tetrachloroethlene, toluene), NO_2 (nitrogen dioxide), SO_2 (sulfur dioxide), and O_3 (ozone). The locations of the stationary and mobile sources of these pollutants were mapped and examined in light of their spatial correspondence to areas of high asthma hospitalization rates.

Proximity: Analysis with GIS

This study accounts for exposure to air pollution burdens by using proximity analysis to create impact zones around the TRI facilities (TRIs) and other listed major stationary point sources (SPSs) as a proxy for areas of elevated air pollution, as shown in Figure 5.3. Exposure to the pollution from truck traffic is accounted for by the creation of impact zones surrounding the major truck routes (MTRs), many of which traverse residential neighborhoods. Impact zones were also constructed around limited access highways (LAHs) to represent areas of elevated exposure from other vehicular traffic in addition to trucks.

The impact zones constructed for this study were based on distances established as standards by environmental agencies or used most often by other researchers as the area of greatest potential exposure from sources. One-half mile radius impact zones were constructed around TRI facilities;[56, 57] one-quarter mile radius impact zones around other major stationary point sources of criteria pollutants.[58] In addition, we created a 150-meter impact zone from roadway centerline around both LAHs and MTRs,[59, 60] the "distance within which concentrations of primary vehicle traffic pollutants are raised above ambient background levels."[61] The majority of similar studies found significant associations between traffic-related emissions and respiratory symptoms within the 100 to 200 meter range.[41, 62–64]

Each of these impact zone types constituted a separate layer that was then intersected with the asthma hospitalization layers. A layer of all the impact zones combined was also created and intersected as shown in Figure 5.3. Using the locations of the asthma hospitalization cases, it was possible to determine which cases fell within each of the four different impact zone types, as well as within their sum or "combined" buffer, by "clipping" (i.e., removing all the display elements that lie outside the boundary) the asthma layer by each of the five impact zone layers. The clip function was performed for total asthma hospitalization cases as well as for each of the age cohorts separately.

Rates based on the five-year average were calculated for the portions of the block groups within each type of impact zone and the combined impact zone. Because the locations of the asthma hospitalization cases are pinpointed with accuracy by latitude and longitude and are not aggregated by census tract or block group, it is possible to

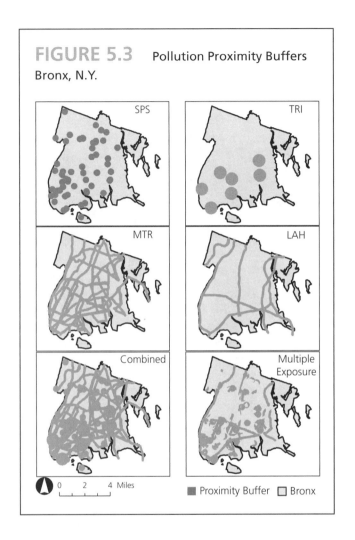

FIGURE 5.3   Pollution Proximity Buffers
Bronx, N.Y.

derive rates for the block groups that can be differentiated by whether the portion of the block groups is in or out of the buffer, as shown in Figure 5.4. This would not be possible using data aggregated by enumeration unit (i.e., census tract) and is only feasible because individual patient record-level data were used.

To develop and compare rates inside and outside the impact zones, an interpolation process called "areal weighting" was performed on the census block groups. The boundaries of census block groups are not coincident with the buffer areas, and therefore, the population data for each tract or block group must be recalculated based on the portion of the tract or block group that falls within the impact zone. The census block groups that fall partially, but not totally, within a certain impact zone are weighted by the proportion of the area that falls within.[65, 66] For instance, if a tract or block group

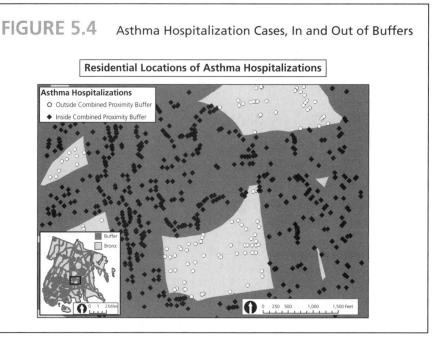

FIGURE 5.4   Asthma Hospitalization Cases, In and Out of Buffers

Each dot represents the residence of one Bronx person admitted to the hospital for asthma in 1999. Some dots represent multiple admissions of the same person or multiple people admitted from the same address. The multiple cases are not shown as individual dots on the map, but have been included in statistical calculations. There were 8,188 hospital admissions in 1999: 5,876 of them from within the areas of the combined buffers and 2312 of them from the areas outside the buffers. Overall in 1999, a Bronx resident was 27 percent more likely to be admitted to the hospital for asthma if living within a buffer area than if living outside a buffer area.

Important note: the patient address locations shown on this map are derived from hypothetical data and do not represent actual addresses. Because of patient confidentiality requirements, the actual address locations could not be shown in a document for public dissemination, and this map is intended to illustrate only the methods used in the analysis. Actual address locations were, however, used by the researchers in the spatial analyses to derive the in- and out-of-buffer rates, odds ratios, and other statistical tests. The researchers were permitted to show only aggregated data (as opposed to record-level data) in any maps available to the public.

Data source: hypothetical data.

is exactly half within the impact zone, the ratio would be 0.5. These ratios are then applied to the population variables to get a reasonable estimate of the population within the impact zones.

The set of demographic and socioeconomic characteristics that we were interested in were quantified and mapped for the within-buffer population and compared to the outside-of-buffer population. The proportion of each variable within the impact zone is based on the proportion of area within the impact zone. Thus, the underlying assumption in this method is that the data for entire unit of analysis (in our case, the block group) are homogeneous, with its population spread evenly throughout, which obviously may not be the case, a limitation of this method. For instance, a large housing project in one corner of the tract would affect the accuracy of areal weighting, as would a large part of the tract being parkland or water, where people are unlikely to live.

Asthma hospitalization rates were developed by using the actual number of cases in each portion of the block group within the impact zones divided by the number of people estimated by areal weighting in that portion of the block group within the impact zones. As noted earlier, this is a simplification; however, considering the small areal extent of the typical Bronx block group, it appears to be reasonably accurate. Rates in and out of impact zones were calculated for the total population and the age cohorts separately, for each of the five years, and then calculated based on the five-year average.[67]

In general, the smaller the unit of data aggregation, the greater the likelihood of homogeneity and the more reliable the method of areal weighting. However, data disaggregation methods exist for obtaining more precise locations of populations, and these can be utilized to calculate better rates in and out of buffers, although these methods are more computationally demanding, time consuming, and require more detailed ancillary data. These data disaggregation methods are referred to as "dasymetric mapping." We developed a new population-mapping technique to improve the "denominator" to calculate more accurate rates.

The Cadastral-based Expert Dasymetric System (CEDS) is a model that uses both an expert system and dasymetric mapping to disaggregate population data (e.g., from the census) into much higher resolution data, giving a more realistic depiction of population locations and densities.[68] Dasymetric mapping entails using ancillary data sets to refine and redistribute the locations of some phenomena (e.g., population) to reflect their distribution more accurately. CEDS, for instance, uses data sets that mask off the areas where people tend not to live (e.g., parks and water bodies) and then redistributes the census populations throughout only the known inhabited areas rather than throughout the entirety of the census unit area (which often includes uninhabited areas). CEDS then uses tax-lot (cadastral) data, which in NYC is on average 150 times finer resolution than the census block group data, to further disaggregate the census population data, as described below.

The expert system is a computerized decision-making program, which has been instructed to "decide," based on heuristic rules and expert judgment, which among several variables in the tax-lot data set to use for disaggregating the census data to calculate the optimally accurate tax-lot-level population. CEDS can be used to reliably disaggregate population data as well as subpopulations such as racial/ethnic groups, age cohorts, income/poverty groups, and those with differing educational attainment levels. We recalculated our rates and analyses based on this more precise population denominator obtained by using CEDS and found more pronounced increases in hospitalization rates in impact zones.[68, 69]

FINDINGS

The results of the proximity and other GIS analyses are instructive in guiding our future research directions. The most noticeable visual aspect of the impact zones that were created around major air pollution sources is the extent to which the Bronx is covered. Approximately 66 percent of the Bronx's landmass falls within the impact zones (excluding major parkland and water bodies). Because the impact zones in this study represent those areas most affected by air pollution, a majority of the Bronx population may be exposed. According to calculations based on the areal weighting script, 88 percent of the people within the impact zones are minorities, and 33 percent are below the federal poverty level. In contrast, outside the impact zone, 79 percent are minorities and 25 percent are below the poverty level. Even though the impact zones cover so much of the Bronx, there is still a disparity between the characteristics of the populations inside and outside the impact zones, indicating the likelihood of disproportionate environmental burdens.

In addition to the differences seen in poverty and minority status inside and outside the impact zones, there is also a difference in asthma hospitalization rates inside and outside the impact zones. Calculating odds ratios for the rates, we found that people living within the combined impact zones are 30 percent more likely to be hospitalized for asthma than people outside the impact zones, as shown in Table 5.2. Within some of the individual impact zones, such as TRI and major stationary point sources, asthma hospitalization rates were 60 and 66 percent higher, respectively, compared to areas outside the impact zones. The odds ratios, in general, are higher for adults 16 years and older than for children 0 to 15 years. This is true for every type of impact zone and for nearly every year of the five years analyzed.

TABLE 5.2.   **Odds Ratio Ranges for the Five-Year Study Period 1995–1999**

Buffer type	Adults	Children	Total population
Combined	1.28–1.30*	1.11–1.17*	1.25–1.29*
Toxic release inventory	1.29–1.60*	1.14–1.30*	1.33–1.49*
Stationary point sources	1.26–1.66*	1.16–1.30*	1.23–1.32*
Major truck routes	1.07–1.17*	1.00–1.09	1.10–1.15*
Limited access highways	0.90–0.93	0.83–0.99	0.86–0.93

* Indicated results are statistically significant at $p < 0.01$.

Although the analysis found that people within the impact zones were much more likely to be hospitalized for asthma than those living outside the impact zones, the risks vary depending on the source of air pollution. Living within toxic release inventory and major stationary point source impact zones poses a higher risk than living within the limited access highway and major truck route impact zones according to the proximity and odds ratio analyses.

In looking at the number of observed cases versus the number of expected cases, based on the overall Bronx five-year average asthma hospitalization rate, the observed cases within the combined impact zones are higher than expected, and those in the areas outside the combined impact zones are lower than expected. A Standardized Incidence Ratio (SIR) was calculated by dividing the observed number of asthma hospitalizations by the expected number of asthma hospitalizations for each subpopulation as defined by impact zone state (inside or outside impact zone) and further refined by age cohort (all ages, 0–15, and 16+). The overall Bronx hospitalization rates were calculated by dividing the total number of asthma hospitalizations by age cohort by the appropriate susceptible populations of the Bronx. The resultant rates were then multiplied by each of the subpopulations to arrive at the expected numbers of hospitalizations. Our analysis confirmed that there was a statistically significant higher incidence of asthma hospitalizations within the impact zones than outside them for each age cohort examined.

Based on our initial analyses, the highways and truck routes seemed to have a protective nature regarding the likelihood of being hospitalized for asthma. This was counterintuitive to the findings of previous studies as well as to anecdotal information given to us by the community partners. Based on further "ground-truthing" type information given to us by the community partners, we realized that the results for these pollution sources might be an artifact of incomplete knowledge of where the population was actually located, and hence arriving at incorrectly high denominators in these areas, resulting in artificially lower rates. By correcting this inaccurate denominator using the CEDS method described earlier, we were able to show more realistic results that more closely conformed to prior studies and the community's experience with these areas.

IMPLICATIONS OF FINDINGS

The increased asthma hospitalization rates for both children and adults living in impact zones suggests that local microenvironments and individual exposures are important in understanding the asthma epidemic and developing public health interventions that will reduce the adverse health effects of outdoor air pollution. The phases of our research have sought to improve the accuracy of our estimates of the asthma hospitalization rates for those exposed to stationary and mobile air pollution sources using proximity as our proxy for exposure. Each phase has made the odds ratios comparing the risk of asthma hospitalization for those residing within impact zones to those living outside them both larger and more significant. Controlling for poverty and minority status diminished but did not eliminate the added risk arising from residential proximity to the four categories of air pollution. Future studies measuring individual exposure and asthma symptoms, using portable sampling equipment and locating its specific measurements, could serve to confirm our findings.

Limitations of Data and Analyses

Several data limitations are encountered when integrating health data in GIS. A basic data quality issue is data accuracy, and this takes two forms: positional accuracy and attribute accuracy. Both have substantial ramifications for the asthma and air pollution study. Positional accuracy refers to how close the location of a data point in a GIS reflects its true position in the real world. The incorrect identification of a data point's location can occur at the time of original measurement of the location or in subsequent data processing, such as change of projection and overlay analyses, and can result in erroneous data aggregation and spatial analysis. Attribute accuracy refers to how closely the data values describe the real-world entity's true attributes. Errors and inaccuracies in attribute data can occur due to inconsistencies in health event definitions and diagnoses as well as population indicators such as race or ethnicity.[70]

There are also data limitations more specific to this study, in addition to the general data limitations mentioned in the preceding paragraph. First, the asthma hospitalization data set contains only hospital discharges and not emergency room or office visits, asthma incidence, or asthma prevalence, so only the most severely ill and poorly managed proportion of the total population affected by asthma is represented in the analysis. Second, the locations of the major pollution sources are obtained from national databases and potentially have inaccuracies with locational attributes as well as nonspatial attributes because much of the information within these data sets is self-reported. Third, the demographic and socioeconomic data are derived from the U.S. Census, and there have been reports of serious undercounting of various populations, especially in dense urban areas. Such inaccurate population counts and locations have the potential to render inaccurate the disease rates developed from the census data. Additionally, the time periods of the data on environmental conditions and asthma hospitalization were not necessarily the same, primarily due to real-world difficulties involved in data acquisition. Table 5.3 provides information on data sources, variables, data processing methods and time periods for the variables of interest.

General study limitations include the issues associated with ecological-level analyses. To avoid the ecological fallacy, we cannot infer any individual outcomes based on community or neighborhood characteristics. Also, the environmental data used (i.e., major air pollution sources) do not translate very well to individual exposures, and the spatial correlations found in the analysis do not imply causality, merely an association or relationship. Lastly, as mentioned earlier, asthma hospitalization data are not a proxy for asthma incidence, and hospitalization for asthma may reflect a failure to manage the disease or lack of access to primary and preventive care. Because of these limitations, community advocates have now secured the inclusion of emergency

TABLE 5.3.   **Data Sources for GIS Analysis**

Data or variables	Source	Data processing method	Year
Asthma hospitalization data	New York State Dept. of Health SPARCS database	Geocoded	1995–1999
Toxic release inventory facility (TRI)	U.S. Environmental Protection Agency	Geocoded	2000
Other major stationary point sources (SPS)	U.S. Environmental Protection Agency	Geocoded	2002
Limited access highways (LAH)	U.S. Bureau of the Census	Selected street segments	2000
Major truck routes (MTR)	NYC Dept. of Transportation/Traffic Rules and Regulations	Selected street segments	2002
Zoning and land use	Lot Info by Space Track and NYC Dept. of Finance, RPAD (Real Property Attribute Data)	Spatially joined with property tax lots	2002
Demographic and socioeconomic data	U.S. Bureau of the Census	Spatially joined with census boundaries	2000
Street segments	U.S. Bureau of the Census	N/A	2000
Water bodies, parks, and other boundaries	U.S. Bureau of the Census	N/A	2000
Digital Orthophoto of NYC	NYC Department of Environmental Protection, NYCMAP	N/A	2000

room visits in the SPARCS database so that future analyses can consider both hospitalizations and emergency room visits.

Organizational Challenges

Power Differentials in the Partnership   The asymmetry created by a large medical center and community-based organization (CBO) forming a partnership is exacerbated by the grant structure when the larger organization is also the grantee and the CBO is a subcontractor. For SBEJP, this has resulted in a significant power differential between MMC and FABB, reflected most dramatically in the process of distributing funds rather than in the amount of funds (which is now equally shared between FABB, Lehman, and MMC). Funds are transferred from NIEHS to MMC electronically, but several administrative steps are then required before FABB or Lehman can receive funds, including establishing internal fund numbers; generating, negotiating, and signing the subcontract; and invoicing MMC for services. Because grant funds constitute a large proportion of FABB's total operating budget, delays in the process have a profound impact on its staff and its cash flow. Attending to the bureaucratic paperwork consumes a disproportionate amount of precious staff time with the CBO always as "supplicant." Another example was the principal investigator's decision to ask the institutional partners (Lehman and Montefiore) to absorb a 10 percent funding cut without consulting FABB, which FABB viewed as paternalistic.

Differences in Foci or Interest, Time Commitments, and Investments   FABB's staff are fully devoted to environmental justice efforts, although its SBEJP subcontract represents only one of FABB's funding sources. MMC and Lehman staff have only part-time commitments to SBEJP and, therefore, have many other time commitments. Although interest in academic publication is shared by all partners, FABB writes educational brochures, newspaper columns, and for magazines that reach the public, other CBOs, and EJ organizations, whereas Lehman and MMC are mainly interested in professional journals in their staff's various disciplines. Writing and publishing also compete with other, often more pressing organizational and political priorities.

Agenda Setting and Project Conceptualization   The community partner was crucial in project conceptualization and in developing the initial working hypothesis that outdoor air pollution makes asthma worse, based on their long-term and immediate experiences. Historically, asthma researchers have focused on allergies and indoor air pollution, whereas FABB emphasized the importance of the multiple burdens in the community. As noted in Table 5.1, each partner contributed to the development and evolution of the study.

Integration of Local Knowledge Bases and Street Science with GIS Analysis   Street science is defined as "a new framework for environmental health justice that joins local insights with professional techniques."[71] In this definition, traditional assessment methods and nonscientific contributions are not seen as mutually exclusive, but each is necessary for the complete realization of the other. By integrating local knowledge bases and community-specific ways of knowing with traditional analytic methods, both can be considerably improved, yielding not only more substantive results but results that will more likely be accepted by the community as their own.[72]

One kind of participatory research consists, in part, of nonscientist stakeholders informing the research in such a way that would not be possible by outside "experts" alone conducting the analyses. This is generally accomplished by community members providing intimate knowledge of the community or issue at hand, posing questions and gathering data that are particular or unique to the area, which would be virtually impossible for outsiders to obtain. Participatory research also involves all stakeholders together developing analytic methods that are appropriate to the community forming the geographic focus of the study. The ideal collaborative research goes beyond a *participatory* paradigm and addresses deeper institutional power dynamics and the hierarchy of knowledge that labels one body of knowledge and experience as nonscientific and another as scientific and recognizes the political and social context. For instance, the community partners suggested that we use GIS to examine not only the correspondence of individual pollution sources to asthma hospitalizations but also the impact of living within close proximity to more than one pollution source, which we did in the multiple exposure analysis. This analysis demonstrated even higher than expected hospitalizations among those residents living close to two or more pollution sources.

Data Collection and Analysis   Community members provided important local knowledge and helped to collect sensitive data about the community in several ways, as shown in Table 5.4. Many of these local knowledge bases have been incorporated into the analysis of our asthma and air pollution study. Each phase of the analysis has been instructive in guiding our subsequent research directions and demonstrating the gaps and uncertainties that need further explanation and examination in our future research.

FABB also participated in meaningful ways in our analysis of GIS findings, not only with the review and critique of data collection and analytic methods but also with interpreting the results, giving guidance and offering tentative explanations based on local knowledge about anomalous findings from the research. FABB sought more discussion regarding the institutional and political implications of GIS research, the power dynamics of GIS research methodologies, and how CBPR and interdisciplinary research could be better tools for community empowerment and integrating historical, social, political, and economic perspectives.

Dissemination of Research Results   One of the challenges in disseminating the results of our study is that publishing the findings in only academic and professional journals will not suffice. We must also find ways to present our results so that members of the affected community and other communities affected by high rates of asthma and

TABLE 5.4. **Community Contributions to Data Collection and Analysis**

Variable of interest	Community contribution and impact on study
Truck routes	Databases obtained from the official sources, such as the Department of Transportation, were incomplete, according to community members who often witnessed trucks on local residential streets not designated as truck routes. Although suggested by FABB, resources did not permit enumeration of off-route trucking volume.
Active/inactive pollution sources	Of the stationary point sources of pollution that appeared on the federal lists, residents knew that some of the facilities were no longer active, and others were not properly reported as to emissions.
Actual location of residential areas within a block group	Areal weighting script used to calculate populations in portions of census block groups was based on the assumption of homogeneity of residential populations. The community had more specific knowledge of densities within block groups, such as the location of major housing projects, which influence the disease rates in and out of impact zones, and led to the dasymetric mapping phase of the study.
Buffer distances for highways	Standard guidelines for impact assessment assume that highways are at grade level, yet many highways in the Bronx are either elevated or below grade in cuts. Residents' knowledge of the differential impact of highway grade on the pollution that entered their house or street led us to reconsider standard buffer distances assigned to highways because grade affects the distance typical traffic-related pollutants travel.

air pollution can understand and act on our findings. This includes developing culturally and linguistically appropriate maps, tables, charts, and risk communication materials, media, and a Web site for community presentations of these GIS findings to promote education and dialogue on appropriate public health and regulatory responses. Also of critical importance is communication of the study's findings to policy- and decision-makers and other government officials. We began this process with other

New York asthma researchers, environmentalists, and asthma advocates at a community forum at the New York Academy of Sciences in January 2007. We intend to organize similar forums in affected communities in the Bronx.

Making the Connection Between Environmental Justice and Environmental Health

This analysis found that people residing within the impact zones were not only much more likely to be hospitalized for asthma than those living outside the impact zones but also more likely to be minority and poor than those outside the impact zones. Previous research has suggested that socioeconomic status itself plays a role in diseases and deaths associated with air pollution.[73, 74] High asthma hospitalization rates reflect both minority and poverty status and high exposures to environmental pollution, and these factors are inextricably entwined.[75, 76] In hierarchical regression analysis, even after controlling for potential confounding factors, such as race/ethnicity and poverty status, the correlation between asthma hospitalization and proximity to air pollution sources remains significant. For instance, in examining the multiple exposure buffers, although race/ethnicity and poverty status account for most of the variance in the model, proximity to multiple sources of pollution remains significant ($R^2 = .429$; $p < .001$). Proximity to any major pollution source (residence within the combined buffers) yields similar results ($R^2 = .452$; $p < .05$).[77]

Poor people, those lacking access or means to health services, support, or resources, may be more likely admitted to the hospital for asthma because they may not receive ongoing preventive or disease management services. Regular access to doctors and medicine might reduce emergency room visits and hospital admissions for asthma, although the impact may vary by cultural background, educational attainment, or level of affluence, further illustrating the multiple determinants of asthma outcomes.

Although further analyses will clarify to what extent high asthma hospitalization rates are correlated with high environmental burdens, the fact remains that the populations in the Bronx in closest proximity to air pollution sources are also those with higher risk of asthma hospitalization and higher likelihood of being poor and minority. Regardless of whether the high asthma hospitalization rates are due to environmental causes or result primarily from poverty and other sociodemographic factors, the findings of this research point to a health and environmental justice crisis.

LESSONS ON INTERDISCIPLINARY APPROACHES TO URBAN HEALTH RESEARCH

Benefits and Challenges of the Partnership

As we have described, a major benefit of the interdisciplinary and organizational collaboration is the complementary knowledge, skills, and perspectives that each partner brings to the effort, none of whom could accomplish the research or its translation into public policy effectively on their own. Partners regularly share information that originates in disciplines, advocacy networks, and professional circles that enrich and broaden the perspective of all parties. We function as each other's eyes and ears in many forums where we would otherwise be unlikely to participate. Each partner brings different organizational and institutional resources that support the collaboration, not always in stereotyped roles, particularly as FABB staff have considerable expertise and training in environmental science, food justice, and endocrine disruptors, whereas the academic and clinical professionals have little knowledge and experience in these areas. The community partners keep the academic and clinical professionals up to date on major environmental justice controversies and challenges well before they reach the mainstream media and have risen to leadership positions in citywide coalitions, such as the New York Asthma Partnership. Despite the differences between partners, described previously, mutual respect and trust have developed over time, permitting more debate, problem solving, and reflection. The partnership is still far from achieving the ideal, and time for reflection and discussion remains a precious and limited resource.

Perspectives of the Stakeholders and Lessons Learned

Each organization contributes a unique perspective to the partnership. Lehman College, for example, brings an academic perspective that combines activism with teaching and research. SBEJP has provided an avenue to expand available support to conduct GIS research. Lehman staff arranged for FABB staff to receive formal training in a GIS certificate program, and the partnership has supported the development of a master's degree program in public health at Lehman College and a master's degree in GISc, focusing on environmental and health spatial sciences. The physicians and faculty of the Albert Einstein College of Medicine are both clinical and academic partners in SBEJP and are employed by Montefiore Medical Center. Most of SBEJP's efforts address environmental aspects of public health and, therefore, broaden the clinician's perspective beyond caring for individual patients and families. Our community partner FABB offers an ongoing dialogue with the Bronx community served by the medical center and its staff. Our clinicians are challenged by how to incorporate into practice and public policy our findings about the increased risk for asthma hospitalizations posed by geographic proximity to sources of stationary and mobile air pollution.

Within the community, SBEJP provides resources, both financial and intellectual, for the growth and development of FABB, which also maintains a community-academic partnership with the Mailman School of Public Health of Columbia University. The two partnerships are quite different and enrich FABB's capacity and community impact in different ways.

Like so many CBOs in impoverished communities, FABB suffers with being underresourced and understaffed in trying to address all of the aspects of environmental justice that face the South Bronx. FABB has sought to break the cycle of underfunding that affects community-based organizations, but this remains an unrealized goal. FABB has been eager to assure that "street science" is respected for its superior local knowledge as well as its desire to better integrate community expertise with more traditional forms of expertise. FABB has invested heavily in youth internships, teaching in neighborhood schools, and collaborating with other South Bronx organizations to promote its broad environmental justice agenda and has greatly influenced SBEJP's overall direction, activities, and research.

CONCLUSION

An interdisciplinary partnership has conducted important research with significant findings that should help focus attention on reducing stationary point and mobile sources of air pollution in urban areas. The work undertaken collaboratively in the partnership, especially regarding advances in technical methods, resulted in more robust findings, which became substantively more accurate in all four categories of major pollution sources investigated. The partnership contributed to an ongoing, iterative, and developmental process for improving the methodology and only began to integrate the local knowledge and expertise of community residents and advocates. Only if the findings of this research are incorporated into public policies at the community, neighborhood, borough, and citywide levels will we have achieved the community empowerment sought through such collaboration and CBPR.

SUMMARY

In this chapter, we examined the interdisciplinary research process and outcomes in a study of air pollution and asthma in economically distressed, mixed land-use neighborhoods in the Bronx, New York. We analyze how the unique contributions of our academic, medical, and community partners successfully integrated geographic information science, clinical epidemiology, and street science to reach a more robust understanding of the impact of local microenvironments and individual exposures on asthma rates. Results showed that people residing within high-impact pollution zones (especially stationary sources) were more likely to be hospitalized for asthma and to be minority and poor, even after results were controlled for sociodemographic characteristics and despite the limitations of data sources and methodologies. We discussed the challenges of, and lessons learned by, working in an intersectoral partnership (e.g., differing mandates, resources, and power) and the need for research findings and collaborative processes to be incorporated into neighborhood and citywide policy making to reduce pollutant sources and improve health care.

DISCUSSION QUESTIONS

1. What is the added value of studying childhood asthma from a biomedical and environmental perspective compared to either perspective alone?

2. What are the contributions and limitations of geographic information science (GISc) to increasing scientific understanding of the relationships between exposures or risk factors and disease?

3. In the case history the authors present, what roles did each participating organization play in the research? What unique contributions did each make to the research? What were some of the key challenges they faced, and how did the research team work to overcome them?

4. What are the contributions and limitations of community-based participatory research to solving environmental health problems facing urban communities?

ACKNOWLEDGMENTS

This research was partially supported by grant number 2 R25 ES01185-05 from the National Institute of Environmental Health Sciences. The National Oceanic and Atmospheric Administration's Cooperative Remote Sensing Science and Technology Center (NOAA-CREST) also provided critical support for this project under NOAA grant number NA17AE162. The statements contained within this chapter are not the opinions of the funding agency or the U.S. government but reflect the authors' opinions. This research was also supported in part by the George N. Shuster fellowship, the PSC-CUNY Faculty Research Award, and Montefiore Medical Center's Medical Geography Award.

We also thank all the individuals belonging to member organizations of the South Bronx Environmental Justice Partnership, who understood the relevance of this project to environmental health justice and gave their unstinting encouragement and assistance in the effort.

The very interdisciplinary team members who contributed to various portions of this project are Holly Porter-Morgan, PhD, Lehman College; Andrew Maroko and Jun Tu, PhD candidates, Earth and Environmental Sciences, CUNY Graduate Center; Dellis Stanberry and Juan Carlos Saborio, Environmental, Geographic, and Geological Sciences Department, Lehman College, CUNY; Carlos Alicea, director, For a Better Bronx; Marian Feinberg, For a Better Bronx; Jason Fletcher, biostatistician, Albert Einstein College of Medicine.

NOTES

1. Yen, I. H., and Syme, S. L. The social environment and health: A discussion of the epidemiologic literature. *Annual Review of Public Health,* 20 (1999): 287–306.

2. Goldman, B. A. *Not Just Prosperity: Achieving Sustainability with Environmental Justice.* Washington, D.C.: National Wildlife Foundation, 1993.

3. Maantay, J. A. Mapping environmental injustices: Pitfalls and potential of geo-graphic information systems (GIS) in assessing environmental health and equity. *Environmental Health Perspectives,* 110, Suppl 2 (2002): 161–171.

4. Northridge, M. E., and Shepard, P. M. Environmental racism and public health. *American Journal of Public Health,* 87, no. 5 (1997): 730–732.

5. National Institutes of Environmental Health Sciences. *Strategic Plan for the Elimination of Health Disparities.* Research Triangle Park, NC, National Institutes of Environmental Health Sciences, 2004.

6. Viswanathan, M., Ammerman, A., Eng, E., et al. *Community-based Participatory Research: Assessing the Evidence: Summary.* Evidence Report/Technology Assessment, No. 99. Rockville, Md.: Agency for Healthcare Research and Quality, August 2004.

7. Israel, B. *The value of community-based participatory research. Community-based participatory research: Conference summary.* Agency for Healthcare Research and Quality, Conference on Community-Based Participatory Research, November 27–28, 2001, Rockville, MD. Available at www.ahrq.gov/about/cpcr/cbpr/cbpr1 .htm Published November 27, 2001. Accessed January 31, 2009.

8. Israel, B., Schulz, A. J., Parker, E. A., and Becker, A. B. *Community-based participatory research: Engaging communities as partners in health research.* Talk given at the annual conference of Community-Campus Partnerships for Health, Washington, D.C.: April 29–May 2, 2000.

9. Israel, B. A., Schulz, A. J., Parker, E. A., and Becker, A. B. Review of community-based research: Assessing partnership approaches to improve public health. *Annual Review of Public Health,* 19 (1998): 173–202.

10. Goldberger, J., Wheeler, G. A., and Sydenstrycker, E. A study of the relation of family income and other economic factors to pellagra incidence in seven cotton mill villages of South Carolina in 1916. *Public Health Reports,* (1920) 35: 2673–2714.

11. Sampson, R. J. Neighborhood-level context and health: Lessons from sociology. In I. Kawachi and L. F. Berkman, eds., *Neighborhoods and Health,* pp. 132–146. New York: Oxford University Press, 2003.

12. Wilson, W. J. *The Truly Disadvantaged: The Inner City, the Underclass, and Public Policy.* Chicago: University of Chicago Press, 1987.

13. Wilson, W. J. *When Work Disappears.* New York: Knopf, 1996.

14. Robert, S. Community-level socioeconomic status effects on adults' health. *Journal of Health Social Behavior,* 39 (1998): 18–37.

15. Robert, S. Socioeconomic position and health: The independent contribution of community socioeconomic context. *Annual Review of Sociology,* 25 (1999): 489–516.

16. Katz, L., Kling, J., and Liebman, J. Moving to opportunity in Boston: Early impacts of a housing mobility program. *Quarterly Journal of Economics,* 116, no. 2 (2001): 607–654.

17. Becker, K., Glass, G., Braithwaite, W., and Zenilman, J. Geographic epidemiology of gonorrhea in Baltimore, Maryland, using a geographic information system. *American Journal of Epidemiology,* 147, no. 7 (1998): 709–716.

18. Bowman, J. D. GIS model of power lines used to study EMF and childhood leukemia. *Public Health GIS News and Information,* 32 (2000): 7–10.

19. Bullen, N., Moon, G., and Jones, K. Defining localities for health planning: A GIS approach. *Social Science & Medicine,* 42, no. 6 (1996): 801–816.

20. Chakraborty, J., and Armstrong, M. P. Using geographic plume analysis to assess community vulnerability to hazardous accidents. *Computers, Environment and Urban Systems,* 19, no. 5–6 (1995): 1–17.

21. Chen, F., Breiman, R., Farley, M., Plikaytis, B., Deaver, K., and Cetron, M. Geocoding and linking data from population-based surveillance and the U.S. Census to evaluate the impact of median household income on the epidemiology of invasive *Streptococcus* pneumonia infections. *American Journal of Epidemiology,* 148, no. 12 (1998): 1212–1218.

22. Cromley, E. K. Case study of the use of GIS to inventory and understand the pattern of traffic accidents in Connecticut. In K. Clarke, ed., *Getting Started with Geographical Information Systems,* 3rd ed. (pp. 257–261). Upper Saddle River, N.J.: Prentice Hall, 2001.

23. Devasundaram, J., Rohn, D., Dwyer, D., and Israel, E. A geographic information system application for disease surveillance. *American Journal of Public Health,* 88, no. 9 (1998): 1406–1407.

24. Glass, G., Morgan, J., Johnson, D., Noy, P., Israel, E., and Schwartz, B. Infectious disease epidemiology and GIS: A case study of Lyme disease. *GeoInfo Systems,* 2 (1992): 65–69.

25. Guthe, W., Tucker, R., and Murphy, E. Reassessment of lead exposures in New Jersey using GIS technology. *Environmental Research,* 59, 2 (1992): 318–325.

26. Ihrig, M., Shalat, S., and Baynes, C. A hospital-based case-control study of stillbirths and environmental exposure to arsenic using an atmospheric dispersion model and a geographical information system. *Epidemiology,* 9, no. 3 (1998): 290–294.

27. Kingham, S., Gatrell, A., and Rowlingson, G. Testing for clustering of health events within a geographical information systems framework. *Environmental Planning A,* 27, no. 5 (1995): 809–821.

28. Kohli, S., Sahlen, K., Lofman, O., et al. Individuals living in areas with high background radon: A GIS method to identify populations at risk. *Computer Methods and Programs in Biomedicine,* 53, no. 2 (1997): 105–112.

29. Kulldorff, M., Feuer, E., Miller, B., and Freedman L. Breast cancer clusters in the northeast United States: A geographical analysis. *American Journal of Epidemiology,* 146, no. 2 (1997): 161–170.

30. Love, D., and Lindquist, P. Geographical accessibility of hospitals to the aged: A geographic information systems analysis within Illinois. *Health Services Research,* 29, no. 6 (1995): 629–651.

31. Parker, E., and Campbell, J. Measuring access to primary medical care: Some examples of the use of geographical information systems. *Health Place,* 4, no. 2 (1998): 183–193.

32. Pine, J., and Diaz, J. Environmental health screening with GIS: Creating a community environmental health profile. *Journal of Environmental Health,* 62, no. 8 (2000): 9–15.

33. McMaster, R. B., Leitner, H., and Sheppard, E. GIS-based environmental equity and risk assessment: Methodological problems and prospects. *Cartography and Geographic Information Systems,* 24, no. 3 (1997): 172–189.

34. Sheppard, E., Leitner, H., McMaster, R. B., and Hongguo, T. GIS-based measures of environmental equity: Exploring their sensitivity and significance. *Journal of Exposure Science and Environmental Epidemiology,* 9 (1999): 18–28.

35. Tobler, W. Cellular geography. In S. Gale and G. Olsson, eds., *Philosophy in Geography,* pp. 379–386. Dordrecht, The Netherlands: Reidel, 1979.

36. United States Bureau of the Census. Census 2000 Summary File 1, New York State. Washington, D.C.: U.S. Government Printing Office, 2001.

37. Maantay, J. A. Zoning law, health, and environmental justice: What's the connection? *Journal of Law and Medical Ethics,* 3 (2002): 572–593.

38. Maantay, J. A. Zoning, equity, and public health. *Am J Public Health,* 91, no. 7 (2001): 1033–1041.

39. Jackson, K., ed. *The Encyclopedia of New York City.* New Haven, Conn.: Yale University Press, 1995.

40. Guo, Y., et al. Climate, traffic-related air pollutants, and asthma prevalence in middle-school children in Taiwan. *Environmental Health Perspectives,* 107, no. 12 (1999): 1001–1006.

41. Edwards, J., Walters, S., and Griffiths, R. C. Hospital admissions for asthma in pre-school children: Relationship to major roads in Birmingham UK. *Archives of Environmental Health,* 49 (1994): 223–227.

42. English, P., Neutra, R., Scalf, R., Sullivan, M., Waller, L., and Zhu, L. Examining associations between childhood asthma and traffic flow using a geographic information system. *Environmental Health Perspectives,* 107 (1997): 761–767.

43. Friedman, M. S., Powell, K. E., Hutwagner, L., Graham, L. M., and Teague, W. G. Impact of changes in transportation and commuting behaviors during the 1996 summer Olympic games in Atlanta on air quality and childhood asthma. *JAMA,* 285, no. 7 (2001): 897–905.

44. Neutra, P. Examining associations between childhood asthma and traffic flow using a geographic information system. *Environmental Health Perspectives,* 107, no. 9 (1999): 761–767.

45. Romieu, I., Menese, F., and Sienra-Monge, J. J. Effects of urban air pollutants on emergency visits for childhood asthma in Mexico City. *American Journal of Epidemiology,* 141 (1995): 546–553.

46. Schwartz, J., Slater, D., and Larson, T. V. Particulate air pollution and hospital emergency room visits for asthma in Seattle. *Am Rev Respir Dis,* 147 (1995): 826–831.

47. Studnicka, M., Hackl, E., Pischinger, J., et al. Traffic-related NO_2 and the prevalence of asthma and respiratory symptoms in seven year olds. *European Respiratory Journal,* 10 (1997): 2275–2278.

48. Sunyer, J., and Spix, C. Urban air pollution and emergency admissions for asthma in four European cities: The APHEA Project. *Thorax,* 52 (1997): 760–765.

49. Green, R. S., Smorodinsky, S., Kim, J. J., McLaughlin, R., and Ostro, B. Proximity of California public schools to busy roads. *Environmental Health Perspectives,* 112, no. 1 (2004): 61–66.

50. New York City Department of Health. *Asthma facts,* 2nd ed. Available at www.nyc.gov/html/doh/downloads/pdf/asthma/facts.pdf. Published 2003. Accessed January 31, 2009.

51. New York State Department of Health Statewide Planning and Research Cooperative System [SPARCS]. *Technical Documentation.* New York State Department of Health, Albany, N.Y.: 2002.

52. United States Environmental Protection Agency, Office of Environmental Information. The Emergency Planning and Community Right to Know Act Section 313 Release and Other Waste Management Reporting Requirements. Washington, D.C.: U.S. EPA, 2001.

53. Maantay, J. A. Race and waste: Options for equity planning in New York City. *Planners Network,* 145, no. 1 (2001): 6–10.

54. Brunekreef, B., Dockery, D. W., and Krzyzanowski, M. Epidemiologic studies on short-term effects of low levels of major ambient air pollution components. *Environmental Health Perspectives,* 103, Suppl 2 (1995): 3–13.

55. Delfino, R. J., Gong, Jr., H., Linn, W. S., Pellizzari, E. D., and Hu, Y. Asthma symptoms in Hispanic children and daily ambient exposures in toxic and criteria air pollutants. *Environmental Health Perspectives,* 111, no. 4 (2003): 647–656.

56. Neumann, C. M., Forman, D. L., and Rothlein, J. E. Hazard screening of chemical releases and environmental equity analysis of populations proximate to toxic release inventory facilities in Oregon. *Environmental Health Perspectives,* 106, no. 4 (1998): 217–226.

57. Chakraborty, J., and Armstrong, M. P. Exploring the use of buffer analysis for the identification of impacted areas in environmental equity assessment. *Cartography Geographic Information Systems,* 24, no. 3 (1997): 145–157.

58. New York City Mayor's Office of Environmental Coordination. *City Environmental Quality Review (CEQR) Technical Manual,* 2001.

59. Hitchins, J., Morawsaka, L., Wolff, R., and Gilbert, D. Concentrations of submicrometer particles from vehicle emissions near a major road. *Atmosphere and Environment,* 34 (2000): 51–59.

60. Zhu, Y., Hinds, W. C., Kim, S., and Sioutas, C. Concentration and size distribution of ultrafine particles near a major highway. *Journal of the Air & Waste Management Association,* 52 (2002): 1032–1042.

61. Venn, A. J., Lewis, S. A., Cooper, M., Hubbard, R., and Britton, J. Living near a main road and the risk of wheezing illness in children. *American Journal of Respiratory and Critical Care Medicine,* 164 (2001): 2177–2180.

62. Livingstone, A. E., Shaddick, G., Grundy, C., and Elliot, P. Do people living near inner city main roads have more asthma needing treatment? Case control study. *British Medical Journal,* 312 (1996): 676–677.

63. Nitta, H., Sato, T., Nakai, S., Maeda, K., Aoko, S., and Oho, M. Respiratory health associated with exposure to automobile exhaust. Results of cross-sectional studies in 1979, 1982, and 1983. *Archives of Environmental,* 48 (1993): 53–58.

64. Wilkinson, P., Elliott, P., Grundy, C., et al. Case-control study of hospital admission with asthma in children aged 5–14 years: Relation with road traffic in northwest London. *Thorax,* 54, no 12 (1999): 1070–1074.

65. Flowerdew, R., and Green, M. Areal interpolation and types of data. In S. Fotheringham and P. Rogerson, eds., *Spatial Analysis and GIS,* pp. 121–145. Bristol, UK: Taylor and Francis, 1994.

66. Goodchild, M., and Lam, N. Areal interpolation: A variant of the traditional spatial problem. *Geo-Processing,* 1 (1980): 297–312.

67. Maantay, J. A. Asthma and air pollution in the Bronx: Methodological and data considerations in using GIS for environmental justice and health research. *Health & Place,* 13 (2007): 32–56. E-pub November 28, 2005.

68. Maantay, J. A., Maroko, A. R., and Herrmann, C. Mapping population distribution in the urban environment: The Cadastral-Based Expert Dasymetric System (CEDS). *Cartography and Geographic Information Systems,* 34, no. 2 (2007): 77–102.

69. Maantay, J., Maroko, A. R., and Porter-Morgan, H. A new method for mapping population and understanding the spatiality of disease in urban areas: Asthma in the Bronx, New York. *Urban Geography,* 29, no. 7 (2008): 724–738.

70. Cromley, E., and McLafferty, S. *GIS and Public Health.* New York: Guilford Press, 2002.

71. Corburn, J. *Street Science: Community Knowledge and Environmental Health Justice.* Cambridge, Mass.: MIT Press, 2005.

72. Maantay, J., and Ziegler, J. *GIS for the Urban Environment.* Redlands, Cal.: Environmental Systems Research Institute Press, 2006.

73. O'Neill, M. S., Jerret, M., Kawachi, I., et al. Health, wealth, and air pollution: Advancing theory and methods. *Environmental Health Perspectives,* 111, no. 16 (2003): 1861–1870.

74. Schulz, A. J., Williams, D. R., Israel, B. A., and Lempert, L. B. Racial and spatial relations as fundamental determinants of health in Detroit. *Milbank Quarterly,* 80, no. 43 (2002): 677–707.

75. Krieger, N. Embodying inequality: A review of concepts, measures, and methods for studying health consequences of discrimination. *International Journal of Health Sciences,* 29, no. 2 (1999): 295–352.

76. Meliker, J. R., Nriagu, J. O., Hammad, A. S., Savoie, K. L., Jamil, H., and Devries, J. M. Spatial clustering of emergency department visits by asthmatic children in an urban area: South-western Detroit, Michigan. *Ambulatory Child Health,* 7 (2001): 297–312.

77. Fletcher, J. *Report on the Regression Analysis of Asthma Hospitalization Rates and Proximity to Major Air Pollution Sources.* Bronx, N.Y.: Albert Einstein College of Medicine, 2006.

CHAPTER

6

RACIAL INEQUALITY IN HEALTH AND THE POLICY-INDUCED BREAKDOWN OF AFRICAN AMERICAN COMMUNITIES

ARLINE T. GERONIMUS, J. PHILLIP THOMPSON

LEARNING OBJECTIVES

- Describe how prevailing ideological viewpoints on black health (mis)interpret black behavior.
- Describe the biological and social pathways by which racial ideologies and policies may undermine the health of African American populations.

- Present policy alternatives that could help to overcome some of the detrimental impact of racialized ideologies and policies and thereby help to promote the health of African Americans and reduce black/white inequalities in health.

- Discuss the role that democratic movements can play in addressing the detrimental impact of racialized ideologies and creating policies that support health.

The greatest danger lies not in the so-called "problems" of race, but rather in the integrity c national thinkinǫ and in the ethics of national con- duct.

—W.E.B. Du B

INTRODUCTION

Young through middle-aged adults in high-poverty urban African American populations have a high probability of dying or becoming disabled long before they are old.[1,2] Figure 6.1 shows that in Harlem or Chicago's South Side, one-third of African American girls and two-thirds of boys who reach their fifteenth birthdays do not live to celebrate their sixty-fifth. In contrast, only 10 percent of girls and about 25 percent of boys nationwide fail to live to age sixty-five. Indeed, African American youth in some urban areas face lower probabilities of surviving to age forty-five than white youth nationwide do of surviving to old age.[2,3]

Stress-related chronic diseases are the primary reasons for this excess mortality in urban African American populations,[3,4] and evidence indicates that their negative impact on life expectancy may be growing. For example, excess deaths attributed to circulatory disease or cancer each *doubled* among young and middle-aged men in Harlem from 1980 to 1990.[4] In contrast, the more publicized homicide rates began to decline. As a general rule, racial differences in health tend to widen after age twenty-five and become most pronounced among those aged thirty-five to sixty-four.[5-9] Although racial differentials in infant health are also stark, they often reflect differences in the health of reproductive-age women,[10] substantial percentages of whom already suffer from stress-related diseases that can complicate pregnancies.[1]

African American men and women in high-poverty urban areas also have rates of health-induced disabilities at ages thirty-five and fifty-five that are comparable to the national averages for fifty-five- and seventy-five-year-olds, respectively.[2] These disabilities in young and middle adulthood limit capacity to work, often necessitate caregiving, and lead to premature death. Rates of death or disability are shown in Figure 6.2, illustrating stunning inequalities between African American residents of

---

Note: An earlier, longer version of this chapter appeared in the *DuBois Review,* 1 (2004): 247–279. *Epigraph.* Reprinted with the permission of Cambridge University Press.

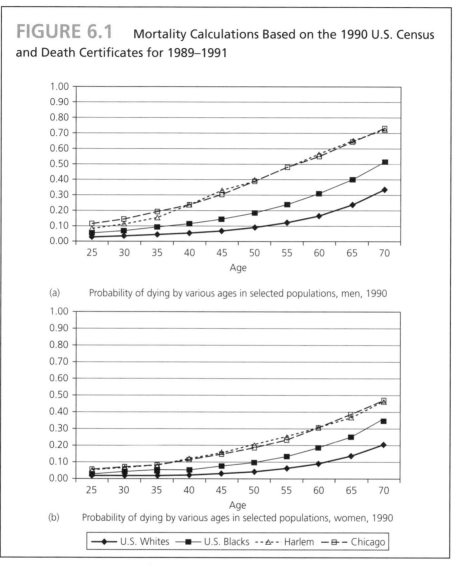

FIGURE 6.1   Mortality Calculations Based on the 1990 U.S. Census and Death Certificates for 1989–1991

(a)   Probability of dying by various ages in selected populations, men, 1990

(b)   Probability of dying by various ages in selected populations, women, 1990

◆— U.S. Whites   ■— U.S. Blacks   --△-- Harlem   --◻-- Chicago

Note: In the these graphs, *Harlem* comprises African American residents of the Central Harlem Health Center District in New York City; *Chicago* comprises African American residents of the South Side community areas of Near South Side, Douglas, Oakland, Fuller Park, Grand Boulevard, and Washington Park in Chicago, Illinois.

Harlem or Chicago's South Side and whites or blacks nationwide. Only 30 percent of teenage girls and 20 percent of teenage boys residing in these urban areas can expect to be alive and able-bodied at age sixty-five.

Reducing the size of these and other racial inequalities in health has been a high-priority, national public health policy objective for more than two decades. Yet racial

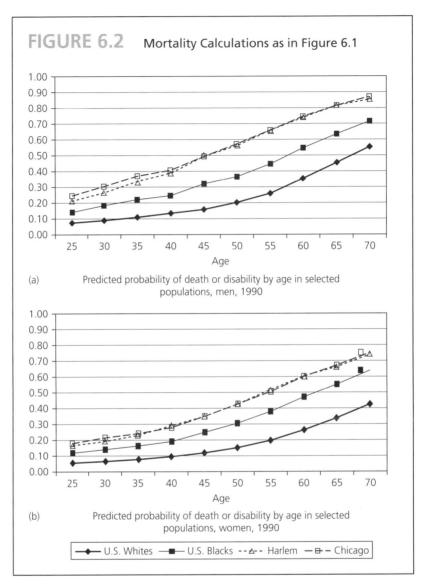

FIGURE 6.2 Mortality Calculations as in Figure 6.1

(a) Predicted probability of death or disability by age in selected populations, men, 1990

(b) Predicted probability of death or disability by age in selected populations, women, 1990

◆ U.S. Whites   ■ U.S. Blacks   --△-- Harlem   --⊟-- Chicago

Note: Disability calculations are based on 1990 U.S. Census data, using public use microdata areas (PUMAs) that most closely approximate mortality areas for Central Harlem Health Center District in New York City and Chicago's South Side community areas of Near South Side, Douglas, Oakland, Fuller Park, Grand Boulevard, and Washington Park in Chicago, Illinois.

disparities in important health indicators have persisted and, in some cases, grown.[11] This is true even for some health disparities that have been energetically targeted for reduction, such as infant mortality rates. This failure is notable and, we argue, a major indictment of public policies aimed at African American communities. In this chapter, we examine the causes and consequences of inequities in health between African

American and other urban communities and assess the role of policy in creating and perpetuating these differences. By drawing on a broad range of disciplinary approaches, we demonstrate the value of examining health inequities from a variety of perspectives, including biological, sociological, psychological, and political.

At least since 1971, when William Ryan coined the phrase "blaming the victim,"[12] a raft of literature has criticized public policies that concentrate on encouraging individuals to change their behavior instead of on creating structural changes in the social environment.[13-23] More recently, Bruce Link and Jo Phelan[21, 22] have argued that failures to eliminate disparities in health result from undue emphasis on ameliorative approaches that target the risk factors linking socioeconomic position to health in a particular context but not on altering the context itself.

From this "fundamental cause" perspective, the only effective way to reduce or eliminate differentials in health is to address the underlying "social inequalities that so reliably produce them."[22] This is a formidable challenge that requires going beyond the usual health policy discourse. Toward this end, we start by noting that racial inequalities in health are the predictable manifestation of linkages among prevailing racialized ideologies, political and economic structural inequalities that follow, the personal and social coping mechanisms adopted to manage dominant ideologies and structural inequalities, and the physiological effects of these coping efforts.

Thus, before classifying policies according to their emphasis on individual behavioral change or on political-economic structural change, we ask whether premises that undergird *both* perspectives misinterpret black health problems and whether they are harmful to black health. We illustrate below that current policy ideas and proposals rely on specific social and moral viewpoints that are racially biased toward white norms and behavior and that these viewpoints, in and of themselves, have negative implications for black health. They stimulate race-related stress that can "weather" the cardiovascular, metabolic, and immune systems, fueling the development or progression of disease.

RACIALIZED IDEOLOGIES: DEVELOPMENTALISM, ECONOMISM, AND THE AMERICAN CREED

Racialized ideologies influence social science's interpretation of black health problems and of blacks themselves. Here we identify and then critique three central and mutually reinforcing American ideologies that inform common understandings of the production of health inequality: developmentalism, economism, and the American Creed.

Developmentalism

Developmentalism[24-28] is the most widely used model for interpreting the relationships between age and health and among age, identity, and social expectations in the United States. Linked to the acquisition of abilities necessary to take personal responsibility, it is an individualistic and economistic model. It assumes that people's lives unfold in three biological and psychosocial stages—birth through adolescence, full maturity, and gradual senescence—in which children, adolescents, and the elderly face fairly predictable age-related health and mortality risks. Childhood risks stem from biological and psychological immaturity, which is generally outgrown. Adolescents are also expected to outgrow their psychosocial vulnerability to engage in risky behaviors.[29–31] The elderly face the inevitable physiological deterioration that culminates in death and that for many people—although not for many African Americans—has recently been compressed into the very end of life.[2, 32, 33]

Economism

Economism is rooted in the assumption that all adult human beings know their own needs and wants, are essentially self-interested and competitive, and are mainly motivated by economic considerations. Economism elevates a particular version of individual agency—or "personal responsibility"—into a general social definition of what it means to behave responsibly. In this view, markets are the arbiters of social exchange; individuals can shape their placement in the social hierarchy by choosing to invest in their human capital to best position themselves to engage the market and fulfill their personal responsibilities. Economism thus divorces material context from culture,[34] and it privileges material well-being over other contributors to human health and wholeness.

The American Creed

The American creed combines the values of equality and personal responsibility. Equality is expressed in the creed's promise of equal rights and opportunity for all citizens, but the creed is not an ideology of equal outcomes. Instead, individual outcomes depend on personal responsibility. Thus, inequality is expected, and poverty is considered a just consequence of poor effort.[35] The American creed has a strong transcendent quality that is firmly rooted in the American psyche. It unites an imagined community of virtuous seekers of the American dream—people who work hard, play by the rules, and stoically suffer the consequences if they do not. The creed is connected to what makes many white citizens believe that they are good and decent people—and that many blacks are not.

The creed underlies the universalism that ignores fundamental differences in the life circumstances of whites and blacks. The creed also underlies the imaginary "level playing field" of the economistic perspective. The creed is not only a dominant ideology but also hegemonic.[36] Robert Dahl has asserted that "To reject the American creed is in effect to refuse to be an American. As a nation we have taken great pains to insure that few citizens will ever want to do anything so rash, so preposterous—in fact, so wholly un-American."[37]

The Effects of Prevailing Ideologies on Interpretations of Black Health Problems

Developmentalism, economism, and the American creed are all racialized ideologies. They ignore or, worse, denigrate African American historical, social, and moral perspectives, and they disrupt African American coping mechanisms. This, in turn, induces poor health and exacerbates illness.

Developmentalism frames health as a universal process of biological unfolding that is only undone or impeded by accident or by poor behavioral choices. On closer inspection, development actually reflects biological potential nurtured through a combination of resources and values that are largely restricted to members of the dominant group (whites). The developmental understanding of the relationship between age and health expresses dominant cultural ideals, values, and age-graded social expectations. Centrally, developmentalism and rigid cultural commitment to the nuclear family ideal are mutually reinforcing. Healthy development can proceed because parents are charged with supervising, supporting, and protecting children and adolescents. Cultural and parental competence is measured by the extent to which young people can separate from their parents and establish independent identities at the appropriate time: They are expected to break away from their primary reliance on parents for support, and parents are expected to "let go."

In these ways, the dominant cultural scenario for the life course identifies the proper objects of attachment (first to parents and then to spouse and other peers) and identity development (always as an individual, first in the context of the nuclear family of origin and later in the context of peers), and it outlines the cadence of life-course demands along the axes of dependence and responsibility. Dependents (youth and the elderly) are relatively free from family (or "personal") responsibility, whereas young through middle-aged adults are expected to be both independent and highly responsible.[5]

Through the developmental prism, it is difficult to appreciate that some cultural groups may value group self-sufficiency over individual self-sufficiency or that family structure itself is historically and culturally variable. For instance, African American urban populations often recognize an extended and multigenerational definition of family. Here, families comprise kin who may or may not be biologically related but are part of networks of reciprocal obligations that fulfill functions the dominant ideology would reserve for nuclear families.[38–41] Indeed, the extreme economic need, social exclusion, and early health deterioration that characterize African American families in high-poverty areas require a degree of multigenerational connectedness and familial responsibility and reliance throughout the life span that makes aspects of the dominant developmental ideology untenable. In high-poverty black communities, children, youth, and adults participate actively in fulfilling domestic responsibilities; individuals hold allegiance to multigenerational collectives of community or kin.

In this context, the dominant cultural understanding of psychosocial development is not sensible. Instead, maintaining active family ties, cooperation, and support is especially salient to blacks in high-poverty areas and takes priority over self-reliance and independence. African American adults often do not feel the same responsibility as their white counterparts to "let go" of youthful family members—both because they rely on their cooperative efforts and because they view society as neither level nor welcoming for African American youth. For their part, poor black teens cannot take a moratorium from family responsibility or, with death and disability all around, are they likely to view themselves as invincible. These teens have ample reason to protect the ties they have to their elders because the intergenerational perspectives provided by their parents help them make sense of ongoing social, political, and economic exclusion.[42]

Interconnections among members of social or kin networks help participants feel valued and provide practical and caring support. Both contributions can promote health. By feeling part of a collective that stands in opposition to the dominant culture, members of the collective are able to contest the dominant culture's images of themselves as morally marred or culturally deficient. This has positive health consequences.[43–49] The positive impact of social integration and social support on health is said to rival the detrimental impact of such known biomedical risk factors as cigarette smoking, obesity, and high blood pressure.[50] Social support that serves as a buffer against race-related stress,[51] stigmatization,[52] lifestyle incongruity,[53–55] or culturally incompetent medical care[43,56] reaps critical advantages for black health. This is especially true where residential and school segregation are an omnipresent physical representation to both blacks and whites of black inferiority.

Thus, the relatively longer, healthier lives of whites are conditioned not only on greater access to material resources but also on the psychic benefits of having their values honored in public discourse and institutional structures and timetables. Explanations for racial health inequality must encompass the impact of pervasive insults to the personal and collective integrity of African Americans. We are here suggesting that cultural oppression is as important a structuring force in black health as economics.[57]

Although material resources contribute to health in a critical way, populations vary in their strategies for achieving economic security or social mobility. The most promising avenues for any population are ones that are environmentally adaptive, responsive to socioeconomic opportunities and constraints, and culturally mediated.[58–60] Moreover, health also comes from a sense of rootedness in and affirmation of cultural values, practices, affective ties, and beliefs that give life purpose and meaning.[43,50] These psychosocial resources may be especially important in averting stress-related disease.[43] The economistic approach is problematic when considering racial disparities in health not only because it promotes "victim blaming" or "ameliorative" interventions but also because it ignores the culturally mediated psychosocial aspects of health. As we discuss later, this perspective can lead to policies that are counterproductive or to structural interventions that have limited effect.

Even social epidemiologists and policy advocates who focus on structural issues unduly limit their thinking to economic interventions and metaphors. Few pay any attention to the impact of affective ties and social identity on health. They see the ultimate goal of social research and policy as providing access to material resources (e.g., income, health insurance, food stamps, good housing) or to other forms of "capital" that are commutable in a market economy (including human capital investment opportunities such as education or social capital development). This reflects the large degree to which economistic assumptions about human behavior have permeated cultural discourse.

A recent explication of the "*essential nature* of social stratification" (emphasis added) with a view toward determining "an ideal socioeconomic status (SES) measure for public health research"[61] offers insights into the centrality of economism in the thinking of investigators interested in the *social* determinants of health. Oakes and Rossi locate the definition of SES, or social structure, in "differential access (realized and potential) to desired resources." They draw on Coleman's social theory, which they note "is rooted in the *purposive action of an individual agent,*" (emphasis added) and identify three types of capital: material, human, and social.

Furthermore, they assert, "Human capital is a critical component of SES since it is a resource that may be used to acquire socially valued goods. It is fungible in a market economy." And finally, even social capital is stripped of affective ties and social identity: "social capital stands for the ability of actors to secure benefits by virtue of membership in social networks and other social structures. Examples include increased educational achievement, social mobility, employment opportunities, decreased welfare dependency, and low levels of teenage pregnancy."[61]

Note that this highly individualistic, acquisitive, and materialistic discussion is made not by researchers who primarily advocate individual behavior change but by those who "believe that a narrow focus on individuals outside of historical, social, and biophysical contexts limits the understanding of disease etiology, health, and intervention modes."[61]

Economism misunderstands black health problems by ignoring cultural oppression. Similarly, unequal racial opportunity is commonly defined in narrow economistic terms as unequal access to the material resources and social contacts needed for individual advancement. The problem with racial segregation, in this view, is not that it represents overwhelming cultural ostracism of blacks and a colossal moral failure to rectify the nation's horrendous racial history but simply that it limits blacks' access to contacts and resources or, in health terms, exposes them to noxious social and physical environments. This economistic understanding of segregation skirts the moral and institutional impact of America's racial history on its current social hierarchy, imposing an individualistic and decontextualized viewpoint on black health problems that few African Americans share.

We believe that economism also leads to misunderstandings of the black middle class. The expansion of the black middle class has been identified as a solid sign of economic progress and as a precursor to eventual widespread black social integration. The dominant view among whites is that although limited racial discrimination persists, African Americans are on a steady path toward full integration and equality with whites.[62–64] The black middle class, however, does not define itself solely by its ability to consume valued material goods; rather, racial identity figures prominently in its view of middle-class social status.[65] The economistic concept of a nonracialized middle class treats African Americans as individuals isolated from their extended family networks, group history, social context, and social identity. It falsely assumes that, like middle-class whites, middle-class blacks feel distanced from the suffering of poor blacks.

Many middle-class blacks are still morally allied and socially associated with the defamed black poor, and most are segregated in the same or proximate neighborhoods.[66] Individual economic or educational success does not bring the same rewards for African

Americans that it does for whites.[67, 68] Crime victimization is a good example of this disproportion. For whites, crime victimization rates decline as income increases, but black victimization rates rise as income increases.[69]

Given this context, it is not surprising that the health of middle-class blacks and whites differs greatly in many regards, especially in prevalence of stress-related diseases.[51, 70–72] Middle-class black populations have only modestly better functional health status than high-poverty black populations, in sharp contrast with the steep economic gradient in functional limitation prevalent among white populations.[2, 9, 32, 73] It also indicates that interventions addressing the acquisition of education, income, or material goods alone will be insufficient to eliminate racial health inequality.

The third ideology, the American creed, asserts the essential fairness of U.S. institutions, thus wiping away fundamental structural inequalities and cultural oppressions. The American creed is basically a white point of view.[74] This difference in group perspective reflects the continuing absence of deep public consideration of slavery, Jim Crow laws, and subsequent forms of racial discrimination in the United States. The U.S. government never instituted a national anti-racist educational program after slavery.[75] Nor did the government institute a full employment "Marshall Plan" to counter the effects of centuries of slavery and segregation, despite black demands for such a program.[76] In thinly coded racial language, Republican Party leaders from Goldwater to Reagan to Bush attacked the 1960s Great Society programs as an unwarranted tax burden on hardworking (white) Americans for (poor black) people who do not want to work.[77]

Allowing human monstrosities of the scale of slavery and legal segregation to pass without deep ethical consideration conceals the questionable legitimacy of today's racially segregated communities and institutions. White Americans evaluate African American demands for justice from the standpoint of the creed morality. Their belief in the essential fairness of U.S. institutions and in the equality of opportunity in social structures leads many whites to the racially prejudiced stereotype that blacks are lazy and culturally disposed toward poverty. In his study of white opposition to welfare, Martin Gilens[78] argued that although some whites may harbor general antipathy for blacks, "for many whites the stereotype of blacks as lazy grows out of the belief that the American economic system is essentially fair, and that blacks remain mired in poverty despite the ample opportunities available to them. These perceptions in turn are fed by media distortions that neglect the 'deserving poor' in general and portray poor blacks in a particularly unsympathetic light."[78]

Thus, as Jennifer Hochschild[63] writes: "many whites see middle-class blacks as making excessive demands and blaming their personal failures on a convenient but nonexistent enemy. Even more whites see poor blacks as menacing, degraded strangers."

Internalizing creed ideology can be harmful to the health of blacks who "play by the rules." Sherman James has identified a predisposition among most African Americans to engage in persistent high-effort coping with social and economic adversity that he calls "John Henryism."[79] Individuals in low-income African American populations who exhibit high levels of John Henryism are the ones most apt to be hypertensive, which directly contradicts notions that fatalism or indolence precipitate cardiovascular disease among low-income African Americans. Those hoping to eliminate racial health inequality must be responsive to the evidence that African Americans of *all* social classes pay a disproportionately high price in stress-related disease for their membership in American society.

Without basic reconstruction of widespread racist stereotypes and essentialist myths regarding the virtues of American democracy, there is little intellectual foundation for scientific investigations of black health problems that take structural and cultural aspects of racism seriously. The creed blames blacks for their condition and thus blocks understandings of broader structural and cultural causes for racial differences as well as broader social responsibilities for persistent racial inequality. Meanwhile, blacks undergo harmful stress from powerful ideological forces valued by whites as common sense.[59, 60]

Racial Ideologies and Black Health

Whether health is construed narrowly or broadly, developmentalism, economism, and the American creed are of limited value to public health policy advocates working to eliminate racial health inequality. The problem of racial health inequality leads us to ask: How do we reconcile the notion that modern Americans have the developmental potential to be healthy at least through middle age with the stark evidence that many young and middle-aged African Americans are not? Adhering to the developmental model limits our perspective, reducing instances of poor health and mortality among relatively young adults to exceptions. Calling such groupwide experiences exceptions to the rule of a long healthy life is an inadequate explanation. It offers little to help explain the rapid health decline of African Americans that becomes detectable in their twenties, even among the middle class.[10]

As an alternative, Geronimus[1, 7] conceptualizes aging as a process of *weathering*. That is, people's health reflects the cumulative impact of their experiences from conception to their current age.[80] The older they are, the more time they have had to experience negative health impact and the greater the opportunity for these experiences to express any (even lagged) health effects or to accumulate or interact with others.

Weathering posits that African Americans experience early health deterioration because they have more serious and more frequent experiences with social and economic adversity relative to whites. On a physiological level, persistent high-effort coping with acute and chronic stressors has a profound effect on health and disease. Although the body's ability to respond to acute stress (the "fight or flight" response) is protective in certain threatening situations, under other circumstances the physiologic systems activated by stress (the allostatic systems) can damage the body.[81] Allostatic systems enable people to respond to changing physical states and to cope with ambient stressors such as noise and crowding as well as extremes of temperature, hunger, danger, or infection. As Bruce McEwen[82] notes, the body's response to a stress-inducing challenge is twofold: turning on an allostatic response that introduces a complex cascade of stress hormones into the body and then shutting off this response when the threat has receded. When the allostatic system is not completely deactivated, however, the body experiences overexposure to stress hormones. Long periods of overexposure result in "allostatic load," which can cause wear and tear on the cardiovascular, metabolic, and immune systems.

Allostatic load may result from exposure to a series of acute stressors (e.g., job loss, eviction, or the death of a loved one) or from long-term exposure to chronic stress (e.g., that associated with social stigma or persistent economic adversity). Black residents of high-poverty urban areas are subjected to environmental and psychosocial stressors, both acute and chronic, beginning in utero. As they move through young and middle adulthood, urban African Americans suffer many health-harmful burdens that persist, accumulate, and interact with one another to exacerbate weathering and increase allostatic load. Examples include persistent material hardship; repeated exposure to environmental hazards and ambient or social stressors in residential and work environments; high psychosocial stress and high-effort coping that increase in young to middle adulthood as family leadership roles are assumed and obligations expand and compete; pressure to adopt unhealthy behaviors as a means to cope with growing stress, uncertainty, or persistent material hardship; early development of chronic conditions and the practical, financial, and emotional difficulties associated with these; lack of medical services or differential treatment by health care providers; and feelings of stigma, frustration, or anger at racial injustice.

Over the life course, weathering and allostatic load can cause the allostatic systems to wear out or become exhausted, leading to cardiovascular disease, obesity, diabetes, increased susceptibility to infection, and accelerated aging. African Americans suffer from these stress-related conditions at greater rates, at earlier ages, and with a higher probability of early death than do whites. They are prominent contributors to racial health inequality.

Individuals can make changes in their lives to mitigate weathering and reduce allostatic load, but only to a small degree. The weathering model suggests that behaviors such as smoking, poor diet, and sedentary lifestyle may be secondary to the constraints or stresses of everyday life or may interact with allostatic load to produce adverse health outcomes. Significant changes in the social, political, and physical environments are required to substantially reduce or eliminate weathering and allostatic load in the black population.

IMPLICATIONS FOR PUBLIC POLICY

New public health and social policy discussions must embrace the dynamic relationship between population health and the needs of family economies and caregiving systems in high-poverty African American communities. Weathering and the pervasive health uncertainty it implies have local social consequences as they enlarge the scope of caregiving needs while simultaneously depleting the pool of caregivers and economic providers. Analysts' casual disregard of the responsiveness of such local institutions as kin networks and their critical function in promoting health and well-being creates racial barriers between public health professionals and those with indigenous knowledge.

Policies that are likely to fragment or impose new obligations on already overburdened networks, that disregard the local cadence of life-course demands or norms of care across and within generations, or that rely on or legitimize demeaning stereotypes will increase allostatic load for the urban poor and, ultimately, further imperil their health.[59] Policies that are informed by uncritical acceptance of developmentalism, economism, and the American creed are likely to have such impacts. In this section, we show that the policy discourse concerning black health outcomes is steeped in dominant ideological perspectives that valorize existing social inequalities and undermine recognition of social and cultural strengths in black communities.

The government's insistence on the value of low-paying work, regardless of social context, is an example of the harmful effects of these racialized ideologies on black communities. Policymakers tend to perceive unemployed young and middle-aged adults as socially atomized individuals rather than active participants in family economies and caregiving systems strained by persistent poverty and pervasive health uncertainty. Whether unemployment is viewed as malingering or as resulting from labor-market discrimination, the perceived remedies revolve around getting the unemployed working, with little concern for ripple effects through kin networks or the impact of increased stress on the health of these "working-age" adults.

According to our analysis, low rates of labor force participation in high-poverty, urban, African American communities represent a combination of structural barriers to employment,[83] high rates of health-induced disability,[84] and collective strategies for seeing to the considerable caregiving needs of multigenerational kin networks.[41, 58, 85, 86] In the context of black communities, where death and infirmity are erratically scattered across the life span, men and women cannot easily maintain secure positions in the work force. Bound, Schoenbaum, and Waidmann[84] found that health differences between blacks and whites can account for most of the racial gap in labor force attachment for men. They found that black women would be substantially *more* likely to work than white women were it not for the marked health differences. In subsequent work, Bound et al.[87] document that working people with health limitations typically earn between 20 percent and 40 percent less than people without such limitations. Finally, they found that health disparities can account for a significant part of the higher participation rates in public assistance programs among blacks (and Native Americans) relative to whites.

Additionally, practical challenges for members of family or social networks who care for the disabled can undermine their efforts to fulfill competing obligations to family and work. In these circumstances, multigenerational families may divide kin network responsibilities among young and middle-aged adults so that some contribute economically by participating in the work force, whereas others focus their energies on the caregiving and other domestic needs of the extended family.[41]

Indeed, a pervasive theme in recent research on welfare reform is that most recipients of welfare assistance share the dominant cultural belief in the dignity of paid work but that the jobs available to them both fail to improve their economic situation and put great strains on their ability to fulfill responsibilities for their extended families.[88]

A general conclusion of recent research is that welfare policy requiring poor people to get paid jobs does little to ease poverty. Meanwhile, Sharon Hicks-Bartlett[38] shows that African Americans in poor communities are so interdependent that when one person gets full-time employment, a cascade of social problems for others may be set in motion. Katherine Newman[89] observes that, given the general level of poverty in Harlem, it is hard for those not on welfare to hold jobs or go to school unless some family members stay on the welfare rolls. Ariel Kalil and her colleagues[90] describe how requiring young black mothers to take paying jobs puts new strains on their relationships with family members and the fathers of their children, consistent with findings of earlier researchers.[39, 41, 85, 91–93]

Another example is the policy pressure for marital childbearing, which is the logical extension of developmentalism and its ties to the nuclear family ideal. Through these lenses, policy advocates see unmarried mothers as lone mothers rather than as participants in kin networks. They focus on policy remedies that encourage marital childbearing or at least paternity support, unaware that such remedies are meager at best or that they undermine complex systems for caregiving and economic provision worked out through kin networks, not nuclear families. Even some who recognize the functional, economic importance of kin network participation often interpret tight social networks as ones that restrain people in poor African American communities. They selectively highlight Carol Stack's[39] original observation that participation in these networks can make it hard for individuals or married couples to make and save money or get ahead financially as nuclear households. Overshadowed by the concern over nonmarital childbearing, the importance to health and well-being of caregiving, risk pooling, or the transmission of shared values is missed. Few people in positions to inform or make public policy see these positive contributions of black norms and social bonds.

Yet Tom DeLeire and Ariel Kalil[94] found critical exceptions to the shibboleth that children raised in married families fare better than others do. Although teens in single-parent, divorced, widowed, and stepfamilies were disadvantaged, teens with divorced mothers in multigenerational families fared no differently from those in married families. Moreover, youth living with their never-married mothers in multigenerational households—most often black teens whose young mothers had low education and income—had social and academic outcomes that were *better* than those in married families. These positive child outcomes are consistent with our thesis that nonmarital childbearing as part of an extended kin network is adaptive in this population.

A third example is fertility timing. Public policy to prevent teen childbearing was both prompted and legitimated by ideas embedded in racialized perspectives of developmentalism and economism. Through the prism of developmentalism, teen mothers are perceived to be lone and immature adolescents rather than young adult members of multigenerational kin networks. They are judged as individuals who made wrong choices with grave personal and social consequences. An additional presumption is that simply postponing childbirth until they are past their teen years would allow them to be better mothers and to accumulate sufficient "human capital" to be successful in the labor market. Although its scientific basis is open to question, this view has gathered great political momentum. It has served as a basis for important policies, including key aspects of national welfare policy.[86]

Despite dramatic reductions in U.S. rates of teen childbearing over the past fifty years, teen childbearing continues to occur disproportionately among low-income African Americans. Indeed, in such high-poverty, urban, African American populations as Detroit, Watts, or Chicago's South Side, the modal age for first childbirth is in the teenage years.[60] According to our analysis, this is because early fertility remains in sync with the needs of local family economies and caregiving systems in high-poverty black communities. Weathering challenges, even threatens, family economies and caregiving systems as it increases the probability of widowhood or orphanhood and prolonged disability.[95] These risks and their adverse effects are reduced when child-bearing occurs early and child rearing is seen as the obligation of a multigenerational kin network rather than of a biological nuclear family.

Children may fare best if their birth and preschool years coincide with their mother's peak health and access to social and practical support provided by relatively healthy kin. This period occurs at a younger age for African American than for white women. In fact, 1990 infant mortality rates for teen mothers in Harlem were *half* those for older mothers, even though the preponderance of "older" first-time mothers in Harlem were only in their twenties.[1] Nor do empirical findings related to child development and school achievement provide consistent endorsement for the political viewpoint that teen childbearing harms children. Moore et al.,[96] for example, found that in their national sample of four- to fourteen-year-olds, black children whose mothers were eighteen or nineteen at their birth performed better in reading and math than those whose mothers were in their early twenties. Geronimus, Korenman, and Hillemeier[97] studied the performance of preschool and elementary school age children of a national sample of sisters who experienced their first births at different ages. They found evidence that children of teenage mothers in high-poverty black populations fare as well as or better than children of older mothers on standard measures of socioemotional development, cognitive development, and school performance. Although these findings on infant health and child development are consistent with others in a methodologically diverse literature that spans two decades,[98–106] few in the broader public seem aware of them, nor have such findings informed interventions to reduce the black-white gap in infant mortality or to improve the school performance or well-being of urban black children.[60] In contrast to the dominant view, qualitative evidence from ethnographies and in-depth interviews suggests that African American residents of high-poverty urban areas have socially situated knowledge of the benefits to child and family health and well-being of early childbearing, child rearing in multigenerational families, and parental respite from the labor force[10, 38, 39, 41, 88, 107] The mismatch between indigenous and authoritative knowledge has made low-income African Americans appear lazy, unable to take personal responsibility, and impervious to sex education and family planning measures, as their rates of unemployment and nonmarital or teen childbearing continue to be what the larger public views as alarming. This alarmist interpretation has fueled public contempt for teen or nonmarital childbearing, including resentment of teen mothers, new theories that question the morality of residents of urban black communities, and new, more punitive ideas about how to solve the "problem that hasn't gone away."

Following developmentalist logic, policymakers discredit black elders in high-poverty urban communities as good parents because of their seeming failure at their supervisory function. Policymakers feel entitled to act in loco parentis to entire communities, in effect discrediting adults in these communities while meting out paternalistic and punitive policies aimed to encourage urban youth to toe the line. The dominant reaction against unmarried parents, teenage mothers, or the unemployed has introduced new and highly publicized sources of stigma for young parents, their children, and their elders.

Such stigma can contribute to weathering. The resulting policies and programs effect perturbations in their protective networks, with the potential to inflict further health harm on African Americans. This developmentalist consensus has been effectively used to undercut support for social safety nets and other antipoverty programs.[108] The Family Support Act of 1988 and the 1996 Personal Responsibility and Work Opportunity Reconciliation Act (PRWORA) placed barriers, even barricades, in the way of urban teen mothers who hoped to pursue educational or career opportunities. Bush administration proposals to reauthorize PRWORA's time limits, while increasing the number of hours mothers on welfare are required to work and expending resources on promarriage policies and increased abstinence programs, would exacerbate this trend in the wrong direction. But these approaches are the logical results of uncritical acceptance of developmentalism, economism, and the creed.

Our analysis also has implications for policy interventions that are perceived as "structural." So-called structural interventions usually do not challenge the boundaries of larger political-economic-spatial structures, and they tend to ignore fundamental issues of racial identity and black marginalization. One example is the focus of many progressives on increasing the minimum wage. Arguments for and against increasing the minimum wage are usually debated in social management terms. The main dispute in the scholarly economic literature is whether increasing the minimum wage would reduce poverty and encourage workers to enter the market or whether it would inadvertently increase unemployment among the very groups it intends to help.[109, 110] This debate is technical and inconclusive. What is of interest here are the contours of the debate. It is framed in the economistic and utilitarian terms of whether raising the minimum wage would help more people than it harms *in terms of income*.[111] The debate over the minimum wage, however, is just as much a collective moral and political debate over the kind of society that the United States should be. That is, should employment policy be guided by an overarching goal of achieving a more economically and racially equal society? Is it morally and socially acceptable if most blacks are not trained to occupy high-end service jobs and blacks' labor is allowed to become obsolete in the face of globalization? The prevalent economistic orientation of most structuralist approaches leaves them unable to address the bedrock issue of whites' lack of emotional attachment to blacks. Being a racial minority in a racially hostile majoritarian democracy, blacks are left without political safeguards in the midst of a potentially devastating economic transformation.

Another example is the widespread perception that universal health insurance will go a long way toward eliminating health disparities. Leading political advocates still portray universal health insurance as a rallying cry for all uninsured persons.[112] Blacks are more skeptical as health insurance proposals for the most part do not address fundamental health problems in black communities that are connected to racial subordination. Leading proposals for universal health insurance continue to ration health care according to ability to pay, thus providing incentives to health practitioners and insurers to discriminate against low-income blacks.[113] Moreover, few health care providers locate their practices in central cities. In fact, Fossett and Perloff et al.[114, 115] suggest that access to care in high-poverty urban areas is constrained more by the lack of accessible physicians than by the lack of insurance. Thus, although white policy advocates view universal health insurance proposals as a call for major structural change, for blacks they represent a minimum ameliorative policy that leaves basic structures of racial subordination intact.

Another example is the call for housing vouchers and other programs that enable some African Americans to move out of urban ghettos. The premise underlying such programs is that if individual black families are freed of the environmental hazards, ambient stressors, and social and economic constraints imposed by life in racially segregated ghettos, they will find more opportunities to invest in their human capital, find jobs, and avoid stress. Several researchers have examined the relationship between residential segregation and health outcomes and found evidence that segregation is a factor above and beyond the effects of poverty or individual demographic characteristics.[116–118] Among African Americans, segregation is also positively associated with increased rates of all-cause mortality,[119, 120] chronic conditions such as cardiovascular disease,[121] and infectious diseases such as tuberculosis.[122] Current efforts to move ghetto residents into more affluent areas are small and politically fragile, however, as discussed in other chapters in this volume (see Chapters Four and Seven).

All of these examples imply that understanding what factors shape public sentiment on race and how they might be influenced are critical public health and social policy objectives. Embedded racial biases reinforce the urban ghettoization that limits access to municipal services, health care, healthy environments, and educational and employment opportunities.[123–125] They support discriminatory hiring practices[83] and reduce the availability of welfare and other social insurance benefits.[126] Racialized ideologies not only affect clinical judgments to the detriment of black patients[127, 128] and fuel black distrust of health care professionals and public health initiatives[129, 130] but also weaken public support for initiatives to improve the health of poor black (and other minority) populations by framing their problems as self-inflicted. This view leaves unexamined industries' willingness to target marginal communities for environmental hazards or unhealthy consumer products,[131–134] and it creates a mismatch between dominant cultural expectations for acting "responsibly" and family or local community needs.[60, 86] These conditions induce race-related stress that causes wear and tear on the cardiovascular, metabolic, and immune systems, fueling the development or progression of disease. Without neutralizing pervasive racial prejudices embedded in dominant ideologies, sustaining health-enhancing political successes will be difficult, and the biological potential of African Americans to lead long healthy lives will continue to be subverted.

BUILDING A MOVEMENT FOR POLICY REFORM

We agree with analysts who argue that a broad social movement is needed to enact significant health reforms.[135] It is far from clear how to construct such a movement, however.[136] No doubt, numerous scholars will disagree with our support for considerations of racial difference. One familiar critique has been that emphasizing racial (and other) differences leads to divisive and counterproductive identity movements.[137] Critics have argued that movements for community empowerment and demands for the recognition of racial difference are largely discursive and that they have displaced a focus on structural economic inequalities that are at the heart of problems in marginalized communities.

These critics seem discomforted and frustrated by advocacy for greater community empowerment and racial representation. Such advocacy is, indeed, often polarizing, and it may divert attention and resources away from efforts to unify movements of low-income groups against powerful economic and political elites. However, these critiques seem to ignore the seriousness of problems motivating black and other identity advocates in the first place. Black advocates argue that white-led organizations—such as the Democratic Party and labor unions—continue to promote policies that, however salutary for whites, seem unjust and of marginal benefit for blacks, Latinos, and others.

Critics of identity movements make the economistic assumption that poor whites and blacks share common grievances that white leaders of broad-based organizations understand and capably represent. Black struggles, however, are only partially about class issues and are not just a misdirected expression of class grievances. The essence of blacks' race struggle is not against white elites; it is directed against the racism—intentional or institutional—that nonelite and elite whites share.[138] A proper analogy to today's race relations between blacks and whites is not the relationship between slave and slave owner or laborer and employer; it is more like the relationship between an overburdened and angry wife and an abusive and cheating husband. Just as conservative cries for women to strengthen families by rallying behind their husbands seem counterproductive to abused spouses, calls from politicians for a "dampening of sentiments based on group identity"[137] are likely to seem self-serving and undermining to blacks and other marginalized groups. As women's advocates do not place much confidence in movements for family unity that do not address spouse abuse, black advocates are intensely resistant to movements that emphasize moderation in racial advocacy for the sake of cross-racial unity.

Black activists have long recognized the potential benefits of solidarity with non-elite whites and the limits to blacks' capacity to address major social problems on their own. This is why black advocates bother to engage in racial criticism rather than turn entirely inward. Yet interracial solidarity is only a potential, and a long-awaited one at that. Whites' willingness to accommodate racial difference signals a stronger commitment to building interracial solidarity than appeals for blacks to join interracial coalitions based on short-term economic interests. Black advocates have long and unsuccessfully appealed to whites to acknowledge and legitimize struggle against racial subordination rather than merely asking blacks to join what are essentially white-inter-est-based, interracial, economic coalitions. The surest means of reducing divisiveness within movements is to provide marginalized groups with a sense that their well-being is safeguarded by other groups.[139]

The Politics of Building Solidarity

The American creed, we have argued, is based on belief in the essential fairness of cur-rent economic and political arrangements in American society. The creed relegates black experiences, demands, and criticisms to the periphery of politics and actually cultivates racial prejudice by blaming black poverty on a lack of personal responsibil-ity. Although American pluralism is tolerant of diversity in certain private moralities such as religious faith, it is fundamentalist with regard to the basic legitimacy of politi-cal and economic structures. For example, many blacks have argued to no avail that the definition and enforcement of inheritance laws and property rights have legiti-mized ill-gotten wealth from slavery and Jim Crow, while simultaneously perpetuating a false explanation for black economic inequality.[140] Blacks' formal right of dissent has little practical value in challenging such government-, corporate-, and mass media–backed social structures. The economistic view undergirds this kind of shallow pluralism, in which individuals and groups compete for audiences and resources within the context of unquestioned government rules and affirmative ontological boundaries. Economism discourages reforming these rules and boundaries, and in so doing, it reduces interracial trust and the potential for cross-racial political solidarity.

Just as alternative explanations for black health problems are precluded in dominant research paradigms and just as alternative perspectives on American society are margin-alized by belief in the American dream, alternatives for building a movement around public health issues are possible. Rather than accepting rules governing participation and struggling for a redistribution of goods and services within these limits, an alterna-tive is to build a movement for democracy that contests the boundaries of political debate and the rules determining which groups get to participate in the political arena.

A political argument for accepting the procedural status quo is that there is little broad political support for revamping existing rules governing political participation and rethinking conventional policy paradigms, particularly within the white middle class. Radical demands attract narrow political constituencies, and even if they are intensely mobilized, such movements have little hope of passing legislation. Black health advocates are, therefore, encouraged to tailor their demands to what is accept-able to the white middle class and to reforms that will be taken seriously. This kind of pragmatic realism is politically shortsighted. It has produced ineffective policy and maintained racial tensions in the ghetto, handled by an ever-expanding criminal justice system. Framing health problems within the boundaries of traditional political and policy discourse is likely to lose the mobilizing energies of black activists. In addition, a victory using such an approach will likely leave blacks' particularly severe community health problems unaddressed.

Bringing about fundamental policy reform requires imagining (within the realm of the possible) a movement for democracy that is both broadly appealing *and* intense. We will approach this task in two steps. First, we will discuss what it means to challenge the everyday understanding of black poverty and community participation so that more whites may come to believe that there are valid reasons for sharp racial dissent within society. We think this is an important step both in reducing white resentment of black criticism and in redefining the social problems that government must solve. Then we will propose changing the rules governing electoral participation as a possible approach for a democracy-oriented movement for health reform.

A key aspect of racial difference is that blacks tend to have a much broader view of the legitimate bounds of political reform than whites do. Blacks see their health problems as rooted in the economy, in racial segregation, in a racist political culture, and in black political powerlessness. From this point of view, healthy black communities would require fundamentally restructured housing and environmental conditions, good jobs, political reform, and preceding all of this, major changes in racial discourse.

Although the black perspective poses strategies and demands that are far removed from mainstream white opinion, there are political advantages to taking such a broad view. One is that it is highly motivating for many blacks; it connects with their sense of justice, history, and deeply felt aspirations in a way that a narrow economistic framing of black health problems does not. It also brings the power of intense protest, a power that, for example, the Clinton health initiative sorely lacked. Protest is a part of deepening pluralism—making it more inclusive of marginalized groups. Despite the discomfort it may cause, it encourages social learning and moral repositioning by groups unfamiliar with radically different perspectives on U.S. history and public policies. In so doing, it opens up political space for broader reform. Such space is desperately needed.

We believe that a logical and promising strategy for building a movement for progressive health reform would be to change the rules governing political participation to include groups likely to support radical health reforms. For example, both immigrants and citizen slum dwellers are frequently discounted in political calculations because most immigrants cannot vote and many slum dwellers are former felons who also cannot vote. Because immigrants tend to be poor and live in neighborhoods with native poor people, these areas lose voting power in relation to wealthy areas having fewer immigrants. In short, immigrant disenfranchisement weakens the capacity of the native-born poor to secure support for their schools and neighborhoods in state and local budget contests. The immigrant vote could aid low-income citizens in poor communities to win funding needed for health and social services. Although enfranchising immigrants may seem like an impossibility in the present political climate, it may become more attractive as their numbers continue to swell and as municipal leaders consider the implications of having huge numbers of poor city residents with no representation in the political process.

A second means of expanding suffrage would be to extend the vote to ex-felons. An estimated 3.9 million formerly incarcerated U.S. citizens are disfranchised, including 1 million who have fully completed their sentences. The large scale of felony disfranchisement among the black population is mainly the result of state drug laws and harsh sentencing policies that have been disproportionately imposed on blacks. About 1.4 million African American men are disfranchised. In Alabama and Florida, more than 30 percent of African American men are permanently disfranchised. In Mississippi and Virginia, one in four black men is permanently disfranchised.[141]

This restricted franchise implies that democracy is a privilege awarded to noble citizens who respect moderation and consensus. Ironically, this view of democracy excludes those who need the power of representation the most, and it disarms democracy as a means of ameliorating potentially explosive social conflicts. If not through political participation, how will excluded groups identify themselves or be identified as part of their communities? This question becomes pointed and poignant when applied to specific health problems, such as HIV/AIDS, that are increasingly concentrated[125] among those excluded from political participation. How can communities work cooperatively with ex-felons and immigrants to generate greater awareness and public support for combating HIV/AIDS when they cannot participate in local politics? History has shown that extending voting rights to blacks, for example, was crucial for strengthening other movements of marginalized groups, as well as the responsiveness of political structures to poverty and discrimination. Adopting progressive social policies to eliminate the political exclusion of immigrant noncitizen taxpayers and ex-felons could have similarly beneficial impacts today.

Working within the constraints of the American creed has fueled intolerance between these mainstream and marginalized groups. Black demands are increasingly viewed as unjust to many low-income and middle-class whites, for example.[142] How did that happen? When black civil rights advocates moved from demands affecting southern whites to demands affecting northern white liberals, such as school desegregation and full employment, they lost much of their white liberal support. Rather than engage in contentious political argument with their liberal white allies, frustrated civil rights groups and black political leaders settled for partial concessions, such as affirmative action, as a pragmatic accommodation to white mainstream opinion.[143] Because these programs provided limited help for the black poor, however, black organizations lost much of their black grassroots support, intensity, and mobilization capacity. In their weakened state, black civil rights advocates were unable to successfully challenge the conservative movement that attacked even minimal affirmative action programs as discriminatory against whites. As a consequence, black leaders today are faced with a demobilized black public still saddled with the problems of slums and a more hostile white public. Their defense of even the minimal compensatory reforms they settled for in the past are now denounced by some white liberals as divisive and morally repugnant.

By agreeing to a shallow pluralist approach rather than sticking with their broadly framed, more contentious agenda, black advocates now find themselves in a much weaker position.[76]

After decades of avoiding the central problem of ideological and political disputes over the nature of black poverty in favor of narrowly framed ameliorative programs, we have seen some clear results in public health. Dramatic improvements in black health outcomes that became evident during the late 1960s[144] are now stalled. The absence of vigorous contestation of the defamation of black ghetto communities has resulted in increasing vilification, making even ameliorative interventions stingier.

We have argued that public health failures to date stem, in part, from ideologically driven and poorly informed policy discussion about the lives of the African American poor. Given the context in which they find themselves, to accept the values or roles of economistic individuals would be self-defeating for many African Americans. The rub is that, increasingly, public policy is uncharitable to those who do not accept economistic values or roles. This creates a disconnect between larger societal expectations, policies, programs, or laws on the one hand and family or local community needs on the other. This disconnect feeds health-threatening stigmas against urban African Americans and intensifies their material hardship by leading to policies, programs, and laws that undermine the work of social and kin networks. As we have shown, these approaches leave poor black urbanites with fewer resources to meet increasing needs while also undermining their efforts to provide social support, identity affirmation, or pool economic risk to avert the worst consequences of material hardship.[42, 59, 145] All of this has the potential to increase allostatic load and exacerbate weathering, leading to chronic or infectious disease, comorbidity, and death.

With a fundamentally new type of policy discussion, not only within the public health community but also within the broader social welfare and antipoverty policy communities, we can lift the veil over taken-for-granted cultural processes that shape policies and programs in ways that harm African Americans.[146] Without a new type of policy discussion that questions rules of exclusion and raises unpopular racial criticisms, we have little hope of generating the power, intensity, or deep interracial solidarity needed to produce fundamental health reform.

Thus, black health analysts and advocates today confront a choice similar to that faced by black social advocates in the mid- to late-twentieth century. Should they pursue an incremental, shallowly pluralist approach that will be more popular and more easily winnable within the confines of existing white middle-class opinion? Or should they encourage substantive reform and intense political and policy debate, engaging in the risky work on the edges of our weakly pluralist democracy?

SUMMARY

In this chapter, we show that prevailing ideological viewpoints on black health misinterpret black behavior, and that dominant racial ideologies themselves have negative health effects on African American communities. Second, we show that public policies and practices reflecting prevailing ideological viewpoints harm African American communities. Together, these ideologies and policies undermine black health by adversely affecting the immune, metabolic, and cardiovascular systems, fueling the development or progression of infectious and chronic diseases. Third, we argue that health reform pursued within the same prevailing ideological viewpoints that misinterpret black health problems have limited effectiveness. We argue for culturally appropriate public policies that value African American social perspectives and coping mechanisms. We suggest that substantive health reform is best pursued through a democratic movement that challenges dominant ideological commitments.

DISCUSSION QUESTIONS

1. What are some of the reasons that black adults have higher mortality rates than whites?

2. Define the three racialized ideologies that the authors describe: developmentalism, economism, and the American creed. Explain how these ideologies influence the risk of specific diseases and health conditions.

3. What does the concept of "weathering" refer to as it affects the health of African Americans? How does it affect individual health and intergenerational susceptibility to poor health?

4. What are the implications of weathering for the development of health-promoting public policies? What kinds of policy interventions might reduce weathering?

ACKNOWLEDGMENTS

The authors gratefully acknowledge financial support from the Robert Wood Johnson Foundation through an Investigator in Health Policy Research Award to Dr. Geronimus. We are also indebted to Sylvia Tesh, Sherman James, Martin Rein, Rachel Snow, Alice Furomoto-Dawson, Dayna Cunningham, and John Bound for helpful discussions and comments on previous drafts; to Meghen Fennelly for research assistance; and to N. E. Barr and Diane Laviolette for help with the preparation of the manuscript. The views expressed are our own.

NOTES

1. Geronimus, A. T. Understanding and eliminating racial inequalities in women's health in the United States: The role of the weathering conceptual framework. *Journal of American Medical Women's Association,* 56, no. 4 (2001): 133–136.

2. Geronimus, A. T., Bound, J., Waidmann, T. A., Colen, C. G., and Steffick, D. Inequality in life expectancy, functional status, and active life expectancy across selected black and white populations in the United States. *Demography*, 38, no. 2 (2001): 227–251.

3. Geronimus, A. T., Bound, J., Waidmann, T. A., Hillemeier, M. M., and Burns, P. B. Excess mortality among blacks and whites in the United States. *N Engl J Med*, 335 (1996): 1552–1558.

4. Geronimus, A. T., Bound, J., and Waidmann, T. A. Poverty, time and place: Variation in excess mortality across selected U.S. populations, 1980–1990. *J Epidemiol Community Health*, 53, no. 6 (1999): 325–334.

5. Adler, N. E., Boyce, W. T., Chesney, M. A., Folkman, S., and Syme, S. L. Socioeconomic inequalities in health: No easy solution. *JAMA*, 269 (2003): 3140–3145.

6. Elo, I. T., and Preston, S. H. Educational differentials in mortality: United States, 1979–85. *Soc Sci Med*, 42 (1996): 47–57.

7. Geronimus, A. T. The weathering hypothesis and the health of African American women and infants: Implications for reproductive strategies and policy analysis. In G. Sen and R. C. Snow, eds., *Power and Decision: The Social Control of Reproduction*, pp. 77–100. Cambridge, Mass.: Harvard University Press, 1994.

8. Geronimus, A. T., and Bound, J. Black/white differences in women's health status: Evidence from vital statistics. *Demography*, 27, no. 3 (1990): 457–466.

9. House, J., Kessler, R., Herzog, R., Mero, R., Kinney, A., and Breslow, M. Age, socioeconomic status, and health. *Milbank Q*, 68 (1990): 383–411.

10. Geronimus, A. T. Black/white differences in the relationship of maternal age to birthweight: A population based test of the weathering hypothesis. *Soc Sci Med*, 42, no. 4 (1996): 589–597.

11. Pappas, G., Queen, S., Hadden, W., and Fisher, G. The increasing disparity in mortality between socioeconomic groups in the United States, 1960 and 1986. *N Engl J Med*, 329 (1993): 103–109.

12. Ryan, W. *Blaming the Victim*. New York: Pantheon Books, 1971.

13. Gusfield, J. R. The Culture of Public Problems: Drinking-Driving and the Symbolic Order. Chicago: University of Chicago Press, 1981.

14. Gusfield, J. R. The control of drinking-driving in the United States: A period of transition? In M. Laurence, J. R. Snortum, and F. E. Zimring, eds., *Social Control of the Drinking Driver*, pp. 109–135. Chicago: University of Chicago Press, 1988.

15. Bookchin, M. *The Philosophy of Social Ecology: Essays on Dialectical Naturalism*. New York: Black Rose Books, 1990.

16. Bookchin, M. *Our Synthetic Environment,* rev. ed. New York: Harper & Row, 1974.

17. Fitchen, J. M., Heath, J. S., and Fessenden-Raden, J. Risk perception in community context. In B. B. Johnson and V. T. Covello, eds., *The Social and Cultural Construction of Risk: Essays on Risk Selection and Perception,* pp. 31–54. Dordrecht, The Netherlands: Reidel, 1987.

18. Crawford, R. You are dangerous to your health: The ideology and politics of victim blaming. *International Journal of Health Services,* 7 (1977): 663–680.

19. Rose, N. E. Scapegoating poor women: An analysis of welfare reform. *Journal of Economic Issues,* 34, no. 1 (2000): 143–159.

20. Tesh, S. N. *Hidden Arguments.* New Brunswick, N.J.: Rutgers University Press, 1988.

21. Link, B. G., and Phelan, J. C. Social conditions as fundamental causes of disease. *Journal of Health and Social Behaviors,* 36 (1995): 80–94.

22. Link, B. G., and Phelan, J. C. Understanding sociodemographic differences in health: The role of fundamental social causes. *American Journal of Public Health,* 86 (1996): 471–473.

23. Saegert, S. C., Klitzman, S., Freudenberg, N., Cooperman-Mroczek, J., and Nassar, S. Healthy housing: A structured review of published evaluations of U. S. interventions to improve health by modifying housing in the United States, 1990–2001. *American Journal of Public Health,* 93, no. 9 (2002): 1471.

24. Berzonsky, M. D. Theories of adolescent development. In G. Adams, ed., *Adolescent Development: The Essential Readings,* pp. 7–8. Oxford: Blackwell, 2000.

25. Muuss, R. E. Friendship patterns and peer group influences: An ecological perspective based on Bronfenbrenner, Kandel, and Dunphy. In R. E. Muuss, ed., *Theories of Adolescence,* 5th ed., pp. 300–319. New York: McGraw-Hill, 1988.

26. Muuss, R. E. *Theories of Adolescence,* 6th ed. New York: McGraw-Hill, 1996.

27. Patterson, S. J., Sochting, I., and Marcia, J. E. The inner space and beyond: Women and identity. In G. R. Adams, T. P. Gullotta, and R. Montemayor, eds., *Adolescent Identity Formation,* pp. 9–24. Newbury Park, Cal.: Sage, 1992.

28. Steinberg, L. *Adolescence,* 3rd ed. New York: McGraw-Hill, 1993.

29. Burt, M. R. Reasons to invest in adolescents. *Journal of Adolescent Health,* 31 (2002): 136–152.

30. Brown, J. D., and Witherspoon, E. M. The mass media and American adolescents' health. *Journal of Adolescent Health,* 31 (2002): 153–170.

31. Furstenberg, F. F. The sociology of adolescence and youth in the 1990s: A critical commentary. *Journal of Marriage & Family,* 62, no. 4 (2000): 896–910.

32. Hayward, M. D., and Heron, M. Racial inequality in active life among adult Americans. *Demography,* 36, no. 1 (1999): 77–91.

33. Rowe, J. W., and Kahn, R. L. *Successful Aging.* New York: Pantheon Books, 1998.

34. Goodwin, J., and Emirbayer, M. Network analysis, culture, and the problem of agency. *American Journal of Sociology,* 99, no. 6 (1994): 1411–1454.

35. Katz, M. B. Reframing the "underclass debate." In M. B. Katz, ed., *The "Underclass Debate": Views from History.* Princeton, N.J.: Princeton University Press, 1993.

36. Rein, M. Dominance, contest, and reframing. In A. Ben-Arieh and J. Gal, eds. *Into the Promised Land? Issues Facing the Welfare State,* pp. 213–238. Westport, Conn.: Praeger, 2000.

37. Dahl, R. A. *Who Governs: Democracy and Power in an American City,* p. 317. New Haven, Conn.: Yale University Press, 1961.

38. Hicks-Bartlett, S. Between a rock and a hard place: The labyrinth of working and parenting in a poor community. In S. Danizer and A. C. Lin, eds. *Coping with Poverty: The Social Contexts of Neighborhood, Work and Family in the African-American Community,* pp. 27–51. Ann Arbor: University of Michigan Press, 2000.

39. Stack, C. B. *All Our Kin.* New York: Harper & Row, 1974.

40. Stack, C. B. *Call to Home.* New York: Basic Books, 1996.

41. Stack, C. B., and Burton, L. M. Kinscripts. *Journal of Comparative Family Studies,* 24 (1993): 157.

42. Ward, J. V. *The Skin We're In.* New York: The Free Press, 2000.

43. James, S. Racial and ethnic differences in infant mortality and low birth weight: A psychosocial critique. *Annals of Epidemiology,* 3 (1993): 130–136.

44. Guendelman, S. Health and disease among Hispanics. In S. Loue, ed., *Handbook of Immigrant Health,* pp. 277–301. New York: Plenum Press, 1998.

45. Guendelman, S., Gould, J. B., Hudes, M., and Eskenazi, B. Generational differences in perinatal health among the Mexican-American population: Findings from HHANES 1982–84. *American Journal of Public Health,* 80, Suppl (1990): 61–65.

46. Landale, N. S., Oropesa, R. S., Llanes, D., and Gorman, B. Does Americanization have adverse effects on health? Stress, health habits, and infant health outcomes among Puerto Ricans. *Social Forces,* 78, no. 2 (1999): 613.

47. Rumbaut, R., and Weeks, J. Unraveling a public health enigma: Why do immigrants experience superior perinatal health outcomes? *Research in the Sociology of Health Care,* 13 (1996): 335–388.

48. Sundquist, J., and Winkleby, M. A. Addictive substances, including tobacco—cardiovascular risk factors in Mexican American adults: A transcultural analysis of NHANES III, 1988–1994. *American Journal of Public Health,* 89, no. 5 (1999): 723.

49. Stern, M., and Wei, M. Do Mexican Americans really have low rates of cardiovascular disease? *American Journal of Preventative Medicine,* 29, no. 6 (1999): S9.

50. James, S., Schultz, A. J., and van Olphen, J. Social capital, poverty, and community health: An exploration of linkages. In S. Saegert, J. P. Thompson, and M. R. Warren, eds., *Social Capital and Poor Communities,* pp. 165–188. New York: Russell Sage Foundation, 2001.

51. Williams, D. Race, socioeconomic status, and health: The added effects of racism and discrimination. *Annals of the New York Academy of Sciences,* 896 (1999): 173–188.

52. Jones, C. P. Levels of racism: A theoretic framework and a gardener's tale. *American Journal of Public Health,* 90, no. 8 (2000): 1212–1215.

53. Dressler, W. W. Modeling biocultural interactions: Examples from studies of stress and cardiovascular disease. *Yearbook of Physical Anthropology,* 38 (1995): 27–56.

54. Dressler, W. W. Hypertension in the African American community: Social, cultural, and psychological factors. *Seminars in Nephrology,* 16, no. 2 (1996): 71–82.

55. Dressler, W. W. Modernization, stress, and blood pressure: New directions in research. *Human Biology,* 71, no. 4 (1999): 583–605.

56. Scribner, R., and Dwyer, J. H. Acculturation and low birthweight among Latinos in the Hispanic HANES. *American Journal of Public Health,* 79 (1980): 1263–1267.

57. Lamont, M. Colliding moralities between black and white workers. In E. Long, ed., *Sociology to Cultural Studies,* pp. 263–285. New York: Blackwell Press, 1997.

58. Geronimus, A. T. On teenage childbearing and neonatal mortality in the United States. *Population and Development Review,* 13, no. 2 (1987): 245–279.

59. Geronimus, A. T. To mitigate, resist, or undo: Addressing structural influences on the health of urban populations. *American Journal of Public Health,* 90 (2000): 867–872.

60. Geronimus, A. T. Damned if you do: Culture, identity, privilege and teenage childbearing in the United States. *Social Science & Medicine,* 57 (2003): 881–893.

61. Oakes, J., Rossi, M., and Rossi, P. H. The measurement of SES in health research: Current practice and steps toward a new approach. *Social Science & Medicine,* 56, no. 4 (2003): 769–784.

62. Bobo, L. D., and Kluegel, J. R. Perceived group discrimination and policy attitudes: The sources and consequences of the race and gender gaps. In C.T.A.

O'Connor, C. Tilly, and L. D. Bobo, eds., *Urban Inequality: Evidence from Four Cities,* pp. 163–198. New York: Russell Sage Foundation, 2001.

63. Hochschild, J. L. *Facing Up to the American Dream: Race, Class, and the Soul of the Nation.* Princeton, N.J.: Princeton University Press, 1995.

64. Kluegel, J. R., and Bobo, L. D. Status, ideology, and dimensions of whites' racial beliefs and attitudes: Progress and stagnation. In J. K. Martin and S. A. Tuch, eds., *Racial Attitudes in the 1990s: Continuity and Change,* pp. 93–120. Westport, Conn.: Praeger, 1997.

65. Dawson, M. C. *Behind the Mule: Race, Class, and African American Politics.* Princeton, N.J.: Princeton University Press, 1994.

66. Charles, C. Z. The dynamics of racial segregation. *Annual Review of Sociology,* 29 (2003): 167–207.

67. Kaufman, J. S., Cooper, R. S., and McGee, D. L. Socioeconomic status and health in blacks and whites: The problem of residual confounding and the resiliency of race. *Epidemiology,* 8 (1997): 621–628.

68. Sikes, M., and Faegin, J. *Living with Racism.* Boston: Beacon Press, 1994.

69. Kennedy, R. Racial trends in the administration of criminal justice. In N. J. Smelser, W. J. Wilson, and F. Mitchell, eds., *America Becoming: Racial Trends and Their Consequences,* Vol. 2, pp. 1–20. Washington, D.C.: National Academy Press, 2001.

70. James, S., Keenan, N., Strogatz, D., Browning, S., and Garrett, J. Socioeconomic status, John Henryism, and blood pressure in black adults: The Pitt County Study. *American Journal of Epidemiology,* 135, no. 1 (1992): 59–67.

71. Light, K., Brownley, K., Turner, J., Hinderliter, A., Girdler, S., Sherwood, A., and Anderson, N. Job status and high-effort coping influence work blood pressure in women and blacks. *Hypertension,* 25, no. 4 (1995): 554–559.

72. Williams, D., Yu, Y., Jackson, J., and Anderson, N. Racial differences in physical and mental health: Socioeconomic status, stress, and discrimination. *Journal of Health Psychology,* 2 (1997): 335–351.

73. House, J., Lepkowski, J., Kinney, A., Mero, R., Kessler, R., and Herzog, A. Social stratification of aging and health. *Journal of Health and Social Behaviors,* 35 (1994): 213–234.

74. Dawson, M. C. *Black Discontent: The Report of the 1993–1994 National Black Politics Study.* Chicago: University of Chicago Press, 1996.

75. Feagin, J. R. *Racist America: Roots, Current Realities, and Future Reparations.* New York: Routledge, 2000.

76. Hamilton, D. C., and Hamilton, C. V. *The Dual Agenda: The African American Struggle for Civil and Economic Equality.* New York: Columbia University Press, 1997.

77. Edsall, T. B., and Edsall, M. D. *Chain Reaction: The Impact of Race, Rights, and Taxes on American Politics.* New York: W. W. Norton, 1991.

78. Gilens, M. *Why Americans Hate Welfare.* Chicago: University of Chicago Press, 1999.

79. James, S. John Henryism and the health of African Americans. *Culture, Medicine and Psychiatry,* 18, no. 2 (1994): 163–182.

80. Kline, J., Stein, Z., and Susser, M. *Conception to Birth: Epidemiology of Prenatal Development.* New York: Oxford University Press, 1989.

81. Sapolsky, R. M. *Why Zebras Don't Get Ulcers: An Updated Guide to Stress, Stress Related Diseases, and Coping.* New York: W. H. Freeman, 1998.

82. McEwen, B. S. Protective and damaging effects of stress mediators. *New England Journal of Medicine,* 338 (1998): 171–179.

83. Wilson, W. J. *When Work Disappears: The World of the New Urban Poor.* New York: Knopf, 1996.

84. Bound, J., Schoenbaum, M., and Waidmann, T. A. Race differences in labor force attachment and disability status. *Gerontologist,* 36 (1996): 311–321.

85. Geronimus, A. T. Clashes of common sense: On the previous childcare experience of teenage mothers-to-be. *Hum Organ,* 51, no. 4 (1992): 318–329.

86. Geronimus, A. T. Teenage childbearing and personal responsibility: An alternative view. *Political Science Quarterly,* 112, no. 3 (1997): 405–430.

87. Bound, J., Waidmann, T., Schoenbaum, M., and Bingenheimer, J. B. The labor market consequences of race differences in health. *Milbank Quarterly,* 81 (2003): 441–474.

88. Edin, K. J. The myths of dependence and self-sufficiency: Women, welfare, and low-wage work. *Focus,* 27, no. 2 (1995): 1–9.

89. Newman, K. S. Hard times on 125th Street: Harlem's poor confront welfare reform. *Am Anthropol,* 103, no. 3 (2001): 762–778.

90. Kalil, A., et al. Mother, worker, welfare recipient: Welfare reform and the multiple roles of low-income women. In S. Danizer and A. C. Lin, eds., *Coping with Poverty: The Social Contexts of Neighborhood, Work and Family in the African-American Community,* pp. 201–223. Ann Arbor: University of Michigan Press, 2000.

91. Billingsley, A. *Climbing Jacob's Ladder: The Enduring Legacy of African American Families.* New York: Simon & Schuster, 1992.

92. McAdoo, H. P. Black mothers and the extended family support network. In L. F. Rogers-Rose, ed., *The Black Woman,* pp. 125–144. Beverly Hills, Cal.: Sage, 1980.

93. Hogan, D. P., Hao, L., and Parish, W. L. Race, kin networks, and assistance to mother-headed families. *Social Forces,* 68 (1990): 797–812.

94. DeLeire, T., and Kalil, A. Good things come in threes: Single-parent multigenerational family structure and adolescent adjustment. *Demography,* 39, no. 2 (2002): 393–413.

95. Geronimus, A. T., Bound, J., and Waidmann, T. A. Health inequality and population variation in fertility-timing. *Social Science & Medicine,* 49, no. 12 (1999): 1623–1636.

96. Moore, K., Morrison, D. R., and Greene, A. D. Effects on the children born to adolescent mothers. In R. Maynard, ed., *Kids Having Kids,* pp. 145–173. Washington, D.C.: Urban Institute Press, 1997.

97. Geronimus, A. T., Korenman, S., and Hillemeier, M. M. Does young maternal age adversely affect child development? Evidence from cousin comparisons. *Population and Development Review,* 20, no. 3 (1994): 585–609.

98. Geronimus, A. T. The effects of race, residence, and prenatal care on the relationship of maternal age to neonatal mortality. *American Journal of Public Health,* 76 (1986): 416–1421.

99. Geronimus, A. T. Weathering Chicago. *International Journal of Epidemiology,* 32, no. 1 (2003): 90–91.

100. Geronimus, A. T., and Korenman, S. Maternal youth or family background? On the health disadvantages of infants with teenage mothers. *American Journal of Epidemiology,* 137, no. 2 (1993): 213–225.

101. McCarthy, J., and Hardy, J. Age at first birth and birth outcomes. *Journal of Research on Adolescence,* 3 (1993): 373–392.

102. Rauh, V. A., Andrews, H. F., and Garfinkel, R. S. The contribution of maternal age to racial disparities in birthweight: A multilevel perspective. *American Journal of Public Health,* 91 (2001): 1815–1824.

103. Rich-Edwards, J., Buka, S. L., Brennan, R. T., and Earls, F. Diverging associations of maternal age with low birthweight for black and white mothers. *International Journal of Epidemiology,* 32 (2003): 83–90.

104. Levine, J., Pollack, H. A., and Comfort, M. Academic and behavioral outcomes among the children of young mothers. *Journal of Marriage & Family,* 63, no. 2 (2001): 355–369.

105. Moore, K. A., and Snyder, N. O. Cognitive attainment among firstborn children of adolescent mothers. *American Sociological Review,* 56 (1991): 612–624.

106. Rothenberg, P. B., and Varga, P. E. The relationship between age of mother and child health and development. *American Journal of Public Health,* 71, no. 8 (1981): 810–817.

107. Burton, L. M., and Whitfield, K. E. "Weathering" towards poorer health in later life: Comorbidity in urban low income families. *Public Policy and Aging Report,* 13 (2003): 13–18.

108. O'Connor, A. *Poverty Knowledge: Social Science, Social Policy, and the Poor in Twentieth-Century U.S. History.* Princeton, N.J.: Princeton University Press, 2001.

109. Ellwood, D. T., and Bane, M. J. *Welfare Realities: From Rhetoric to Reform.* Cambridge, Mass.: Harvard University Press, 1994.

110. Sessions, D. N., and Stevans, L. K. Minimum wage policy and poverty in the United States. *International Review of Applied Economics,* 15, no. 1 (2001): 65–75.

111. Levin-Waldman, O. M. Minimum wage and justice? *Review of Social Economy,* 58, no. 1 (2000): 43–62.

112. Reich, R. B. The case (once again) for universal health insurance. *The American Prospect.* Available at www.prospect.org/cs/articles?articleId=4701. Published April 22, 2001. Accessed July 30, 2008.

113. Stone, D. How market ideology guarantees racial inequalities. In *Healthy, Wealthy and Fair: Health Care and the Good Society.* New York: Oxford University Press, 2007.

114. Fossett, J. W., Perloff, J. D., Peterson, J. A., and Kletke, P. R. Medicaid in the inner city: The case of maternity care in Chicago. *Milbank Quarterly,* 68, no. 1 (1990): 111–141.

115. Fossett, J. W., and Perloff, J. D. *The "new" health reform and access to care: The problem of the inner city.* Report prepared for the Kaiser Commission on the Future of Medicaid, December 1995.

116. LaVeist, T. A. Linking residential segregation to the infant-mortality race disparity in U.S. cities. *Sociol Soc Res,* 73 (1989): 90–94.

117. Polednak, A. P. Segregation, discrimination and mortality in U.S. blacks. *Ethn Dis,* 6 (1996): 99–108.

118. Williams, D. R., and Collins, C. Racial residential segregation: A fundamental cause of racial disparities in health. *Public Health Reports,* 116 (2001): 404–416.

119. Cooper, R. S., Kennelly, J. F., Durazo-Arvizu, R., Oh, H-J., Kaplan, G., and Lynch, J. Relationship between premature mortality and socioeconomic factors

in black and white populations of U.S. metropolitan areas. *Public Health Reports,* 116 (2001): 464–473.

120. Jackson, S. A., Anderson, R. T., Johnson, N. J., and Sorlie, P. D. The relation of residential segregation to all-cause mortality: A study in black and white. *American Journal of Public Health,* 90 (2000): 615–617.

121. Cooper, R. S. Social inequality, ethnicity and cardiovascular disease. *International Journal of Epidemiology,* 30 (2001): S48–S52.

122. Acevedo-Garcia, D. Zip code-level risk factors for tuberculosis: Neighborhood environment and residential segregation in New Jersey, 1985–1992. *American Journal of Public Health,* 91 (2001): 734–741.

123. Kelley, R. D. G. Playing for keeps: Pleasure and profit on the postindustrial playground. In Lubiano, W., ed. *The House That Race Built,* pp. 195–231. New York: Pantheon Books, 1997.

124. Newman, K. S. *No Shame in My Game: The Working Poor in the Inner City.* New York: Knopf/Sage, 1999.

125. Wallace, R., and Wallace, D. Socioeconomic determinants of health: Community marginalisation and the diffusion of disease and disorder in the United States. *British Medical Journal,* 314 (1997): 1341.

126. Bound, J. The health and earnings of rejected disability insurance applicants. *American Economic Review,* 79 (1989): 482–503.

127. Chasnoff, I. J., Landress, H. J., and Barrett, M. E. The prevalence of illicit-drug or alcohol use during pregnancy and discrepancies in mandatory reporting in Pinellas County, Florida. *New England Journal of Medicine,* 322 (1990): 1202–1206.

128. Schulman, K. A., Berlin, J. A., Harless, W., et al. The effect of race and sex on physicians' recommendations for cardiac catheterization. *New England Journal of Medicine,* 340, no. 8 (1999): 618–626.

129. Dalton, H. L. AIDS in blackface. *Daedalus,* 118 (1989): 205–223.

130. LaVeist, T. A., Nickerson, K. J., and Bowie, J. V. Attitudes about racism, medical mistrust, and satisfaction with care among African American and white cardiac patients. *Medical Care Research and Review,* 57, Suppl (2000): 146–161.

131. Davis, R. Current trends in cigarette advertising and marketing. *New England Journal of Medicine,* 316 (1987): 725.

132. LaVeist, T. A., and Wallace, J. M. Health risk and inequitable distribution of liquor stores in African American neighborhoods. *Social Science & Medicine,* 51 (2000): 613–617.

133. Mohai, P., and Bryant, B. Environmental injustice: Weighing race and class as factors in the distribution of environmental hazards. *University of Colorado Law Review,* 63 (1992): 921–932.

134. U.S. Department of Health and Human Services. *Healthy People 2010: Understanding and Improving Health.* Washington, D.C.: U.S. Government Printing Office, 2000.

135. Kilbreth, E. H., and Marone, J. A. Power to the people? Restoring citizen participation. *Journal of Health Politcs, Policy and Law,* 28 (2003): 2–3.

136. Nathanson, C. A. The skeptic's guide to a movement for universal health insurance. *Journal of Health Politcs, Policy and Law,* 28, no. 2–3 (2003): 443–472.

137. Fainstein, S. S. Can we make the cities what we want? In S. Brody-Gendrot and R. Beauregard, eds., *The Urban Moment: Cosmopolitan Essays on the Late 20th Century City,* pp. 249–272. Thousand Oaks, Cal.: Sage, 1999.

138. Kelley, R.D.G. *Freedom Dreams: The Black Radical Imagination.* Boston: Beacon Press, 2002.

139. Pettit, P. *The Common Mind: An Essay on Psychology, Society, and Politics.* New York: Oxford University Press, 1993.

140. Dawson, M. C., and Popoff, R. Reparations: Justice and greed in black and white. *Du Bois Review,* 1, no. 1 (2004): 47–91.

141. Project, T. S. *Losing the Vote: The Impact of Felony Disenfranchisement Law.* Available at www.sentencingproject.org/tmp/File/FVR/fd_losingthevote.pdf. Published October 1999. Accessed July 30, 2008.

142. Kinder, D. R., and Sanders, L. M. *Divided by Color: Racial Politics and Democratic Ideals.* Chicago: University of Chicago Press, 1995.

143. Skrentny, J. D. *The Ironies of Affirmative Action: Politics, Culture, and Justice in America.* Chicago: University of Chicago Press, 1996.

144. Almond, D., Chay, K., and Greenstone, M. Civil rights, the war on poverty, and black-white convergence in infant mortality in Mississippi. Unpublished manuscript, 2003.

145. Mayer, S., and Jencks, C. Poverty and the distribution of material hardship. *Journal of Human Resources,* 24, no. 1 (1988): 88–112.

146. Kleinman, A. K., and Kleinman, J. The appeal of experience; the dismay of images: Cultural appropriations of suffering in our times. In A. Kleinman and M. Lock, eds., *Social Suffering,* pp. 1–24. V. D. Berkeley: University of California Press, 1997.

CHAPTER

7

AN INTERDISCIPLINARY AND SOCIAL-ECOLOGICAL ANALYSIS OF THE U.S. FORECLOSURE CRISIS AS IT RELATES TO HEALTH

SUSAN SAEGERT, KIMBERLY LIBMAN, DESIREE FIELDS

LEARNING OBJECTIVES

- Describe the multiple pathways through which housing and health are related in the case of the foreclosure of housing.
- Define several explanatory models, including the epidemiological model, the social-ecological model, and the more specific housing niche model.

- Evaluate the authors' choice of methods for studying connections between foreclosure and health and suggest other methods that would add different kinds of knowledge.

- Explain the implications for health interventions related to the foreclosure crisis in at least three levels.

HOUSING AND HEALTH: WHAT'S THE CONNECTION?

The history of public health is replete with concern about the quality and availability of adequate housing, especially in cities where working class and poor neighborhoods were filled with dilapidated, crowded, and unsanitary housing.[1] Indoor plumbing, proper ventilation, occupancy codes, lead paint regulations, and standards for heating and cooling are but a few examples of the important housing improvements motivated by threats to health and public health activism.[1-3] Concerns about the negative effect of poor housing on health remain.[1,4] Substandard housing still exists as well as homelessness. Both are associated with exposure to infectious diseases via pests, unsanitary conditions, crowding, and in the case of homeless people, lack of housing at all or crowded temporary shelters. Dampness, cold, and mold, as well as pests, are related to chronic diseases. Homes also can be the sites for exposure to stored toxins, lead, and other dangerous chemicals. Home accidents are frequent and related to design features, appliances, and maintenance. Numerous housing conditions from crowding through dampness have been associated with negative mental health effects.[1,5] All of the health effects of housing just described have been uncovered through epidemiological analyses that trace exposures to a health hazard to disease outcomes. Given this epidemiological paradigm, there is very little reason for public health experts to have been interested in the relationship between foreclosure and health.

We became involved with the issue of foreclosure as a result of our work on the consequences of homeownership for low- and moderate-income households.[6] Even though Saegert has written about the relationship between health and housing,[7] health was not initially a focus of the research reported in this chapter. Rather, our national survey of 759 low- and moderate-income homeowners had revealed substantial satisfaction and benefits associated with homeownership but also vulnerability to financial difficulty over time. Those homeowners who contacted a nonprofit homeownership counselor were able to find their way out of their difficulty, but those who failed to do so more often fell into mortgage delinquency and were fearful of foreclosure.

As a result of that finding, we worked with a group of national and local housing and financial institutions to craft a study that would help us understand the motivators, facilitators, and barriers to seeking help with mortgage delinquency. The research began in the spring and summer of 2006 before the mortgage foreclosure crisis in the United States dominated newspaper headlines. However, early warning signs were evident in the form of homeownership preservation initiatives and working groups on foreclosure at community development organizations and efforts by states to pass antipredatory lending laws. The close interrelationship between health and foreclosure only became apparent as we began to talk to homeowners in danger of foreclosure.

The paradigms employed by researchers, financial agents, and policymakers to explain, prevent, or study the consequences of foreclosure also do not recognize a connection to health. In 2008, U.S. mortgage delinquencies and foreclosures were at an all-time high and do not show signs of slowing. In May 2008, U.S. foreclosure filings set a record with one in every 483 households entering foreclosure. This is a 48 percent increase since May of 2007 and a 7 percent increase from the previous month.[8] Although stakeholders take varying positions in their assessments of the causes and solutions to this problem, popular media accounts emphasize the role of the subprime mortgage market and the targeting of less informed consumers for bad loans and irresponsible borrower behavior as causes. As evidenced by the 2008 multibillion-dollar bailout of the investment firm Bear Stearns, government intervention has been on the side of industry. Homeowners, particularly those with low and moderate incomes are left to grapple with rising costs of food and other necessities, increased responsibility for health care costs, stagnant wages, and rising unemployment. The stress alone could make one sick. But health and illness remain absent from most discussions of the U.S. foreclosure crisis.

The framing of the foreclosure problem around the flow of capital on the one hand and individual homebuyer's decisions on the other reflects the dominance of the discipline of economics in housing studies and policy. Policymakers accept that some buyers in any market will make bad decisions and suffer losses. The problem of housing foreclosures became a matter for intervention only when the stability of major financial institutions and the flow of capital into the economy started to be threatened. In analyzing the causes of foreclosure, housing specialists have applied an economic analysis based on rational choice theory that emphasizes the calculated trade-offs between risk of financial loss and chance of gain.[9] Even within this framework, analyses of predatory lending practices that lure low-income buyers with low short-term adjustable interest rates while hiding the long-term costs are often absent. Health problems are typically viewed as one cause of lost income referred to as a "trigger event." Health consequences of foreclosure are not discussed but would be considered as part of the potential cost calculations the homebuyer should have made within the rational choice model. The potential for stress from financial obligations or threat of foreclosure, as well as lack of money for medical care, food, and other necessities, should figure into the buying decision in the first place. Or when these costs become apparent, the homebuyer should sell or possibly default and go into foreclosure; both actions have the potential for negative personal consequences for homeowners but are rational from an economic perspective.

In this chapter, we use the social-ecological model (see also Chapter Four in this volume) to explore the role of health as both a cause of foreclosure and a consequence. We begin by examining the disciplinary paradigms that had prevented either health or housing research from making these connections. In the rest of the paper, we discuss (a) the social-ecological model that allows a more complex analysis of the relationship of housing and health; (b) the multiple methodologies implied by the nature of the relationship; (c) how our findings from fourteen focus groups of low- and moderate-income homeowners threatened with foreclosure led us to a concern for the health aspects of foreclosure; (d) interpretive frameworks appropriate to the findings; and (e) implications for interventions at multiple levels. We draw on Link and Phelan's concepts of "contextualizing risk factors" and "fundamental causes"[10] to understand how both mortgage foreclosure and poor health in the United States fall most heavily on minority (especially African American) populations, lower income households, and other more vulnerable groups. We look beyond health care costs and discuss the consequences of lost income, mental and physical health as both cause and consequence of foreclosure, homeownership and ontological security, and social networks and the sharing of vulnerability to health risk. Understanding the nuances of these connections is an essential step in locating windows of opportunity for policy interventions. Our conclusions reconsider the role of social policy as a determinant of health and as a possible route of intervention for the U.S. foreclosure crisis.

THE SOCIAL ECOLOGY OF FORECLOSURE

We believe that foreclosure is a particularly useful context for examining the relationship between housing and health. The processes of purchasing a home, falling behind on one's mortgage, and eventually losing a home present an opportunity to look at health and housing in a social-ecological context and examine the social policies and processes that are part of these events. Looking at health and housing through the lens of foreclosure also deepens our understanding of the risks and benefits of homeownership. This is particularly important in the United States where homeownership is popularly conceived of as the American dream and from a policy standpoint believed to be the solution to multiple problems facing poor communities. Also, across nations, there appear to be spatial patterns of foreclosure concentration along lines of race, class, and local economic conditions. This leads us to further believe that the U.S. foreclosure crisis, absent strong state intervention on behalf of homeowners, may exacerbate already existing racial/ethnic and income-based health disparities.

Health and Housing in Context

Sometimes called the "new" public health, a social-ecological approach views "environment" broadly defined as a central determinant of health and thus a focal point for interventions aimed at promoting health and health equity. Social policies emerge as widely influential and potentially cost-effective strategies for promoting health compared to individualized interventions focused on specific risk factors. Identifying social policy reforms that can positively influence upstream determinants of health is an essential challenge within this approach. In this chapter, we aim to meet this challenge by using the social-ecological framework to look at the roles of social policy in shaping experiences of illness, mortgage delinquency, and foreclosure in the United States.

Link and Phelan[10] emphasize the role of upstream determinants of health and argue for public health research focused on social conditions as fundamental causes of disease. They criticize the almost exclusive focus of many public health interventions on proximal causes such as behavior or individual characteristics because, they claim, even when a particular proximal cause is eliminated, the underlying social conditions that led particular people to be exposed to it will manifest themselves in new but similarly unequal ways. Thus, effective policies to improve population health must address the role of social conditions, which they broadly define as "factors that involve a person's relationship to other people" (p. 81). To do this effectively, policymakers need research that helps them understand how people are put "at risk for risk."

The context for understanding housing and health includes the physical properties of homes, their function as settings for social life, and the markets that distribute them. Housing also fixes people in particular neighborhoods, communities, states, and regions, which all have implications for access to opportunities and resources. The fact that the same populations experience more housing and foreclosure problems and poorer health leads us to look farther upstream for even more fundamental social conditions that distribute both. These include individual characteristics like age, education, and employment that affect social and economic relationships; group qualities like social capital, neighborhood, and poverty; as well as macrosocial determinants such as social and economic policies and practices and racism (e.g., targeting predatory lending to African American communities).

Saegert and Evans[7] introduced the concept of housing niches to describe the way that multilevel social processes channel people with particular financial, social, and human assets (including health) into particular locations and housing stocks. The location of a household in a particular housing niche is the consequence of personal choice, actions, knowledge, and social structures and policies that differentially distribute assets. These include racism, class reproduction, market functioning, and public policies. Once a household is in a particular niche, the exposures to hazards, social and economic conditions, and opportunities within a particular housing unit and area affect the health of the household and members' ability to accumulate assets. The health and asset accumulation of the generation that first occupies a housing niche affect the health and asset bundle of the next generation.[7]

The main contribution of the niche model is to place the usual focus on proximal causes of poor health (lifestyle etc.) and foreclosure (reckless taking on of debt) in the larger context of the factors that contribute to class, race, and other differences in the probability of these behaviors and to look for policy and institutional causes of the problem, not just individual behaviors or exposures. Using the rise of subprime borrowing to explain race and income-based differences in foreclosure is analogous to cultural behavioral explanations of health disparities. This logic emphasizes blaming the poor judgment or profligate lifestyle of individuals for the bad consequences that befall them, whether it be poor health or foreclosure. In contrast, proponents of the niche model as well as some public health scholars have argued that it is necessary to examine the social structural conditions that provide incentives for such behavior and block access to opportunities that would promote more positive outcomes.[10, 11, 12] Distributions of individual-level risk factors for disease, such as smoking, diet, and exercise, and their relationship to disparities fall into this model. Regarding foreclosures, borrowers' bad credit is seen as a preexisting condition related to individual spending, saving, and earning habits. In this light, the subprime industry can be viewed as providing a needed service to borrowers who would otherwise not be able to access credit and buy homes.

However, it has been shown that in the United States, geographic patterns of subprime lending cannot be explained by borrower characteristics alone. This suggests the existence of racial and neighborhood targeting by this segment of the lending industry.[13] Similarly, the food, alcohol, and tobacco industries target poor and nonwhite communities with advertising for disease-promoting products.[14] Considered together, a picture emerges where these contextual factors that put people *at risk for risk* are stacked in communities already struggling with the life and health consequences of low socioeconomic status.[10] The social-ecological framework connects these pools of risk and allows us to look at both individual- and group-level factors influencing health and housing. When we approached the problem of understanding how low- and moderate-income homeowners took more financial risks than they could afford in purchasing their home, we were not yet aware of the links between poor physical and mental health and foreclosure. However, because of our use of a social-ecological model, we began with an understanding of risk as generated both by individual behavior and by contextual factors. This attention to context led us to discover the role of health as both cause and consequence of mortgage delinquency. It also directed our attention to the social policies that put low- and moderate-income households at risk for foreclosure and for poor health.

THE RESEARCH AND ITS CONTEXT

When we began this research, the mortgage foreclosure crisis in the United States had not yet been recognized. There were early warning signs and concerns about subprime loans, but most of the housing finance industry saw these as primarily the problems of individual homeowners.[15] We became involved with the topic of mortgage delinquency as a result of a 2004–2005 national survey by the Housing Environments Research Group at the Center for Human Environments at City University of New York. The study, conducted among low-income homeowners who received nonprofit prepurchase homeownership education, revealed that many homeowners faced financial challenges as time went on. If they did not seek help from a nonprofit housing counseling agency, then fear of foreclosure and the number of late mortgage payments increased.[6] Research conducted in 2005 at Freddie Mac indicated that half of homeowners in delinquency on mortgage payments were not in contact with their mortgage lenders and suggested ways to encourage these homeowners to contact their lenders.[16] The funders of our study included banks, insurance companies, and other financial institutions, as well as a foundation concerned with asset building and the quasi-governmental agency charged with increasing access to credit in underserved communities. Their goal was to understand why homeowners do not seek help for mortgage delinquency and how they understand their financial plight.

Choosing a Method

The first decisions we had to make were whom we were going to study and how we were going to contact them. The study needed to be national in scope, yet the budget was limited and the time frame for completion was one year. The sample needed to, in some convincing way, represent the "universe" of low- and moderate-income homeowners in danger of foreclosure. Our previous experience with mail surveys reminded us that even though they are accepted within many practical contexts, the low response rates heighten the possibility of obtaining a biased sample. In addition, the homeowners threatened with foreclosure were likely to be hard to reach. They had every reason to avoid and ignore calls and letters. They were being hounded by creditors and were in a potentially embarrassing and stressful situation that they might not want to discuss. Indeed, the one survey study that became available in preprint about the medical causes of home mortgage foreclosures mailed 2,000 surveys that had been laboriously selected from four states. In the end, the researchers received 128 responses from 1813 valid postal addresses.[17]

One of the lessons we learned by venturing into a field dominated by financial institutions was that much of the research and data on the topic were proprietary. For example, the Roper study that showed absence of seeking help among half of borrowers who went into foreclosure was the property of Freddie Mac. A detailed report that would have allowed us to understand how they got their sample and more about how the study was conducted was never made available. In addition, data on mortgage delinquencies and foreclosures from which to draw a sample frame or even target our sites for study were hard to obtain. There are Web sites that provide data on foreclosures, but they were reputed among banks and financial institutions to be unreliable. The most reliable data from Mortgage Brokers of America were expensive to buy and less current than the accessible but reputedly less reliable data sources. Foreclosure information is not easily tracked and measured.[12] In addition, some authors have presented evidence that nondisclosure of information by the lending industry serves the purpose of obscuring the targeting of more problematic loan products to minority populations.[18] And finally, the legal and regulatory frameworks for foreclosures are determined at the state, not the federal, level. We discovered considerable variation in the timeline and legal process of foreclosure across states. Such variation would complicate developing a survey about experiences with foreclosure. Given the time frame and budget, these considerations led us to look for ways to select study participants who would be typical even if the sample was not drawn in a statistically representative manner.

The nature of the research question led us to favor a qualitative method. In the previous quantitative survey, we had established that there was a problem with mortgage delinquency when low- and moderate-income homeowners did not seek help with financial problems. Now our task was to find out *why* some didn't seek help and *how* others did. Because we didn't know the answer, we needed to ask open-ended questions. We reviewed our options for obtaining qualitative data and eventually decided that a focus group methodology would best help us understand how homeowners in trouble viewed their situations and made decisions about what to do.

Other methods we considered include interviews and participant observation. Interviews would have allowed us to gather in-depth stories about individual cases but would limit our ability to understand how these stories are socially constructed as similar or different from other people's experiences in the same community. Participant observation would have required us to live and/or work alongside people going through foreclosure and the professionals helping them. This method would have been prohibitively time consuming because our phenomenon of interest takes months, if not years, to unfold. Although we did not elect to use this method for conducting our research with homeowners and nonprofit staff, we view our four years of engagement with the nonprofits and lending institutions we partnered with as a form of participant observation. We drew on this experience and these relationships while interpreting and analyzing our data as well as relating it to industry policies and practices.

The conversational format of focus groups proved particularly appropriate for understanding how a problem like foreclosure is defined and approached because it allows people to question, challenge, agree with, and disagree with each other. Establishing trust and rapport with participants is critical to gathering useful data with all of these methods. As it turned out, the opportunity for homeowners faced with foreclosure to talk with others in their situation also increased their willingness to discuss how they got into their situation, what they did to cope, and how these efforts were working.

Foundation for Further Research

From a policy standpoint, however, focus groups would be the first stage of a research program that would provide a more solid representation of the populations affected and wider geographic coverage of populations. A larger, more representative sample would also allow the comparisons of different subgroups among homeowners threatened with foreclosure. The insights we gained from the focus groups can provide the basis for developing a closed ended survey instrument that could be distributed to a large sample and analyzed quantitatively. Such a study would require a longer time frame and a larger budget. However, since by this time more quantitative research has been done on foreclosure, it is possible that sample frames have already been assembled that could be used to draw the survey sample. In addition, the depth and breadth of the foreclosure crisis are putting pressure on financial institutions for more transparency, which might include easier access to proprietary information for the purposes of policy research and evaluation.

Because research has shown that mortgage arrears/foreclosures are geographically clustered, there is reason to believe that community- and state-level factors are operating beyond the aggregation of particular population characteristics. For example,

Newman and Wyly[13] have shown that borrower characteristics did not predict sub-prime loans as strongly as institutional practices targeting particular geographic areas. Thus, multilevel regression modeling would be appropriate to distinguish the effects of being in a particular community from the effects of household demographic traits such as race, income, and credit history. By employing geographic information systems as these authors did, it is possible to overlay multiple address-linked data sets to provide a more complete picture of the contextual aspects of communities threatened with foreclosure.

Methods and Sample

The sites for the focus groups were selected to represent a mix of market, geographic, economic, and demographic factors to yield locally and nationally relevant results about the experience of mortgage delinquency among low- and moderate-income homeowners. In combination with census data, state per capita foreclosure rates, the prevalence of high-interest subprime loans by Metropolitan Service Area (MSA), survey data from 2004–2005 documenting incidence of ever being behind on mortgage payments or making late payments, and fear of foreclosure[6] guided the site selection process. Together, these indicators helped us identify sites where low- and moderate-income homeowners might be especially vulnerable to becoming delinquent on their mortgages. The availability of nonprofit foreclosure intervention, other homeowner education resources, and antipredatory lending campaigns was an additional selection criterion used to narrow potential study sites to those where delinquent homeowners had the opportunity to seek assistance for their financial difficulties. The final sites for the focus group research were New York, N.Y.; St. Louis, Mo.; Hamilton, Oh.; Duluth, Ga.; and Waco, Tex.

To learn about how low-income homeowners responded to mortgage delinquency and their experiences with seeking assistance for this problem, we used mixed and multiple methods that included focus groups, videos, questionnaires, and field notes. At each research site, we partnered with a nonprofit group to aid in our recruiting efforts. We chose this strategy because we had worked with a network of nonprofit housing organizations in our mail survey and found that relationship improved our access to local homebuyers. In addition, the partnerships led these nonprofits to be interested in the findings and quick to make programmatic changes to respond to problems we identified. Because delinquent homeowners were likely to be hard to reach, it was helpful that nonprofits sent focus group invitation mailings to their clients, especially those who they had reason to believe might be facing financial strain. We supplemented this approach by placing newspaper advertisements in three cities. The advertisements and the letters of invitation gave a toll free number to call for delinquent mortgage holders wanting to participate in a focus group. In all, we screened 200 potential participants to obtain our sample.

We conducted nine focus groups and two individual interviews with a total of 88 homeowners and five focus groups with a total of 39 nonprofit professionals; in all,

127 people participated in this study. The majority of participants (70 percent) were female. Across all groups, the majority of participants were African American, with English-speaking Latinos (30 percent) and whites (16 percent) representing smaller portions of our sample. Homeowner participants may be characterized as moderate- or low-income people. A protocol guided the focus group questions by giving the researchers a script with stem questions and a guide for probes and follow-up questions.

The topics covered included

The difficulties they encountered as homeowners that resulted in their becoming delinquent on their mortgages

Whether they received homeownership counseling before buying or since then

How they first knew they were in trouble and questions about their financial conditions

Their emotional reaction to the situation, how they tried to cope with their problems, and what options they considered

Whether or not they contacted their lender or anyone else and what experiences they had when they sought help

What information they would have liked to have, and what they would do differently if they could do it over again

At the end, they were asked if they would like to videotape a one-minute message to anyone they wished (other buyers in trouble, prospective buyers, lenders, housing counselors, or others).

FOCUS GROUP ANALYSIS AND THE EMERGENCE OF HEALTH AS AN ISSUE

Focus group experiences and transcripts were analyzed using a combination of methods to ensure thoroughness and the reliability of findings. These included on-site reflection written by focus group facilitators immediately after the groups, debriefing with nonprofit staff, listening to recordings in groups to develop coding categories, coding, creating matrices of data, and multiple refinements of this process. All focus groups and interviews were professionally transcribed.

Our analyses of the interrelation of health problems and the threat of foreclosure grew out of the broader analysis of how participants became delinquent, the consequences of this problem for participants and their households, and how they coped with this problem. Initial review of our field notes and audio recordings of the focus groups revealed that issues associated with medical problems, health care, and medical expenses were consistently implicated in the cascade of trouble leading up to mortgage delinquency and that the experience of delinquency translated into health consequences for both participants and members of their households. Having identified these issues and their resonance with the social-ecological model of housing and health, we conducted an intensive review of transcripts for personal accounts of how health factors were involved in the cascade of trouble; experiences of illness, injury, and access to health care in the wider social and economic context and their relationship to the threat of foreclosure; and the stories relating the impact of mortgage delinquency on household physical and mental health.

These findings have been presented in three forms: short case studies present a detailed narrative of health's role in the cascade of trouble for an individual homeowner; illustrative quotes communicate key ideas about health and mortgage delinquency in the neoliberal policy context; and exchanges among participants demonstrate the social construction of the experience and consequences of mortgage delinquency that emerged within the focus groups.[15]

The Cascade of Trouble

In every focus group, health problems emerged as part of the story of how homeowners became delinquent on their mortgages. Often, an accident at work, surgery for cancer, a heart attack, and even a pregnancy or the birth of a child started what we began to call "the cascade of trouble." These incidents led to loss of income, medical debt, and loss of capacity to work and handle daily life. Sometimes, the health problems that tipped homeowners into debt were not their own but rather those of a child, spouse, and parent or other kin. Other times, health problems were interwoven with a divorce, missed child support payments, layoffs, hours cut back at work, a car that broke down, which all increased financial and emotional distress. The efforts to cope were complicated by increased demands on time, hours of work lost, dipping into savings, running up new debts, missing mortgage and other debt payments, being subject to late payment fees and higher interest rates, and seeking help with the problem itself and with debts but finding no help. Eventually, a letter from the bank would arrive saying that the homeowner's property was going into foreclosure. Sometimes, homeowners would find a way to work out a payment plan and get caught up. Other times, they had to leave their homes. For many, the situation was still unresolved.

The following dialogue typifies the discussions around health. JoAnn (all names are changed to protect anonymity) began by explaining what happened when she found out she had cancer and had to undergo radiation and chemotherapy.

> *I knew I was in trouble when I had that first dose of chemo and radiation. I'm like, Oh God, I can't go to work. But I was going, but I was late, and I was sick and just. . . . so I knew then, oh my goodness. And when I went into the hospital and actually had to stop working, and I got that last paycheck, and I'm like, okay, Lord, what am I going to do?*

She contacted her lender who said she could not help her until she was at least thirty days behind.

She had taken a budgeting class to prepare to buy a home. She put her knowledge into use to try to figure out how to meet her obligations, but with no income, it was impossible. She knew that if her credit score dropped by the time the bank would work with her, she would not be eligible for help in the form of a loan forbearance, modification, or refinance. It took four months for her to get disability payments, so she refinanced at what she thought was a better interest rate. But when she started getting the bills, the interest rate was much higher, and the lender took no responsibility, blaming it on the broker who had taken a fee and disappeared. Eventually, she found a nonprofit housing counselor who helped her get current, and she found a lawyer to sue the broker. But she still can't work and regards her future as precarious.

At this point, Jerome interjected that his story was similar. Constant medical bills were put on his credit card, and he got behind on other bills. Then his credit score went down, he could not refinance, and as a result of missing payments, his interest rate went way up. Then Sarah joined in to explain that her troubles started when her son was killed. He had helped her out in many ways, but without him, she got behind on bills, including the mortgage. Her credit score dropped, and then her options, like her income, were limited. Jack said his problems began when his two young children became very ill for six months. His wife had to quit her job, and the loss of income put them behind on their bills.

Later in the group, talk turned to the emotional consequences of their experiences. JoAnn spoke of how her daughter's mental health was affected by the stress at home over her cancer, the chemotherapy, and the threat of losing their home. The school counselor called to report:

She's not the same old child, she's not energetic, . . . and I talked to her and I asked her, you know, is everything okay at home, and she just broke down.

JoAnn concluded by saying,

And so it affects everybody . . . my mom was depressed, my daughter was depressed and my sisters were depressed and, you know, my boyfriend . . . everybody around me, it just affects everybody.

Another woman spoke for the consensus in the group:

Depression, frustration, tears, anger, I mean, you name it; you feel the whole spectrum. It's, like, first you're depressed because you know it's going to happen. Then when you try to get help and you don't, well, try this, and try that, and try this, so you feel like you're bouncing in every direction, trying to pull things together. You feel the whole spectrum of negative emotions; there's no particular one that will satisfy you.

The conversations were much the same in every group, but often, health problems were embedded in a larger web of institutional and family crises. For example, Sandra described how her daughter had cancer of the eye; she then lost the child's disability payment when regulations were tightened, and the stress led her husband to leave the family, cutting household income and leaving her without a car. She lives paycheck to paycheck doing telemarketing on commission and is underinsured. Thus, she is not reimbursed for her daughter's $100 a month asthma medicine. Despite all this, her life is more stable than most of her relatives, so she took in her nephew who was getting into trouble. She saw him through high school and into a military career but also incurred higher household costs while he lived with her. She got behind on mortgage payments and refinanced into what she thought was a fixed rate loan that turned out to be adjustable rate with quickly escalating payments. Through working with a housing counselor, she got caught up but felt that her situation was precarious for the foreseeable future.

The extremity of the risks faced by low-income homeowners and the precariousness of all aspects of life are the theme that runs through these focus groups. Poor health is a very prominent "trigger event" that brings down the fragile edifice of many homeowners' hold on security and solvency. For most people we talked to, the threat of foreclosure also had negative mental health consequences, including depression serious enough to interfere with daily life tasks and even leading to consideration of suicide. Family relationships were often collateral damage in these cases, with accounts of divorce and strain between parents and children being frequent. Experts on housing finance understand foreclosure as a risk people took that didn't work out. Foreclosure only becomes a crisis when whole markets collapse, as in Ohio, or the financial system itself is threatened, as was the case in the United States in 2008.

Public health professionals usually address the problems recounted in our focus groups with calls for universal health care or at least health insurance for the uninsured. But the many aspects of life that come tumbling down as a consequence of poor health exceed the problem of medical debt. The loss of housing to foreclosure is just one of these. Children who were headed for college cannot go, marriages come apart, savings are depleted, credit ratings are ruined, bankruptcies are declared, and people lose the equity that they worked hard to accumulate and leave to the next generation. The mental health consequences of this cascade of trouble are hardly ever discussed, and much less is assistance offered.

In the next section, we analyze the lessons we learned from the focus groups and develop a theoretical framework to understand the "fundamental causes" that put the people we spoke with "at risk for risk." Then we discuss the implications for intervening at different levels.

FORECLOSURE AND PUBLIC HEALTH

Our findings on the precariousness of all aspects of the lives of homeowners threatened with foreclosure echo those of a UK research team who offered an analysis of foreclosure as a public health issue in the wake of the mortgage repossession crisis in the United Kingdom during the 1990s. Nettleton[19] situates mortgage repossession in the literature on health inequalities by examining this phenomenon in the context of psychosocial determinants of health and efforts to develop "healthy public policies."

This and subsequent discussions of the public health consequences of mortgage delinquency and foreclosure emphasize stress, emotionality, uncertainty, and loss of control as dimensions of the experience of losing one's home that negatively affect health.[20] These authors also connect increases in foreclosures to "landscapes of precariousness" and the shifting terrain of risk in society.[20, 21] This new terrain is a consequence of restructured welfare policies, as well as changes to employment security associated with globalization and the turn toward more flexible employment. The uncertainty introduced by these economic and social policy changes is incongruous with the long-term financial commitment of a mortgage. Thus, homebuyers are at increased risk for repossession and its health consequences.[22] This literature focuses mainly on the stresses of delinquency and foreclosure and the consequences these can have for health.

Ford and colleagues[20] draw attention to "upstream" causes of poor health by placing the increasing risk of foreclosure within the context of a globalized economy where deregulation of financial and labor markets has rapidly advanced. The erosion of the welfare state in Britain is a related development. However, they do not examine the role that the precariousness of health plays in bringing about foreclosures, a factor we found to be quite significant in the United States. Perhaps it is less important in the United Kingdom because of the state provision of a safety net for mortgagers who lost all income, plus the UK provision of universal health care, even though post-Thatcher changes in the provision of income loss replacement for mortgagers had weakened that safety net.[20] In fact, in international comparisons of both welfare provisions and good health, the United Kingdom ranks well ahead of the United States.[23, 24]

NEOLIBERALISM, THE FORECLOSURE CRISIS, AND HEALTH CONSEQUENCES

Coburn argues that in countries where neoliberal policies have most thoroughly eroded the social safety net, health inequalities have increased most steeply.[23, 25] The neoliberal philosophy assumes that human needs are best met through markets and that these markets are best supported by a noninterventionist state. It emphasizes individuality over society and endorses inequalities as supportive of markets.[23, 26] Income inequality within and between nations is associated with disparities in health.[27, 28] Using international data, Coburn[23] supports this claim and further argues that these effects are tempered by the presence of social welfare regimes.

These state regimes include safety net provisions, including heath care, emergency food, unemployment insurance, and mortgage insurance. As more responsibility for the risk of conditions such as illness and unemployment shifts to individuals, they become highly vulnerable to shocks in their financial, social, and housing stability. Despite their vulnerability, low- and moderate-income homeowners often have more resources than others in their social networks. They thus try to absorb the impacts of neoliberal policies on not only themselves but also on others in their social networks.

Rooted in the politics of neoliberalism, a broad array of social, financial, and housing policies affects the sustainability of homeownership. Neoliberalism refers both to an ideology and a set of practices.[26, 29, 30] The ideology presumes that free markets unfettered by government intervention are always the best route to achieve the best outcomes for the most people. The actual policies associated with neoliberalism in the United States date from Reagan's election and involve deregulation of the financial industry. This climate has been conducive to the proliferation of exotic mortgages, the absence of regulation that allowed fraudulent practices to flourish, and the expansion of homeownership to markets previously able to afford only rental housing. To accomplish these changes, the rhetoric of neoliberal ideology built on longstanding ideas of homeownership as the American dream to justify housing policies that promoted homeownership to the exclusion of other alternatives such as rental housing owned by nonprofits or local housing authorities. This push for homeownership culminated in George W. Bush's vision of "the ownership society." Thus, as we argue elsewhere,[31] neoliberalism emerges as a "fundamental cause" of not only income and health inequalities but, in the United States, also of foreclosures. Lower income and minority households suffer most from neoliberal housing policies that place them more frequently in poor housing and deprived areas, with the accompanying greater exposure to housing-associated health risks.[7, 32] Recent research also increasingly places the same populations at greater risk for housing debt.[33–36] Housing costs and debt are associated with less money available for basic nutrition and other health necessities.[1]

The widening inequalities Coburn identifies have multiple connections to health disparities in the United States. Beyond income, a health care gap has been identified between high- and low-wage workers.[37] Amassing medical debt has been associated with decreased likelihood of acquiring health insurance later in life and negative financial impacts like bankruptcy, lawsuits, and foreclosure. The stress from these conditions is often compounded by aggressive debt collection efforts.[38] Even workers who have insurance are often underinsured and left vulnerable to acquiring debt in the event they become injured or ill. It is estimated that 42 percent of the U.S. population has no health insurance or inadequate coverage against out-of-pocket health expenses, and that trend has been growing since at least 2000.[39] In the United States, nearly one-fifth of adults report having serious difficulty paying medical expenses.[40] The same low- and moderate-income people who buy homes in part to secure their financial futures are being left exposed to increasingly greater risk for covering the costs of their health care.

This of course has consequences for health, and these are mainly through limited access to care and increased stress. Compared to other developed nations, the United States as a society pays more and gets less from our health care system.[41] A recent study by the Commonwealth Fund[24] found that 37 percent of respondents in the United States reported that high medical costs led them to do at least one of the following: skip doses of medication or not fill prescriptions; have a medical problem and not visit a doctor; or skip treatment, tests, or follow up. In the United Kingdom, by comparison, only 8 percent of respondents reported doing at least one of these cost-saving measures.[24]

Health outcomes data from the Organization for Economic Cooperation and Development (OECD) show that the U.S. health care system has negative impacts on population health. The United States leads other nations in potential years of life lost due to diseases of the circulatory system, diabetes, and diseases of the respiratory system.[42] Looking across six nations, the United States ranked last in health equity and healthy lives, whereas the United Kingdom ranked first in equity and fourth in healthy lives.[41] Again, the burdens of poor health and the high cost of health care are placed disproportionately on poor and minority populations in the United States. These are the same people experiencing the highest rates of foreclosure.

Both the UK work on mortgage arrears and repossession and Coburn's work on the effects of neoliberal policies on health inequality draw on the emerging social-ecological paradigm in public health. They both examine the effects of the "upstream" influence of social policies and economic forces that put particular populations "at risk for risk."[10] Ford, Nettleton, Burrows, and their colleagues[19-22] also explore more than one level of analysis when they join their interviews with individual homeowners and national data on population health and mortgage arrears and repossessions. In their quantitative analyses, they compare different geographic regions and describe the role of a variety of institutions and organizations in promoting unsustainable homeownership and increasing other forms of risk for homeowners, like unemployment and sudden loss of income. When looking at homeowners, they separated those who bought under a British housing program that gave residents of what had been public estates the right to buy their units from homeowners who bought on the regular market. Coburn's work[23,25] provides some detail about variation in the social welfare context across nations and uses that to predict health inequality.

CONCLUSION

The housing niche model,[7] which is a refinement of the social-ecological approach, provided a lens through which we could look more closely at the reciprocal causality and interwoven nature of health and foreclosure. The attention to the many aspects of risk in the particular communities we studied led us to use a method and a set of focus group questions that were sufficiently broad to reveal aspects of becoming threatened with foreclosure that we were not initially seeking. From this broadly defined querying of experiences and context, the role of poor health as both a cause and a consequence of foreclosure emerged, as well as a clearer understanding of how changes in labor markets, energy costs, and the whole financial industry, including credit cards and bankruptcy law, played into the causes and consequences of foreclosure.

The housing niche model also focuses on the dynamics of interpersonal interaction in households and the intergenerational consequences of residing in particular housing niches. In the study, both loomed large in the experiences of homeowners threatened by foreclosure. The cascades of trouble that pervaded the focus group discussions could only be understood from such a contextualized model. The importance of the quality of the interactions of threatened homeowners with financial, governmental, and nonprofit institutions also highlights the significance of causes of foreclosure that were far upstream from borrower behavior. The restructuring of the home mortgage industry and the financial sector around secondary markets and automated loan underwriting are examples of such factors.

Intervention Implications of the Linkage of Poor Health and Foreclosure

Our study indicates that health burdens from normal life events such as medical debt, serious illness and injury, lack of insurance and underinsurance, and caring for extended family can trigger mortgage delinquency and increase the risk for homeowners of foreclosure. The financial and emotional stress of illness is made worse by neoliberal cutbacks of the social safety net. The likelihood of financial distress is also exacerbated by the deregulation of labor, financial, and housing markets. All these factors increase the chances of mortgage delinquency and foreclosure. Then, mortgage delinquency and foreclosure also contribute to poorer physical and mental health as a result of the stress and anxiety of financial hardship. Seeking help when none exists may sometimes worsen prospects for avoiding foreclosure because of delays in responding and the time it takes to seek help unsuccessfully. The stress involved can impair decision making, lead to strain on marriages and parent-child relationships, and contribute to even worse mental health consequences.

These findings and related literature indicate that housing foreclosures and their negative health consequences can be reduced by a social safety net that cushions the risks households face in labor and financial markets and provides health care and income replacement for people who are ill or disabled. Politically in the United States, the barriers to turning that insight into more welfare-oriented public policies are formidable (see Chapter Six of this volume). However, the complexity of the problem means that there are many different potential points of intervention. In keeping with the multilevel nature of the social-ecological model of public health, it is important to find ways to assist individuals with their immediate health and housing problems and to provide education to improve their ability to avoid risk. At the same time, public health and housing experts can work to introduce specific policies that would ameliorate forces that increase the risks that bring about health problems and the threat of foreclosure. At the policy level, health policy must go beyond health care and prevention of disease to include housing policy that assures adequate and secure housing. Housing policy must take into account the housing needs of the temporarily and permanently ill, injured, and disabled people, as well as households presumed to be healthy.

For inspiration, we can turn to the urban health pioneer activists of the nineteenth century who crusaded against unhealthy tenements, lack of sanitation and clean water in dense, often immigrant and working class neighborhoods, and poor urban design that denied less well off city dwellers access to parks and active recreation as well as clean light and air.[43] Clearly, the problems brought about by the confluence of increased mortgage arrears and foreclosure exacerbate the poor health burden in poorer, minority, female-headed households and less educated populations. Many of these populations cluster disproportionately in cities. In addition, as we have ridden and walked through neighborhoods in Baltimore and New York that have suffered from the geographic targeting of risky loans and fraudulent or shady lending practices, we see how foreclosure aggravates other urban health problems like drug use and violent crime, as it also brings about an overall worsening of the quality of the physical environment. These trends have been documented quantitatively by Apgar and Calder[33] as well as the studies of Immergluck and his colleagues.[44] In working with our nonprofit research partners engaged in housing counseling, we heard that in larger cities like New York and Chicago, their staffs are deluged by help seekers often to the point where a triage method of responding was required, leaving many calls for help unanswered. At the same time, these cities were in the forefront of innovative efforts to prevent foreclosure and sustain homeownership in minority and low-income communities.

The problems related to foreclosure and health are clearly interdisciplinary in nature, drawing on diverse fields of economics, mental health, consumer education, public health, law, and many others. But agencies and contexts for policy intervention are often organized by disciplines. It is important both to develop discipline-related policy interventions and to make helping professionals as well as clients aware of the multiple dimensions and sources of assistance for these intertwined cascades of trouble. Public health professionals can advocate for policies to provide universal health care, insure the uninsured, increase the adequacy of existing insurance provisions, and provide income and mortgage support to those who lose income due to ill health. Housing professionals can offer timely and useful foreclosure prevention counseling. They can also advocate for reform and regulation of the housing finance industry that will protect future homebuyers from the volume of risk that has sunk so many current homeowners. In addition, labor security, workman's compensation, unemployment insurance, and living wage policies would all contribute to both better health and less danger of foreclosure. Such efforts would surely include improving housing security of tenure and protections from housing crises related to loss of income that would lessen the likelihood of future foreclosure crises. In short, all efforts to improve the quality of life and living conditions, especially for marginalized populations, will most likely contribute to public health. Thus, housing policy, labor policy, and other domains that affect access to sufficient resources and basic life necessities become concerns of public health.

SUMMARY

In this chapter, we use the social ecological model to explore the role of health as both a cause and consequence of foreclosure. We examine the disciplinary paradigms that had prevented either health or housing research from making these connections in the past. Based on our analysis of 14 focus groups of low and moderate income homeowners threatened with foreclosure, we describe the findings that led us to a concern for the health aspects of foreclosure. We explain how both mortgage foreclosure and poor health in the US fall most heavily on minority (especially African American) populations, lower income households, and other more vulnerable groups in the US. We look beyond health care costs and discuss the consequences of lost income;

mental and physical health as both cause and consequence of foreclosure; home-ownership and ontological security; social networks and the sharing of vulnerability to health risk. Understanding the nuances of these connections is an essential step in locating windows of opportunity for policy interventions at various levels of organization. Our conclusions reconsider the role of social policy as a determinant of health and as a possible route of intervention for the US foreclosure crisis.

DISCUSSION QUESTIONS

1. What are the direct and indirect, "hard" and "soft," kinds of evidence linking housing and health?

2. Why are people who public health studies show to be at greater risk for poor health also more likely to experience mortgage delinquency and foreclosure?

3. How can the qualitative findings suggested by this chapter help to generate further research on the relationship between housing and health? Propose an approach for studying the possible relationships between housing and health, suggested by the authors' findings, using more quantitative measures.

4. Select one example from the stories homeowners told in the focus group that showed the relationships between health and foreclosure and propose three different types of interventions that could address it. In your example, consider both interventions related to the particular homeowner's immediate problems and more "upstream" interventions that might prevent being "at risk for risk."

NOTES

1. Krieger, J., and Higgins, D. Housing and health: Time again for public health action. *American Journal of Public Health,* 92, no. 5 (2002): 758–768.

2. Stewart, J. A review of UK housing policy: Ideology and public health. *Public Health,* 119, no. 6 (2005): 525–534.

3. Szreter, S. The population health approach in historical perspective. *American Journal of Public Health,* 93, no. 3 (2003): 421–431.

4. Matte, T., and Jacobs, D. E. Housing and health—Current issues and implications for research and programs. *Journal of Urban Health,* 77, no. 1 (2000): 7–25.

5. Evans, G., Wells, N. M., and Moch, A. Housing and mental health: A review of the evidence and a methodological and conceptual critique. *Journal of Social Issues,* 59, no. 3 (2003): 475–500.

6. Saegert, S., Justa, F., and Winkel, G. *Successes of Homeownership Education and Emerging Challenges.* New York: Center for Human Environments, Graduate Center, CUNY, 2005.

7. Saegert, S., and Evans, G. Poverty, housing niches, and health in the United States. *Journal of Social Issues,* 59, no. 3 (2003): 569–589.

8. RealtyTrac's Rick Sharga to address foreclosure market issues at Inman Connect San Francisco, July 22, 2008. Available at www.realtytrac.com/Content Management/pressrelease.aspx?ChannelID=9&ItemID=4889&accnt=64847. Cited August 11, 2008.

9. Elmer, P. J., and Seelig, S. A. *Insolvency, trigger events, and consumer risk posture in the theory of single-family mortgage.* FDIC Working Paper 98–3, 1998.

10. Link, B., and Phelan, J. Social conditions as fundamental causes of disease. *Journal of Health and Social Behavior,* (Extra Issue: Forty Years of Medical Sociology: The State of the Art and Directions for the Future), 35 (1995): 80–94.

11. Townsend, P., Davidson, N., and Whitehead, M. *The Black Report and the Health Divide.* Harmondsworth, UK: Penguin Books, 1986.

12. Bartley, M. *Health Inequality: An Introduction to Theories, Concepts and Methods. A Useful Synthesis and Review of the Rapidly Growing Research and Literature on Health Inequalities.* Cambridge, UK: Polity Press, 2004.

13. Newman, K., and Wyly, E. K. Geographies of mortgage market segmentation: The case of Essex County, New Jersey. *Housing Studies,* 19, no. 1 (2004): 53–83.

14. Freudenberg, N. Public health advocacy to change corporate practices: Implications for health education practice and research. *Health Education & Behavior,* 32, no. 3 (2005): 298–319.

15. Libman, K., Saegert, S., and Fields, D. Housing and health: What the U.S. foreclosure crisis reveals. Paper presented at European Network for Housing Research, Dublin, Ireland, July 8, 2008.

16. FreddieMac, *Foreclosure avoidance research.* Published 2005. Available from www.freddiemac.com/service/msp/pdf/foreclosure_avoidance_dec2005.pdf.

17. Robertson, C., Egelhof, R., and Hoke, M. Get sick, get out: The medical causes of home mortgage foreclosures. *Health Matrix,* (2008), 85, 65–105.

18. Wyly, E. K., Atia, M., Lee, E., and Mendez, P. Race, gender, and statistical representation: Predatory mortgage lending and the U.S. community reinvestment movement. *Environment and Planning A,* 39, no. 9 (2007): 2139–2166.

19. Nettleton, S. Losing homes through mortgage possession: A "new" public health issue. *Critical Public Health,* 8, no. 1 (1998): 47–58.

20. Ford, J., Burrows, R., and Nettleton, S. *Home Ownership in a Risk Society: A Social Analysis of Mortgage Arrears and Possessions.* Bristol, UK: Polity Press, 2001.

21. Nettleton, S., and Burrows, R. Families coping with the experience of mortgage repossession in the "new landscape of precariousness." *Community, Work & Family,* 4, no. 3 (2001): 253–272.

22. Nettleton, S., and Burrows, R. Mortgage debt, insecure home ownership and health: An exploratory analysis. *Sociology of Health & Illness,* 20, no. 5 (1998): 731–753.

23. Coburn, D. Beyond the income inequality hypothesis: Class, neo-liberalism, and health inequalities. *Social Science & Medicine,* 58, no. 1 (2004): 41–56.

24. Schoen, C., Osborn, R., Bishop, M., and How, S. *The Commonwealth Fund 2007 International Health Policy Survey in Seven Countries.* New York: The Commonwealth Fund, 2007.

25. Coburn, D. Income inequality, social cohesion and the health status of populations: The role of neo-liberalism. *Social Science & Medicine,* 51, no. 1 (2000): 135–146.

26. Harvey, D. *A Brief History of Neoliberalism.* Oxford, UK: Oxford University Press, 2005.

27. Marmot, M., and Wilkinson, R., eds. *Social Determinants of Health.* Oxford, UK: Oxford University Press, 1999.

28. Wilkinson, R. *Unhealthy Societies: The Afflictions of Inequality.* New York: Routledge, 1996.

29. Brenner, N., and Theodore, N. Cities and the geographies of actually existing neoliberalism. *Antipode,* 34, no. 3 (2002): 349–378.

30. Peck, J., and Tickell, A. Neoliberalizing space. *Antipode,* 34, no. 3 (2002): 380–440.

31. Saegert, S., Fields, D., and Libman, K. Deflating the dream: Radical risk and the neoliberalization of homeownership. *Journal of Urban Affairs,* in press.

32. Acevedo-Garcia, D. A conceptual framework of the role of residential segregation in the epidemiology of infectious diseases. *Social Science & Medicine,* 51, no. 8 (2000): 1143–1161.

33. Apgar, W., and Calder, A. The dual mortgage market: The persistence of discrimination in mortgage lending. In X. S., Briggs ed., *The Geography of Opportunity: Race and Housing Choice in Metropolitan America,* pp. 101–126. Washington D.C.: Brookings Institution Press, 2005.

34. Howell, B. Exploiting race and space: Concentrated subprime lending as housing discrimination. *California Law Review,* 94, no. 10 (2006): 101–147.

35. Williams, R., Nesiba, R., and McConnell, E. D. The changing face of inequality in home mortgage lending. *Social Problems,* 52, no. 2 (2005): 181–208.

36. Wyly, E. K., Atia, M., Foxcroft, H., Hammel, D. J., and Phillips-Watts, K. American home: Predatory mortgage capital and neighborhood spaces of race and class exploitation in the United States. *Geografiska Annaler,* 88B, no. 1 (2006): 105–132.

37. Glied, S., and Mahato, B. The widening health care gap between high- and low-wage workers. New York: The Commonwealth Fund, 2008.

38. Daly, H., Oblak, L., Seifert, R., and Shellenberger, K. Into the red to stay in the pink: The hidden cost of being uninsured. *Health Matrix,* 12 (2002): 39–61.

39. Schoen, C., Collins, S., Kriss, J., and Doty, M. How many are underinsured? Trends among U.S. adults, 2003 and 2007. *Health Affairs,* 27, no. 4 (2008): w298–w309 (published online).

40. Schoen, C., Osborn, R., Bishop, M., Peugh, J., and Murukutla, N. *Toward Higher Performance Health Systems: Adults' Health Care Experiences in Seven Countries.* New York: The Commonwealth Fund, 2008.

41. Davis, K., and Schoen, C. *Mirror, Mirror on the Wall: An International Update on the Comparative Performance of American Health Care.* New York: The Commonwealth Fund, 2007.

42. Cylus, J., and Anderson, G. F. *Multinational Comparisons of Health Systems.* New York: The Commonwealth Fund, 2007.

43. Coburn, J. Confronting the challenges of reconnecting urban planning and public health. *American Journal of Public Health,* 94, no. 4 (2004): 541–549.

44. Immergluck, D. From the subprime to the exotic: Excessive mortgage market risk and foreclosures. *Journal of the American Planning Association,* 74, no. 1 (2008): 59–76.

3

INTERDISCIPLINARY APPROACHES TO INTERVENTIONS TO PROMOTE URBAN HEALTH

CHAPTER

8

TRANSDISCIPLINARY ACTION RESEARCH ON TEEN SMOKING PREVENTION

JULIANA FUQUA, DANIEL STOKOLS, RICHARD HARVEY, ATUSA BAGHERY, LARRY JAMNER

LEARNING OBJECTIVES

- Describe and compare the three types of interdisciplinary collaboration within action research teams: (a) scientific collaborations among research investigators, (b) community problem-solving coalitions in which researchers work with community members to translate scientific knowledge into community problem-solving strategies, and (c) intersectoral partnerships involving representatives of organizations who work together to reduce health problems.

- Identify organizational and individual factors that facilitate or impede interdisciplinary collaboration among different constituencies.

- Describe the value of interdisciplinary action research to reduce the health problems associated with tobacco use.

- Discuss the strategies the Tobacco Policy Consortium used to overcome the organizational problems it encountered.

INTRODUCTION

This chapter presents a case study of transdisciplinary (TD) action research involving a consortium of tobacco scientists at the University of California, Irvine, and community decision makers based in Orange County, California. The participants in this university-community partnership focused their efforts on the growing problem of adolescent tobacco use in urban and suburban settings. The members of this *Tobacco Policy Consortium* (TPC) collaborated closely over a two-year period to produce and disseminate an evidence-based *Research and Policy Brief on Preventing Youth Smoking.*[1] In the ensuing sections of the chapter, we (a) discuss key principles of TD action research and present a selective review of recent literature on TD collaboration in scientific and community settings; (b) describe the goals, organization, and collaborative activities of the TPC; (c) summarize the observational, interview, and survey research methods that were used to study processes of TD action research over the course of the TPC project; (d) present empirical findings concerning important factors that either facilitated or constrained effective collaboration among TPC members; (e) summarize "lessons learned" from the TPC study; and (f) suggest potentially useful research directions that could serve to strengthen the science and practice of transdisciplinary action research in future years.

REVIEW OF TRANSDISCIPLINARY ACTION RESEARCH

Transdisciplinary (TD) action research comprises at least three kinds or phases of collaboration: (a) *scientific collaborations* among research investigators, (b) *community problem-solving coalitions* in which researchers work with community members to translate scientific knowledge into community problem-solving strategies, and (c) *intersectoral partnerships* involving representatives of organizations situated at local, state, national, and international levels, who work together to improve environmental, social, and health problems.[2] The two-year TPC offered participant observers a unique vantage point from which to investigate and evaluate the processes and outcomes of TD action research.

In the 1940s, Lewin[3] called upon fellow psychologists to engage in "action research," or efforts to apply scientific research and knowledge to the resolution of societal problems. As Stokols[2] noted, Lewin believed that psychologists should apply their scientific expertise to the analysis and amelioration of community problems such as racial prejudice and public health problems. Lewin inspired many psychologists to embrace the tenets of action research in their own work, although the vast majority of behavioral scientists continued to pursue more experimental, laboratory-based studies rather than undertake research for purposes of resolving social problems.

During the 1960s and 1970s, psychologists were confronted by growing societal concerns about overcrowding, the depletion of natural resources, environmental degradation, and racial violence in cities like Detroit, Newark, and Los Angeles. Problem-focused research in fields such as environmental, ecological, and community psychology expanded rapidly, and collaborations among behavioral scientists and community members ensued in an effort to ameliorate social and environmental problems.[4-6] Yet, participants in these university-community coalitions found the collaborative process to be quite daunting.[7-8] Among the challenges they faced were team members' divergent and conflicting expectations and goals. Psychologists seemed to be prepared only to educate community members about their findings in short-term collaborations, characterized by Sommer[9] as the "hit and run" model of community partnering. Researchers participating in these coalitions seemed to rely heavily on a model commonly used in science and engineering—that is, take scientific findings and then unidirectionally apply them to solve a problem (without much input from the community partners). This model is contrary to the ideals of community-based participatory research in which university-based scientists work closely and reciprocally with community members (with ongoing discussion between researchers and community partners) to understand and discover the best methods for solving a social problem.[10]

Scholars soon realized that more effective strategies for facilitating action research needed to be developed, especially those that promote nonhierarchical and equitable working relationships among community members and university-based scholars.[11-14] Stokols[2] built upon Lewin's original conceptualization of action research, which focused primarily on psychological science and did not give explicit attention to the logistical and organizational challenges associated with interdisciplinary and/or interprofessional collaboration. Stokols' conceptualization of the science of TD action research has two major themes. It encompasses scientists who are trained in and working in different fields, community decision makers and practitioners, and representatives from multiple sectors of society (e.g., education, public health, academia, local and state government). It also gives explicit attention to the empirical study of factors that facilitate or impede TD collaboration toward the goal of enhancing the effectiveness of ongoing and future collaboration among scientists and nonacademicians.[15]

TRANSDISCIPLINARY ACTION RESEARCH CYCLE

As noted earlier, transdisciplinary action research incorporates at least three kinds of collaboration that occur sequentially over different phases—namely, those involving purely *scientific collaborations* aimed at creating new intellectual products such as novel conceptual frameworks and empirical knowledge; *community problem-solving coalitions* in which researchers from different fields work closely with community members to translate scientific evidence into interventional programs aimed at reducing societal problems; and *intersectoral partnerships* involving representatives of community organizations situated at local, state, national, and international levels, all of whom work together to integrate their expertise drawn from multiple disciplines and professions to design and implement broad-gauged policies for improving environmental, social, and public health outcomes.[2]

Scientific collaborations emphasize the *discovery* of new knowledge, whereas community coalitions and intersectoral partnerships place greater emphasis on the *translation* of scientific findings into new programs and policies for improving community health. When considered together, these different forms of collaboration comprise interrelated facets and sequential phases of a *transdisciplinary action research cycle.*[2] During this cycle, purely scientific collaboration occurs at the outset, often followed by university-community coalitions that translate research findings into evidence-based practices and policies; these, in turn, evolve into broader intersectoral partnerships aimed at designing, implementing, and evaluating evidence-based health promotion policies spanning local, regional, national, and international levels as well as multiple sectors of society. Participants working at each level of a transdisciplinary action research project must coordinate their respective efforts to foster the development of scientific innovations that are translated into social change and health-improvement policies. The different forms and phases of TD action research have been investigated independently, but they have not been conceptually well linked as part of an integrative cycle encompassing multiple phases.

Studying and fostering the TD action research cycle is particularly timely. Societal interest and investment in conducting problem-focused TD research have grown dramatically over the past decade.[16–20] Public agencies and private foundations have come to the realization that many of society's most vexing environmental and social problems require large-scale interdisciplinary teams of scientists to create innovative strategies for ameliorating those problems. Large-scale research networks and centers have been established to investigate topics such as tobacco use, obesity, and environmental correlates and causes of disease. These pervasive health and social problems are seen as insoluble through unidisciplinary research. Instead, the development of effective strategies for resolving societal problems will likely require large-scale collaboration among scientists trained in multiple fields working in concert with community decision makers.

Examples of TD science and training centers established over the past ten years include initiatives such as the Transdisciplinary Tobacco Use Research Centers (TTURC) and Transdisciplinary Research on Energetics Center (TREC) as well as the Centers for Excellence in Cancer Communications and Research (CECCR), the Centers for Population Health and Health Disparities (CPHHD), and the Clinical Translational Science Centers (CTSC), which are funded by government agencies such as the National Cancer Institute, the National Institute on Drug Abuse, and the National Center for Research Resources.[21–25] Similarly, nonprofit organizations such as the Robert Wood Johnson and Keck Foundations have launched large-scale initiatives to promote TD collaboration in science, training, and the translation of knowledge into evidence-based practices and policies.[26,27]

The substantial investments that have been made by public agencies and private foundations to establish large-scale team science initiatives is based on the assumption that TD collaboration is valuable at both scientific and societal levels. Among the benefits often ascribed to TD research, training, and translational initiatives are the following:

1. The higher levels of explanatory power afforded by cross-disciplinary theories relative to reductionist analyses rooted in singular disciplinary perspectives;[28, 29]

2. Higher levels of convergent and discriminant validity that can be achieved through a triangulation of methods and multiple methodologies;[30]

3. Greater opportunities for developing broad-gauged public policies that are less likely to trigger unintended adverse consequences due to the gaps in knowledge that are inherent in monodisciplinary perspectives;[31]

4. The resolution or reduction of complex community health and social problems that require a generalist orientation characterized by the integration of multiple scientific conceptual and methodological approaches.[32]

To date, the situational circumstances that facilitate or impede effective TD collaboration among researchers and community members have not been widely studied or reported in a systematic fashion. However, some retrospective accounts, conceptual analyses, and empirical case studies have been published.[13, 14, 33–37] These studies have identified several factors that influence the effectiveness of transdisciplinary collaboration, including the breadth and diversity of collaborators' fields, the cultivation of social capital among team members, and the interdependence of team members' goals. Empirical case studies, like the one described in this chapter, are especially needed to identify antecedents and processes that facilitate or hinder positive outcomes of transdisciplinary scientists' efforts to collaborate not only across disciplinary boundaries but also across the diverse professional fields and perspectives represented among their community-based partners and within multiple sectors of society.

TRANSLATING TRANSDISCIPLINARY RESEARCH INTO COMMUNITY INTERVENTION AND POLICY

An opportunity to implement TD action research arose following the completion of the UC Irvine TTURC, a five-year NIH-funded Transdisciplinary Tobacco Use Research Center.[1] The Robert Wood Johnson Foundation funded an initiative to facilitate the translation of transdisciplinary tobacco research into tobacco control policy to ensure that the TTURC research would ultimately impact public policy. Some of the authors of this paper (who were TTURC researchers) decided to participate and lead the creation and tracking of the UC Irvine (UCI) Tobacco Policy Consortium (TPC). Established in 2003, the two-year TPC was a university-community collaborative partnership comprised of UCI tobacco use researchers (all faculty members of the

TTURC) and community decision makers, including schoolteachers, school administrators, representatives of government agencies, and directors of nonprofit organizations and private foundations.

Our approach to translating tobacco research into public policy initiatives included organizational strategies focusing on both intellectual and social integration. The findings from earlier studies of scientific collaboration[11, 38, 39] highlight the substantial influence of interpersonal processes on the effectiveness of scientists' efforts to integrate their diverse perspectives and research ideas. Stylistic, cognitive, and status-related differences between researchers and community members can derail a collaboration. Altman[11] discusses a variety of circumstances that can strain relationships between researchers and community members. In general, academics and community collaborators may have different, or even clashing, worldviews, values, and time orientations. Community decision makers tend to require much less data and information before committing to action, and they prefer a shorter time frame for taking action. Community decision makers want to work with information that they can use more immediately to change policies and programs.

Furthermore, a major impediment during the early and later stages of university-community collaborations is perceived status differences between researchers and community members.[11] To achieve more effective, sustained collaborations, status differentials and other potential barriers to effective communication need to be confronted and resolved. Without recognizing and removing these communication barriers, conflict can escalate and impede the productivity of the collaboration.

Conflict appears to be an inherent feature of collaboration, and many scholars have argued that it is a normal prerequisite for achieving collaborative success. Tuckman's storming model[39] describes the role of conflict in small groups as they go through the following developmental stages: forming, storming, norming, and performing. When group members join together (usually as strangers), the group begins by "forming" and orienting to one another and getting to know more about other members. The second stage is the "storming" stage when groups experience conflict and polarization around interpersonal issues (e.g., status resentment and power imbalances), and group members may respond emotionally, rather than rationally, when working on tasks. The "norming" stage occurs when cohesiveness develops, along with an in-group feeling. In this stage, new status roles and performance standards are set. "Performing" is the final stage when group members channel their energy into completing tasks. The group's main issues of structure, leadership, and norms are resolved so that participants can work together more effectively. According to Tuckman, groups may repeat these stages at any point.

Both Altman's and Tuckman's conceptual models, outlined above, informed the programmatic strategies adopted by the Tobacco Policy Consortium. Also, empirical findings from Fuqua[33] suggested that conflict impedes effective, smooth-running collaboration. In the study of two groups of tobacco researchers from the TTURCs, the group with minimal conflict was more effective in achieving positive research outcomes than the group with a great deal of conflict, as described elsewhere.[33, 36] The conflicted group had a general social climate that was more formal and more negative than the nonconflicted group. In general, it is unclear whether a positive social climate is an essential condition for successful intellectual integration and intellectual products. Nonetheless, it seems that positive social integration following a "storming" phase can help a group move toward the "norming" stage and, eventually, a "performing" stage.[39] Note that Tuckman's[39] model implies that simply having a positive social climate without some initial "storming" could be an indicator of a complacent, underperforming group that never realizes its full potential.

Collaborations seem to vary along at least two dimensions: social integration and intellectual integration.[36, 37] As shown in Table 8.1, the low and high levels along these dimensions suggest four types of collaboration: high social integration and high intellectual integration; low social integration and low intellectual integration; high social integration and low intellectual integration; and low social integration and high intellectual integration. The TPC was designed to support both social and intellectual integration of ideas between university researchers and community members with the goal of achieving high levels on both dimensions.

Specifically, the TPC conferences among university researchers and community practitioners were structured to encourage several facets of social integration, including informality, friendliness, building consensus, and mutual trust. Ample time was allotted for introductions among people, unstructured (and structured) discussion, and informal communication during meetings, breaks, and meals. In summary, both the intellectual and social components of the TPC were designed to maximize the potential for intellectual integration of policy ideas and to minimize the potential for any damaging interpersonal conflict. Details of the study design follow.

The next sections provide a summary of the intellectual components of the TPC and the methods with which collaborative processes and outcomes were empirically assessed.

TABLE 8.1. **Types of Collaboration Reflecting Different Levels of Social and Intellectual Integration among Participants**

		Intellectual integration	
		Low	High
Social integration	Low	Social and intellectual nonintegration	Asocial intellectual integration
	High	Social support without intellectual integration	Socially supported intellectual integration

Applying Transdisciplinary Action Research Principles to the Design of Collaborative Conferences

Seven half-day conferences were organized over two years at University of California, Irvine (UCI) to identify ways of translating university-based research into innovative tobacco control policies and programs. At the conferences, UCI TTURC scientists presented their research to participating community members and led discussions about how their research might be translated into effective strategies for preventing teen smoking. For example, one group of researchers presented data about critical periods during early adolescent rat brain development indicating that animals are more susceptible to developing nicotine addiction during adolescence than during early childhood or later adulthood. Other research was presented that examined the physical, social, affective, and dispositional contexts of adolescent smoking behaviors. As part of that research, teens answered questions regarding where, when, and with whom they smoke, as well as regarding their mood states before and after smoking. Anger and depression were reported to be positively related to smoking urges among adolescents. The researchers suggested that prophylactic pharmacotherapy for treating anger and depression (e.g., administering medications to nicotine-susceptible youth) could protect against future tobacco use, especially among adolescents with attention deficit hyperactivity disorder (ADHD) who may be medicating themselves with tobacco products.

During conferences 1, 2, and 3, participants introduced themselves, and overviews of university tobacco research and U.S. tobacco control policies were presented. A large portion of conference time was reserved for discussing the significance of the research as well as for brainstorming possible tobacco control strategies aimed at reducing adolescent substance use. During conferences 4 and 5, four TPC subgroups, comprised of diverse researcher and community member participants, were tasked with developing new strategies for reducing adolescent tobacco use. Drawing on earlier research and their professional expertise, members of each subgroup spent a majority of their time talking about possible tobacco control strategies, refining their ideas, and later presenting their strategies to the consortium at large. Following conference 5, the consortium staff compiled a Program Appraisal Survey designed to measure participants' reactions to and relative preferences for the four tobacco policy proposals that emerged from the subgroup discussions.

During conference 6, consortium participants evaluated the various proposals. Certain disagreements about the proposed policy initiatives surfaced with some consortium members opting out of further meetings. For example, the possibility of administering prophylactic medications to reduce adolescents' susceptibility to nicotine addiction prompted vigorous debate. One group advocated giving adolescents various kinds of psychotherapy and pharmacotherapy, whereas another group strongly disagreed with *ever* providing adolescents with any type of tobacco control medications. Following conference 6, some consortium members expressed their discouragement about these disagreements. The consortium staff developed a proposal for a seventh conference with the goal of regaining the consortium's collaborative momentum. Ultimately, conference 7 was held and two tobacco control initiatives were endorsed by consortium members: (a) the creation of a Grants-in-Aid program, providing funds for local tobacco policy efforts that reflected consortium members' ideas and (b) the development and refinement of a research and policy brief geared toward informing local, state, and national policymakers about recent scientific findings related to teen tobacco use and control.

Discussions at many of the conferences generated comments about the important facilitators of and impediments to tobacco control. Participants' conversations focused on the relevance of the scientific research to the unique tobacco policy concerns of consortium members. As described in greater detail later, consortium members included a diverse array of community practitioners ranging from middle and high school principals and teachers to the leaders of nongovernmental organizations and staff members from the offices of local elected officials. Members' attitudes and thoughts about the links between scientific research and public policy, and about their collaboration in general, were captured using a variety of assessment methods, including participant observation, attitude questionnaires, and personal interviews.

Tracking the Intellectual and Social Developments: Assessment of the Collaboration

Assessments were conducted regularly to record specific collaborative processes, including the attitudinal shifts that occurred among TPC members over the course of the project. There were two foci of assessment: (a) members' *attitudes toward tobacco control strategies* (which were suggested and refined by members during the conferences) and (b) members' shifting *attitudes and reactions to the collaborations* that they engaged in over seven half-day conferences. Several new quantitative and qualitative measures, described next, were developed and administered at repeated intervals to evaluate collaborative processes and outcomes.

Collaborative Activities Index   The Collaborative Activities Index includes seven items to assess how often individual consortium members engage in cross-disciplinary activities such as attending conferences outside their respective disciplines, obtaining new insights into one's own work through discussion with individuals from other fields, and establishing new links with colleagues from different disciplinary orientations that may lead to future collaborative work. The response options range on a 7-point scale from "never" to "weekly."

Perspectives on Transdisciplinary Collaboration   The seven-item Perspectives on Transdisciplinary Collaboration Scale includes 5-point Likert scales that assess individuals' values and attitudes toward transdisciplinary collaboration (e.g., "In my own work, I typically incorporate perspectives from fields and disciplinary orientations that are different from my own"). The scale also assesses attitudes toward the UCI TPC, with items such as "I believe that UCI TPC members are open-minded considering perspectives from fields other than their own" and "I believe that a high level of goodwill exists among the members of the UCI TPC."

Perspectives on Scientific Research and Professional Practice The Perspectives on Scientific Research and Professional Practice Scale includes semantic differential scales that ask one subgroup (community members) to indicate their impressions of the other subgroup (research scientists), and vice versa. To gauge members of the two subgroups' impressions of each other, scale items include pairs of bipolar adjectives such as idealistic-realistic, arrogant-humble, and patronizing-respectful.

Perspectives on Tobacco Control Strategies The Perspectives on Tobacco Control Strategies Scale assesses respondents' reactions to alternative tobacco control strategies, many of which were suggested by consortium members. The first section includes twenty-one strategies such as "pay organizations to ban/limit tobacco use," "provide medication to youth to curb their smoking," "alert parents to their child's tobacco and other substance use," and "utilize teachers to administer an adolescent tobacco use prevention intervention." Participants are asked to rate their receptivity to each strategy on a 5-point scale ranging from 1 ("not at all receptive") to 5 ("very receptive").

The second section assesses consortium members' perceptions of the barriers to and facilitators of various tobacco control strategies. Participants read descriptions of several tobacco control strategies and are instructed to rate the extent to which each strategy was feasible, effective, beneficial, favorable, and likely to have negative effects on a set of 5-point Likert scales. Participants also are prompted to write in any beneficial or detrimental consequences they think might be associated with each of the alternative tobacco control strategies.

Program Appraisal Survey The Program Appraisal Survey assesses consortium members' attitudes toward the four tobacco prevention initiatives that were proposed, discussed, and refined by consortium members during previous conferences. The theoretical framework for the survey is derived from affective-cognitive consistency theory.[40] The theory describes how the perceived benefits and costs associated with a particular concept (e.g., a tobacco control policy such as imposing a cigarette sales tax) combine to determine an individual's overall attitude toward the concept. By assessing how negatively or positively an individual feels about potential outcomes linked to a particular concept as well as how likely those outcomes are, a numerical index of the respondent's overall attitude toward a concept (e.g., cigarette tax) is derived. For example, a potential outcome of "increasing sales tax" might be "the emergence of a strong tobacco black market." An individual may feel that such an outcome is unlikely but so undesirable that he or she develops a strongly negative attitude toward the concept of increasing cigarette taxes.

On the Program Appraisal Survey, individuals are instructed to read and evaluate four 1–2 paragraph consortium-generated proposals and action plans. A sample proposal is "to develop and implement an anger management/hostility reduction/bullying reduction program based on an existing nationally recognized exemplar program and determine its effectiveness for reducing alcohol, tobacco, and other substance use." After reviewing each proposal, respondents assess the likelihood and desirability of potential short-term outcomes (e.g., easy for program administrators to implement), intermediate-term outcomes (e.g., increased program funding), and long-term outcomes (e.g., reduction in risky behaviors). Respondents rate the likelihood of each outcome on a scale ranging from 1 to 7 with 1 being "very unlikely" and 7 being "very likely." They also rate the relative desirability of each outcome on a scale ranging from –7 being "very undesirable" to +7 being "very desirable."

Interim Interview Questions   Individualized interviews were conducted with consortium members by phone or in person at participants' respective offices during the interim periods separating the seven half-day conferences. The qualitative interview questions are designed to assess participants' attitudes toward several topics, including the quality of TPC members' collaboration, personal attributes of their fellow collaborators, particular tobacco control strategies, and potential barriers to and facilitators of tobacco control strategies. Some questions are highly open-ended, such as, "Thinking back on the first conference, what stands out in your memory?" Other questions are more specific to factors influencing tobacco control strategies, such as, "What are the most important barriers to implementing tobacco prevention programs and policies at your local schools/community?" Other questions assess participants' goals and motivations, such as, "At this point in the project, what are you hoping to get out of your involvement? What's going to keep you interested and involved?" Questions about the collaboration include "Has your attitude about this project changed since you first heard about it (neutral, more negative, or more positive)?" and "Has your comfort level interacting with UCI researchers increased, decreased, or stayed the same?" For the latter question, community members are asked about "UCI researchers," and UCI researchers are asked about "community members."

Data Collection Schedule   Measures were administered at various times during the seven conferences and in the interim periods between conferences (Table 8.2).

TABLE 8.2.   Data Collection Schedule

Measure	Purpose	Dates administered
Collaborative activities index	Investigation of individuals' cross-disciplinary and collaborative activities	3 time points: Conference 1, 4, 6
Perspectives on transdisciplinary collaboration	Assessment of thoughts about the consortium and about transdisciplinary collaboration in general	4 time points: Conference 1, 6, and 2 interim time points

(Continued)

TABLE 8.2. *(Continued)*

Measure	Purpose	Dates administered
Perspectives on scientific research and professional practice	Rating of impressions of consortium members (i.e., "researchers" and "community members") using semantic differential scales	5 time points: Conference 2, 4, 6, and Professional Practice and 1 interim time point
Perspectives on tobacco control strategies	Investigation of receptiveness to 21 tobacco control strategies to understand barriers and facilitators of tobacco control	4 time points: Conference 1, 6, and 2 interim time points
Program appraisal survey	Evaluation of attitudes toward four consortium-generated tobacco prevention initiatives, including assessment of the desirability and likelihood of potential outcomes of each initiative	Conference 5
Open-ended interim interviews	Assessment of attitudes toward the consortium, transdisciplinary collaboration, tobacco control strategies, barriers, and facilitators	Between all conferences

FACTORS FACILITATING OR IMPEDING COLLABORATION AMONG TPC MEMBERS

An analysis of the antecedent factors that facilitated or constrained collaboration, as well as the processes and tangible outcomes that occurred over the course of the collaboration, is presented next. This analysis, informed by our empirical case study of the TPC, may help shed light on ways to enhance collaboration effectiveness in future university-community partnerships. Our study of the TPC revealed a number of *antecedent* factors (situational circumstances that were in place at the outset of the collaboration) as well as ongoing collaborative *processes* (which occurred over the course of the two-year TPC project) that may have influenced the collaborative *outcomes* or products of the consortium.

Antecedent Factors

Initial Outlook   Overall, TPC members demonstrated a rather *friendly, optimistic, and enthusiastic outlook toward the collaboration and fellow team members.* Participants were impressed with the expertise, energy, and wealth of knowledge possessed by the members of the group. Survey data indicated that members generally maintained a consistently positive attitude (with some fluctuations over time in both upward and downward directions) and a shared commitment to the TPC collaboration punctuated by occasional expressions of conflict and tension. Perhaps the ways in which individuals were selected for membership in the TPC contributed to the group's generally positive social climate. The consortium coordinator handpicked several community members who were invited to join the TPC based on her positive collaborative experiences with them in prior years (e.g., as fellow employees of the Irvine Unified School District and various nonprofit health promotion organizations in Orange County, California). This selection and invitation process may have strengthened the group's willingness to attend and participate in the seven half-day conferences of the TPC and to accomplish what was expected of them during those meetings.

At the same time, all members throughout the TPC project did not sustain a positive initial outlook. In fact, at the sixth conference, many community members expressed a more negative and pessimistic view (particularly when they left the conference feeling that they had not achieved implementable action plans or other major accomplishments near the end of the project period). These negative feelings, expressed at the end of the sixth conference, were corroborated in follow-up interviews conducted with community members of the TPC between the sixth and seventh conferences. Interestingly, community members' negative appraisal of the TPC's accomplishments following the sixth conference was replaced by a more optimistic evaluation of the team's achievements following the seventh and final conference. The more optimistic view may have arisen because, during their final meeting, TPC members reviewed and approved a Research and Policy Brief on Preventing Teen Smoking and agreed on plans to widely circulate the brief to legislators and health promotion organizations at local, state, and national levels. They also agreed to establish a TPC Grants-in-Aid Program with the remaining project funds to help support local community efforts to implement smoking prevention programs aimed at reducing tobacco use among adolescents.

Disciplinary and Professional Scope   The TPC collaboration was established with a membership composition representing a diversity of disciplines and professions. The UCI TTURC center, which spawned the TPC, encompassed a broad array of scientific disciplines ranging from neuroscience to health policy research. This breadth of disciplinary perspectives within the UCI TTURC created difficulties and challenges for diverse researchers trying to work together across multiple disciplinary boundaries.[33, 37]

When the multidisciplinary members of the TTURC joined forces with even more diverse professionals from the community to establish the TPC, collaborative challenges became even more pronounced. School principals, politicians' staff, funding agents, police officers, medical doctors, and others found themselves trying to understand each other's jargon, values, working styles, and goals. TPC members did not share the same language. For example, statistical methods for analyzing survey data and terms such as *psychopharmacogenetic* approaches to studying nicotine addiction were unfamiliar to many community-based members of the TPC. As another example, when a UCI tobacco scientist presented his research on computer modeling of tobacco use, some community members felt frustrated that they were left without understanding any practical implications of the reported findings.

Researchers Versus Community Members   Experiences of frustration arising from TPC members' attempts to communicate across disciplinary and professional boundaries led some nonuniversity participants to conclude early on that the consortium discussions might be beneficial to researchers but not to community members. At times, there was a feeling that researchers were part of one camp who shared a common perspective (e.g., the importance of basic and theoretical science) and that community members were part of another camp who shared a dissimilar perspective (e.g., the importance of bidirectional discussions leading directly to the application of scientific knowledge to the development of programs aimed at preventing or reducing teen tobacco use in the local community). These contrasting perspectives may have arisen from preexisting attitudes in which community members and researchers did not view each other as "equals" (i.e., as having equivalent status) in the TPC partnership.

Often, members revealed during conference discussions (and in their interview and survey comments) that they did not share agreement on what the TPC's priorities were for tobacco prevention and control, and they also recognized that their views on the group's priorities were dauntingly diverse. Researchers believed that more basic and theoretical research was an important goal and that the dissemination and translation of their findings into smoking prevention programs might take years to develop. In contrast, community members wanted to establish short-term, practically oriented programs based on tobacco use research that would quickly benefit the constituents in their own organizations and geographic region. As an example of these diverse perspectives, a researcher prioritized understanding brain sensitivity to nicotine in rats, whereas a police officer emphasized the need to round up more truant teens and get them back in school because truants are often seen smoking. Over the course of the TPC conferences, researchers' and community members' perspectives on tobacco control priorities became more similar as a result of repeated brainstorming sessions and collective discussions of the TPC's priorities. They began to share views on which directions were the most promising for tobacco control in their local communities and organizations.

Professional Goals   Group members' diverse educational and occupational backgrounds meant that their individual *professional goals* and the criteria for promotion in their own jobs were not interdependent, which made it difficult to develop a shared conceptual and programmatic framework for achieving consortium goals. For example, a neuroscientist, a school principal, and a police officer are rewarded in their workplaces for very different reasons. A university-based scientist is promoted for publishing high-quality research in prestigious academic journals and not for making a difference in the number of teens who smoke. A principal of an elementary or middle school is rewarded for developing innovative educational programs that can be touted to school board members and parents. A tobacco use prevention focus per se is less important than demonstrating gains in students' achievement exam scores. School principals' priorities for tobacco control tended to have an educational slant whereby students would learn about math and biology while working on homework or classroom assignments pertaining to tobacco-related problems. Alternatively, police officers are promoted by their departments for being able to demonstrate how they keep the peace and ensure the safety of community members; for example, focusing on truants and getting them back in school may be their highest priority.

Some consortium members' *professions* do not require or foster *collaborative skills* as a basis for achieving their professional goals. Community members may be more accustomed to collaborative roles as part of their work, whereas academicians are more accustomed to pursuing independence and leadership in their jobs as they administer their own labs and write their own papers.

Lack of Shared Intermediate Goals   A barrier that prevented the TPC from achieving an implied goal of self-sustained collaboration and demonstrable reduction in tobacco use was the *lack of shared "intermediate goals"* (or short-term goals) *in the structure of the consortium.* Members knew that their participation required that they come to conferences (for which they received a small stipend), listen attentively at the conferences (or give a talk if they were researchers), and participate in activities (e.g., brainstorming sessions and discussions of tobacco control strategies). The structure of the collaboration did not require that certain milestones or goals had to be met along the way. There was no accountability for a product, except among the TPC organizers and researchers, who developed activities to ensure achievement of most of the consortium's stated goals. Community-based members of the TPC were not required by their organizations to demonstrate products or report on successes. Although members were expected to work toward the goal of translating tobacco research into evidence-based smoking prevention programs and policies during each of the seven conferences, they were not directly accountable individually for doing so. Only the university-based organizers were responsible and accountable to the funding organization, the Robert Wood Johnson Foundation, for demonstrating positive outcomes (which they did in their yearly reports).

Collaborative Processes

Some members felt that a disconnect existed between the university researchers and the community members, noting disparities in their communication styles, life experiences, and "worldviews." The process by which researchers presented themselves at the TPC conferences may have exacerbated community members' preexisting attitudes about the shortcomings of university-based researchers. Community members commented after the first and sixth conferences that some researchers' style of lecturing and "pontificating" without listening during information sharing was not helpful to the group dynamics. Community members had slightly more negative views of university researchers than the researchers had of community members. Many community members did not feel the collaboration was equitable or bidirectional. Over time, however, they came to view the researchers as more receptive and more progressive, as reflected in the gradual shifts toward more positive attitudes that were observed in the repeated-measures analyses of survey and interview data.

To facilitate the development of strategies for translating tobacco research into policy innovations, a series of structured activities were included in the agenda and format of each half-day conference. As noted previously, there were structured times scheduled for members to listen to reports of UCI studies on nicotine addiction and tobacco use and to engage in extended discussions of the research findings and their possible implications for developing improved tobacco control strategies. Structured time was allocated for members to participate in guided, interactive discussions and activities that fostered a synthesis of the university research findings and the development of tobacco control strategies. Specifically, members were organized into small groups that regularly met in conferences to share their ideas about translating tobacco research into improved smoking prevention policies. Furthermore, unstructured time was provided for informal conversations among team members and the development of social capital. Usually, a meal was provided, and people had time to socialize and get to know one another informally.

These activities and the structure of the consortium involved relatively little conflict compared to some other collaborations involving primarily university scientists.[33,37] The substantive focus and organizational structure of TPC meetings may have fostered the generally positive social climate observed at most of the TPC conferences and as evidenced in participants' survey and interview data. The fact that the discussions never required members to determine how to share resources or give up some of their own resources may have been a facilitator of the cooperative atmosphere of TPC meetings as well.

Yet, as noted earlier, there were times when *frustrations and misunderstandings* occurred. Most noticeably, after the sixth TPC conference, members felt frustrated, and a tone of pessimism was evident in survey responses and interview comments. At this conference, community members were surprised to be asked who would volunteer to continue the collaboration beyond the formal funding period of the TPC project and about who would write grants or otherwise commit to working toward the continuation of TPC activities. They did not expect to commit to additional responsibilities by the end of the sixth conference. Furthermore, members assumed that this conference would be the last one, and they were hoping to feel a collective sense of achievement. Instead, community members seemed to feel confirmation of their original concerns about the "hit and run" style of university researchers—that, after two years, the TPC had not provided them with any "take-home" products and information that they could immediately use in their professional roles and that their time and energy were only benefiting the university scientists.

Several months passed before a seventh TPC conference was convened. The tone at that final meeting, in contrast to the sixth conference, was once again decidedly positive and optimistic as members were invited to work together toward refining a draft of the TPC Research and Policy Brief, which had been drafted by a subgroup of TPC members between the sixth and seventh conferences.[1] Also, a new TPC Grants-in-Aid Program was announced at the seventh conference, and community members of the TPC were invited to apply for consulting funds to be used toward the development and implementation of tobacco control programs initiated by their respective organizations. Thus, by the end of the seventh TPC conference, members began to envision a tangible pathway: the widespread distribution of the Research and Policy Brief to legislators and health policy organizations, through which their collaborative efforts over the two-year project period would be translated into a specific tobacco control strategy.

Collaborative Outcomes

Accomplishment of Stated Goals   Overall, the UCI TTURC Tobacco Policy Consortium (TPC) was successful in accomplishing the major goals of the consortium as outlined in the proposal to the Robert Wood Johnson Foundation. First, the TPC was established and sustained over the two-year project period. Approximately twenty-five community decision makers and five TTURC scientists participated in each of the seven TPC conferences. The consortium was unique in its interdisciplinary, interprofessional, and multisectoral composition with various sectors of the community including educational and public health organizations represented. Second, new research findings emerging from the UCI TTURC were collectively synthesized through TPC discussions and activities designed to facilitate university-community dialogue and collaboration. Novel ideas—some readier for implementation than others—were generated to guide the translation of UCI TTURC research findings into community programs that would benefit adolescents residing in the Orange County region. These collaborative ideas were formulated into specific "targets of translation," which was the fourth goal of the consortium.

In addition, the consortium identified institutional/cultural facilitators and barriers to implementing innovative TD approaches aimed at tobacco use prevention and reduction among adolescents. Specifically, participants were asked the following questions: (a) "What are the most important barriers and facilitators to implementing tobacco prevention programs and policies in your local schools and communities?" (b) "In what ways do you think parents, teachers, students, and others can facilitate or hinder collaborative anti-tobacco efforts?" Despite a wide range of responses, participants overwhelmingly agreed that the most important barriers to implementation were (a) competing educational priorities for schools; (b) limited resources, including money, time, and staff; and (c) limited program evaluation research demonstrating the most effective community strategies for preventing and reducing smoking. Key facilitators of effective collaboration and implementation of innovative policies and programs included (a) highly committed volunteers and leaders; (b) scientific research providing clear and empirically validated insights into the sources of teen smoking; (c) creative partnerships among schools, public agencies, and community organizations for streamlining collaborative efforts; (d) peer-to-peer education about and involvement in tobacco control strategies; and (e) the development of evidence-based and demonstrably effective policies for preventing or reducing teen smoking.

Participants also pointed out several ways in which parents and schools can influence the development and implementation of innovative tobacco control strategies. For instance, parents may hinder implementation because of their beliefs that tobacco is no longer a pressing issue due to the gains made in California statewide tobacco control and that, therefore, their children are not at risk for tobacco use. School districts may hinder implementation of tobacco control programs in the classroom due to the "No Child Left Behind" law, which has raised standards for each child to test well on educational achievement tests and, thereby, has relegated health-related curricula to a much lower priority than instruction in areas such as math, science, and English. Health education is often superficial and inadequate in K–12 schools. At the same time, parents may foster implementation of smoking prevention programs owing to their desire to raise healthy children and their support of schools' efforts to achieve broader educational goals beyond the required standards for enhancing children's academic development. Schools, too, may foster implementation if they support the idea of teaching children to be healthy and if administrators and school districts believe in tobacco control.

Over the course of their collaboration, TPC members identified potential targets of translation for community-based tobacco control strategies, especially those building on and incorporating the scientific findings from UCI TTURC studies of nicotine addiction and tobacco use. The four major targets of translation identified by TPC members for possible implementation in the community are outlined here.

1. Via *DVD or Web site,* provide diagnostic assessment of vulnerabilities to nicotine addiction and tobacco use based on an individual's assets and resources. Based on a decisional algorithm, assign appropriate treatment modules that match individual students' and their family's needs. Create versions for both parents and children.

2. Develop a *consensus statement* such as a research and policy brief to inform various groups (ad/marketing campaigns, schools, legislative bodies) about evidence-based tobacco control strategies. Provide an avenue for youth involvement. Publish the consensus statement in multiple print and electronic venues.

3. Develop an *anger management,* hostility, and bullying reduction program based on an existing exemplary program and evaluate its effectiveness for reducing tobacco use. Offer schools monetary incentives for participation.

4. Develop a *three-pronged approach* to (a) teach children the *best practices* of emotion regulation, impulse control, and decision making; (b) monitor high-risk children and adolescents; and (c) collaborate with community centers that offer health, cooking, life skills, and physical activity programs to develop integrative and effective school health programs.

As an elaboration of the second target of translation just noted, TPC members chose to develop and disseminate a Research and Policy Brief on Preventing Teen Smoking. UCI TTURC research was presented and synthesized, and specific directions for tobacco control policy innovations were presented in the brief.[1] Three thousand briefs were distributed to local, state, and national policy and decision makers. The impact on future smoking prevention policies and programs has not yet been assessed.

Finally, the consortium allocated grants-in-aid funding to support local professionals and decision makers in their efforts to launch and sustain evidence-based programs for preventing and reducing teen smoking. Community decision makers and organizational leaders proposed and implemented a variety of programs supported by the TPC Grants-in-Aid program that they felt would be most useful and effective for their constituents. One program was an education and discussion session series in which counselors and at-risk adolescents discussed positive emotional outlets and alternatives to risk-taking behaviors such as smoking. Another initiative, the "Dude, Where Are My Lungs?" program, devised a plan for high school students to mentor younger students and work together to create an educational play incorporating the findings from UCI TTURC research. Audience members, who would be the tobacco control message recipients, included not only adolescents but also younger students and family members. In addition, a new adolescent smoking prevention research pilot study and related affect management training program based on earlier UCI TTURC research were funded and implemented.

Falling Short of Achieving Full Potential   Still, the consortium fell short of achieving its full potential. Specifically, it did not become a self-sustained collaboration that demonstrated reduced tobacco use among teens. To date, consortium members have not met yet again as a group. The consortium did not demonstrate or achieve its implicit longer term goal: to reduce tobacco use among adolescents in a sustained manner. Why did this not occur? The original goals of the consortium did not explicitly include the long-term goal of sustaining the collaboration, and there were negligible funds, time, and support to do so once the foundation-funded project period ended.

Moreover, the multidisciplinary and professional diversity of team members meant that their individualized and dissimilar professional goals were not conducive to sustaining collaboration once the TPC project formally ended. Community members, understandably, did not commit to doing more to sustain the collaboration beyond the two-year funding period. Without a longer time frame, there was little opportunity to translate research ideas into local community interventions. Perhaps initial expectations should have been set so that members would sustain the collaboration on their own, and more time and funding should have been granted to allow members to continue their multisectoral collaboration.

To promote sustained collaboration, institutional incentives could have been sought for the consortium members. Researchers could have sought administrative buy-in through course releases and greater institutional recognition of the value of interdisciplinary collaboration in faculty promotion processes. For community members, monetary incentives for attending, the potential to be associated with other well-respected people at a major university, and the possibility of gaining firsthand knowledge about the latest research that might help them in their jobs may have prompted community members to attend TPC conferences, but additional incentives were needed to sustain longer term collaboration. Community agencies could have found ways to release their representatives to spend more time on the collaboration. If these had been part of the goals of the consortium, then perhaps it would have been more likely to survive after the Robert Wood Johnson Foundation funding was expended.

Finally, the relatively short time frame of the collaboration (two years) made it difficult for members to make a demonstrable impact on public health. Years, not months, may be required to realize the public health benefits of scientific research that has been effectively disseminated and translated into improved community interventions and outcomes, such as reductions in population levels of adolescent smoking. Perhaps ten, twenty, or more years are needed to recognize the long-term impact on public health.[41,42] The consortium enabled members to begin the process of generating novel ideas that could lead to long-term public health benefits over time, but tracking such ideas and outcomes would require a significantly longer period than two years.

In some ways, the TPC project might be better characterized as a "precollaboration" rather than a fully functioning collaboration. That is, it might be more accurate to characterize the consortium as a group just getting started during the initial phase of collaboration when planning begins but difficult decisions and conflict have not arisen. The TPC was, after all, an informal group whose members did not have to sacrifice much time, funds, or other resources to participate. Members did not spend much time making difficult decisions about whom the leaders would be, how funds would be spent, and whose ideas were worthy of being implemented in the future. TPC participants did not face major concerns about whether individual members were being treated respectfully and fairly, whether individuals were meeting the expectations and norms of the group, or whether they would be willing to devote more of their resources toward continuing the collaboration. Their regular work outside the collaboration was not affected particularly negatively or positively by their participation in the consortium. Members were not required to be accountable, by their employers or the consortium organizers, to achieve positive outcomes. Some time was spent at meetings focusing on creating tobacco control *ideas* collaboratively in subgroups, but most of the collaborative ideas were not translated into new *policies and programs* by the end of the collaboration. There was no requirement to actually implement the TPC members' ideas. In fact, when given an incentive and a quick deadline to submit a grant proposal for funds, members chose to drop the more ambitious ideas they had originally generated in consortium subgroups. Instead, they opted to propose programmatic ideas that would more quickly and directly benefit their unique constituents. For example, instead of pursuing the idea of spending weeks reviewing best practices for tobacco control in school settings, a school principal in the TPC proposed a tobacco control plan that tied in with his/her curriculum goals and that could be implemented immediately during the next semester.

IMPLICATIONS AND ADDITIONAL LESSONS LEARNED FROM THE TPC STUDY

This case study of the UC Irvine Tobacco Policy Consortium (TPC) identifies factors that facilitated or hindered the collaborative efforts of university and community partners working to reduce teen smoking. Presented here are several "lessons learned" that focus on improving future university-community collaborations and enhancing the "science of team science" field in general. Suggestions for further study also are presented.

Cycles of Emotional Storm and Calm Influence Group Motivation and Performance

One lesson learned relates to identifying cyclical affective processes during collaboration. For example, the initial observations of the TPC collaboration were positive, meaning that members rated their attitudes toward the TPC favorably, and informal observations corroborated their positivity. Some later observations, however, were more negative, followed by attitudinal improvements later on, suggesting a cyclical nature to the collaborative process. Times of moving forward or backward for the TPC included initial reports of optimism and enthusiasm at the beginning of the collaboration, followed by frustration and skepticism at the conclusion of the sixth conference, and finally, cycling back to a positive social climate and sense of achievement at the end of the seventh conference emanating from certain tangible collaborative achievements—especially, the completion of the TPC's Tobacco Policy Brief and distribution of the TPC grants-in-aid for selected tobacco control projects. As is evident from our observations of the TPC, there are affective ups and downs that shape or color collaborative processes. Understanding personal as well as group motivations and acknowledging the importance of personal as well as group feelings about specific shared goals are essential for improving team collaborations during the transdisciplinary action research cycle.

Understanding Professional or Academic Jargon Requires Time

A second lesson pertains to the difficulties of learning the *lingua franca* (professional terminology) of co-collaborators who represent diverse disciplines and professional fields. The wide scope of the academic and professional backgrounds covering a broad range of experience levels represented in the consortium made for a rich mix of diverse knowledge and perspectives. With such diversity, it was sometimes difficult to find a common language for understanding tobacco control research. For example, during a nicotine pharmacology research presentation, one TPC community member observed that big "agglutinated" terms like *psychopharmacogenetic* were intimidating and off-putting from a layperson's perspective. Over time, professional terminology and academic disciplinary jargon may be gradually demystified and defined. The extra time it takes to explain new terms may be warranted, however, to reduce the risk of alienating fellow collaborators who feel lost in a sea of jargon. Whereas the TPC members each had time to inquire about terms they did not understand, team collaborations must also consider the type and prevalence of jargon that is used throughout collaborative discussions.

Developing Realistic Expectations Helps
Achieve Intended Group Processes and Outcomes

A third lesson learned relates to choosing carefully the goals as well as the administrative tasks requested of the collaborators. Individuals entered the consortium with certain assumptions about key collaborative goals and administrative tasks. For community members, the assumed goals included developing new tobacco control strategies, and the assumed tasks included meeting over a two-year period to contribute their views about research priorities. For the university members, the assumed goals included developing an understanding of community partners' research priorities, and the tasks included assessing community members' views about those priorities. On the surface, the consortium goals and administrative tasks were obvious and useful. Upon deeper analysis, some community members complained about feeling like a number in a large research study when they were interviewed about their views or asked to complete a variety of surveys during or after each conference. Even though the surveys were framed as being necessary for understanding collaboration between community representatives and university researchers, completing surveys was considered an activity that had less benefit when compared to spending time on generating new tobacco control programs or policies.

Thus, it is important to establish realistic expectations early on about time commitment and how long various components of the collaboration will take to complete in light of members' shared goals. Addressing member expectations about the timeline needed for achieving project outcomes is vital for success in any team science collaboration. TPC members could have been warned, for instance, that part of their time would be spent completing surveys and doing small group brainstorming. Furthermore, they could have been told that it might be difficult to create simple, low-cost tobacco control programs, given the limited duration of the conference. Such forewarning may have resulted in fewer complaints about how much time was devoted to administrative activities and less disillusionment about reaching consensus on tobacco control programs or policies.

Small-Group Activities Foster Shared Views and Build Essential Social Capital

Another lesson learned relates to establishing a structured set of group activities designed for sharing viewpoints, both personal and professional, regarding the value of various tobacco control programs, policy, and research. For example, time was allocated in the TPC for interactive, small group discussions when members talked about ideas for tobacco control strategies. The discussions, coupled with the unstructured time during meals, provided opportunities for sharing and explaining perspectives. Uniformly, the most valued activities were the ones that allowed for developing social capital and establishing a common ground for discourse.[43] Time to foster shared views was necessary due to the differences between the professional goals of the community members and the researchers. During small group sessions, community members focused on practical questions such as, "How do we enroll more students in after school smoking cessation programs?" In contrast, university members often focused on research questions such as, "How do we recruit more students to participate in our research study?" Furthermore, community members did not always appreciate the style of university researchers feeling that they tended to "pontificate" while neglecting practical community needs. Despite their differences, all TPC members reported highly valuing and appreciating the time and activities devoted to getting to know the viewpoints of fellow consortium members. One strong recommendation for fostering collaboration emerging from this case study is to emphasize small group interactions that encourage dialogue and allow ample time for all participants to express their views.

In conclusion, the lessons learned from this case study of the TPC speak to identifying program structures for motivating collaboration when team members have very diverse backgrounds and experience levels. The science of team science should look toward deepening the understanding of transdisciplinary scientific collaboration at all phases of the transdisciplinary research cycle.[2, 44]

FUTURE DIRECTIONS

Antecedent Conditions That Warrant Further Study

Understanding antecedent conditions that exist before a transdisciplinary scientific collaboration begins must include not only identifying the disciplinary backgrounds of team members but also acknowledging their beliefs and feelings about the project at the outset. For example, if team members participate by virtue of their technical skill, yet they are otherwise uninterested in the project as a whole (e.g., they would rather be working on their own project and resent the extra work posed by team activities), acknowledging their feelings about the project becomes an important antecedent condition. This case study did not examine affective attitudes about the project before it began but rather examined feelings about the project after it commenced. Future studies should explore the degree of motivational buy-in before large, expensive projects begin. One suggestion is to survey members of large teams after they drop out to determine the reasons for their departure. Whereas cyclical processes in team member motivation (e.g., affective ups and downs) are expected in any transdisciplinary scientific collaboration, identifying antecedent motivational factors is worthy of future study.

Collaborative Processes That Should Be Further Investigated

In addition to antecedent conditions, several processes should be studied to enhance the success of future TD scientific collaborations. One process that should be studied focuses on the transfer of knowledge from one discipline or professional background to another. For example, how does the basic vocabulary and theoretical perspectives from the discipline of psychopharmacology get transferred to a youth guidance counselor, and vice versa? What activities are most effective in promoting effective exchanges of disciplinary information? Would completing a series of "basic primers" or seminars serve as a test for prospective members' motivation to participate in a large TD collaboration? And after completing some kind of "continuing professional education" seminar or training module on TD collaboration, would prospective team members still want to participate? Any type of collaboration readiness "audit" should assess factors that facilitate or impede collaboration across disciplinary and professional lines. Such an audit should ensure that the collaboration has (a) clearly defined goals, (b) goals that are perceived to be attainable, and (c) participants who are relatively united across various community interests and agendas.[45–47] Incentives for collaboration also should be assessed because groups with individuals who have clear incentives to collaborate (e.g., grants funding, administrative support) may be more likely to do so.[48]

Another collaborative process worth exploring is the amount of time members perceive as necessary for completing the team project compared to the actual time necessary. For example, Buehler, Griffin, and Ross[49] describe the "planning fallacy" in which people routinely underestimate the time required for task completion. Future studies should explore the degree of underestimation in task completion that occurs during transdisciplinary scientific collaborations.

Collaborative Outcomes That Warrant Further Study

Of equivalent importance to the study of collaborative antecedents and processes is the study of how transdisciplinary scientific outcomes are translated into health-promotive community intervention and widely disseminated.[50] For example, how were the scientific outcomes of a large team project made available to lay audiences that included community practitioners and local decision makers? What are the most effective formats of translational presentations (e.g. book chapter, journal article, lecture, executive policy brief)? What is the longer term impact of the information after it has been translated and distributed widely to community groups? Which group (e.g., lay public to expert) reports benefiting most from the information?

Clearly, future studies of team science and transdisciplinary scientific collaboration must consider a wider range of collaborative antecedents, processes, and outcomes than have been studied in earlier investigations. Evaluation of the long-term impact of collaboration on science, public health, and society also should be evaluated.[44] Two years (the duration of the UCI TPC) is not sufficient time for planning, implementing, and tracking public health outcomes, such as a reduction in adolescent tobacco use in the community. Most collaborative teams funded by government agencies and private foundations tend to last five years or fewer, which typically is not enough time to see science translated into positive outcomes in the community. Through these future, longer term research efforts, we will be better able to strengthen the science and practice of transdisciplinary action research.

Expanding the Field of Transdisciplinary Action Research

In general, transdisciplinary action research is underexplored and should be studied in its own right[2] so that innovative scientific research is translated into policies and programs that benefit society. To promote transdisciplinary scientific collaboration, university-community collaboration, and intersectoral partnerships, a number of broadly conceptualized future directions would be helpful.

Continue Initiatives to Support Transdisciplinary Collaboration   Greater attention and funding will enable future research teams to conduct and study transdisciplinary action research. Already, an increasing number of researchers and agencies are recognizing the need for more information in this rapidly expanding field. Although many funding agents and university administrators acknowledge and verbally support transdisciplinary collaboration, some have taken concrete steps to establish initiatives that financially support transdisciplinary endeavors. For example, at a national level, NIH representatives should continue to support transdisciplinary scientific initiatives through intra-agency collaboration, and efforts to translate research should be strengthened by organizations such as Robert Wood Johnson and Keck Foundations, which have launched large-scale initiatives to promote TD collaboration in science, training, and the translation of knowledge into evidence-based practices and policies.[26, 27]

As transdisciplinary action research (or the science of team science) grows, additional efforts to evaluate the transdisciplinary collaborations are even more essential. Determining how to evaluate transdisciplinary scientific collaboration is difficult. Reliable and valid evaluative metrics need to be developed. A greater understanding of how to best track and evaluate ongoing collaboration is needed. Only minimal empirical work has tracked collaborative processes, generated hypotheses, and tested hypotheses, which would then contribute knowledge that can be used to refine future collaborations and health-promotive public policies.

Increase the Knowledge Base   The current knowledge base of information on transdisciplinary scientific collaborations, university-community collaborations, and intersectoral partnerships needs to be augmented in several respects. The relevant literature can be described, for the most part, as nonexperimental and diffuse (i.e., scattered across different fields and disciplines). Scholars working in multiple fields have published papers on one aspect of the problem. For example, librarians have discussed definitions of disciplines, and physicists have provided retrospective memoirs of their experiences in a collaboration using terms from their discipline, such as centripetal forces. Although fields such as organizational psychology and public health have discussed teamwork and community-based participatory research, they haven't been used widely to improve TD science, training, and translation.[15]

Provide Effective Incentives to Increase Scientists' and Community Partners' Participation   Greater incentives for researchers, community policymakers, and other policymakers to participate in TD collaboration are needed. Grant funding is helpful to attract more people interested in TD collaboration, but additional incentives are needed for community members and researchers. Community members might need more time off from their usual job responsibilities. They need to problem solve how to achieve mutually beneficial goals of their organization while meeting the goals of the collaboration. For example, a principal figured out how to merge tobacco science research results into her new program on physical health by creating a program in which the heart is studied, and the tobacco research is discussed along with the heart. University researchers can determine how to share resources to help community members achieve their goals—for example, arranging university student assistants to help them with their needs or enabling them to speak in classes to bolster their résumés and ties with the university.

Researchers could provide incentives such as course release time, reduced administrative committee responsibilities, and perhaps a sabbatical from departmental responsibilities while they participate in labor-intensive collaborative projects. They might also be encouraged to join university-sponsored organized research units (ORUs) rather than remaining spread across different departments. Also, because researchers must publish to be promoted, greater support for collaborative cross-disciplinary publications is needed. Too often, journal editors are the "gatekeepers" who determine the boundaries of their fields, and they are not sufficiently receptive to cross-disciplinary work. In addition, collaborative, multiauthored publications are sometimes viewed by university promotion committees as less important than single-authored publications. To foster transdisciplinarity, public funding agencies and private foundations should follow the lead of the National Institutes of Health in recognizing multiple principal investigators on the same collaborative project as a basis for distributing research credit more equitably among team members.

Provide Educational Training   Graduate students and staff should be trained in principles of conducting TD action research. They need to be exposed to multiple disciplinary mentors and sensitized to the barriers and facilitators associated with interdisciplinary collaboration. Additional funding sources and institutional mechanisms are needed to support such training. Conferences and networks can also be beneficial for fostering knowledge about TD collaboration. National conferences such as those organized by funding agencies are also valuable in this regard. For example, in 2006, the National Cancer Institute organized a Science of Team Science conference focused on transdisciplinarity.[51]

Allow a Longer Time Frame for Collaboration Assessment Two years are not a large amount of time for a collaboration. More time is needed for members to understand the research, contemplate how it could be implemented, implement a program, and demonstrate an impact on public health. Collaboration members and funding agencies may need to realize that ahead of time. Although traditional science may normally take years to be translated into policy, transdisciplinary scientific collaboration may take even longer because of the additional time needed to conduct the work. Thus, it may take ten, fifteen, or even twenty years to see effective translation occur.

This case study highlights some of the facets of transdisciplinary action research that occurred among team members in a tobacco policy consortium. It is likely that the lessons learned from this case study will inform future funding of research into the science of team science. Guiding future scientists and professionals through the multiple phases of team collaborations will improve as we understand more about the workings of TD science, training, and translational initiatives.

SUMMARY

In this chapter, we analyzed the Tobacco Policy Consortium (TPC), a grant-funded transdisciplinary action research consortium of tobacco researchers and community decision makers. The TPC collaborated from 2003 through 2005, with the goals of creating a grant program to support local adolescent smoking prevention efforts and developing and disseminating a research and policy brief for local, state, and national policymakers. Our assessments show that despite initial differences in backgrounds, work styles, and perspectives, TPC researchers and community members gradually came to share views on tobacco control priorities as a result of repeated brainstorming sessions and collective discussions. Although the TPC was successful in accomplishing its major goals, it fell short of achieving its full potential— namely, to become self-sustaining and reduce adolescent tobacco use. Lessons learned include improving future university-community collaborations, enhancing the "science of team science," and incorporating measures for sustaining grant-funded community-research partnerships from the outset.

DISCUSSION QUESTIONS

1. Why did the UC Irvine Tobacco Policy Consortium choose to use an interdisciplinary approach to understand youth tobacco use?

2. What obstacles did the consortium encounter and how did they address them?

3. What steps could the consortium have taken to engage young people themselves in their work? What might have been the advantages and disadvantages of youth engagement?

4. Based on their experiences, what suggestions do the authors make for improving the process and effectiveness of interdisciplinary action research? Do you agree with their recommendations?

ACKNOWLEDGMENTS

The authors thank the Robert Wood Johnson Foundation for its support of the reported research via RWJF grant number 46962. Without this support, this project would not have been possible. We also thank all who participated as members of the UCI Tobacco Policy Consortium. The work described in this chapter was supported by a grant from the National Institutes of Health (NIDA/NCI) to establish the UCI TTURC (NIH award DA-13332). The authors are also grateful for the valuable contributions of Dr. Frances Leslie, Dr. Robin Mermelstein, Dr. Kim Kobus, Dr. Glen Morgan, Kimari Phillips, and Amy Brewer to this research.

NOTES

1. UC Irvine TTURC. *Research and Policy Brief: Prevent Youth Smoking.* Available at www.tturc.uci.edu/UCI_TobaccoPolicyBrf_Aug05.pdf. Published 2005. Retrieved August 1, 2007.

2. Stokols, D. Toward a science of transdisciplinary action research. *American Journal of Community Psychology,* 38, no. 1 (2006): 63–77.

3. Lewin, K. Action research and minority problems. *Journal of Social Issues,* 2 (1946): 34–36.

4. Craik, K. H. Environmental psychology. *Annual Review of Psychology,* 24 (1973): 403–422.

5. Milgram, S. The experience of living in cities. *Science,* 167 (1970): 1461–1468.

6. Proshansky, H. M., Ittelson, W. H., and Rivlin, L. G., eds. *Environmental Psychology: People and Their Physical Settings,* 2nd ed. New York: Holt, Rinehart & Winston.

7. Butterfoss, F. D., Goodman, R. M., and Wandersman, A. Community coalitions for prevention and health promotion: Factors predicting satisfaction, participation, and planning. *Health Education Quarterly,* 23, no. 1 (1996): 65–79.

8. Wandersman, A., Valois, R., Ochs, L., de la Cruz, D. S., Adkins, E., and Goodman, R. M. Toward a social ecology of community coalitions. *American Journal of Health Promotion,* 10, no. 4 (1996): 299–307.

9. Sommer, R. Action research. In D. Stokols, ed., *Perspectives on Environment and Behavior: Theory, Research, and Applications,* pp. 195–203. New York: Plenum Press, 1977.

10. Minkler, M., and Wallerstein, N., eds. *Community-Based Participatory Research for Health*. San Francisco: Jossey-Bass, 2003.

11. Altman, D. G. Sustaining interventions in community systems: On the relationship between researchers and communities. *Health Psychology,* 14 (1995): 526–536.

12. Conner, R. F., and Tanjasiri, S. P. Communities evaluating community-level interventions: The development of community-based indicators in the Colorado Healthy Communities Initiative. *Canadian Journal of Program Evaluation,* 14 (1999): 115–136.

13. Gray, B. *Collaborating: Finding Common Ground for Multiparty Problems.* San Francisco: Jossey-Bass, 1989.

14. Klein, J. T. *Crossing Boundaries: Knowledge, Disciplines, and Interdisciplinarities.* Charlottesville: University of Virginia Press, 1996.

15. Stokols, D., Misra, S., Hall, K., Taylor, B., and Moser, R. The ecology of team science: Understanding contextual influences on transdisciplinary collaboration. *American Journal of Preventive Medicine,* 35, no. 2S (2008): 96–115.

16. Esparza, J., and Yamada, T. The discovery value of "big science." *Journal of Experimental Medicine,* 204, no. 4 (2007): 701–704.

17. Maton, K. I., Perkins, D. D., Altman, D. G., Gutierrez, L., Kelly, J. G., Rappaport, J., et al. *Community-based interdisciplinary research: Introduction to the special issue.* Available at www.springerlink.com/content/l053361v67386016. Retrieved October 10, 2006.

18. Nass, S. J., and Stillman, B. *Large-scale Biomedical Science: Exploring Strategies for Future Research*. Washington, D.C.: National Academies Press, 2003.

19. Stokols, D., Hall, K. L., Taylor, B., and Moser, R. P. National Cancer Institute Conference on the Science of Team Science: Assessing the value of transdisciplinary research, *October 30–31, 2006*. Available at http://videocast.nih.gov/ Summary.asp?File=13474, http://videocast.nih.gov/Summary.asp?File=13471, http://dccps.nci.nih.gov/brp/scienceteam/presentations_day1.html, and http:// dccps.nci.nih.gov/brp/scienceteam/presentations_day2.html. Published 2006. Retrieved August 8, 2007.

20. Wuchty, S., Jones, B. F., and Uzzi, B. The increasing dominance of teams in production of knowledge. *Science Express*, 316, no. 5827 (2007): 1036–1039.

21. National Cancer Institute. *Centers for Population Health and Health Disparities.* Available at http://cancercontrol.cancer.gov/populationhealthcenters. Published 2006. Retrieved September 10, 2006.

22. National Cancer Institute. *Health communication and informatics research: NCI Centers of Excellence in Cancer Communications Research.* Available at

http://cancercontrol.cancer.gov/hcirb/ceccr. Published 2006. Retrieved October 5, 2006.

23. National Cancer Institute. *Transdisciplinary Research on Energetics and Cancer Centers.* Available at www.compass.fhcrc.org/trec. Published 2006. Retrieved September 15, 2006.

24. National Cancer Institute. Transdisciplinary Tobacco Use Research Centers. Available at http://dccps.nci.nih.gov/tcrb/tturc. Published 2006. Retrieved October 1, 2006.

25. National Center for Research Resources. Clinical and translational science awards to transform clinical research. Available at www.ncrr.nih.gov/ncrrprog/roadmap/CTSA_9-2006.asp. Published 2006. Retrieved on October 11, 2006.

26. National Academy of Sciences. *The NAS/Keck initiative to transform interdisciplinary research.* Available at www.keckfutures.org. Published 2003. Retrieved July 18, 2003.

27. Robert Wood Johnson Foundation. Active living research. Available at www.activelivingresearch.org/about. Published 2006. Retrieved February 13, 2009.

28. Jessor, R. The problem of reductionism in psychology. *Psychological Review,* 65 (1958): 170–178.

29. Stokols, D. Conceptual strategies of environmental psychology. In D. Stokols and I. Altman, eds., *Handbook of Environmental Psychology,* pp. 41–70. New York: John Wiley, 1987.

30. Campbell, D. T., and Fiske, D. W. Convergent and discriminant validation by the multitrait-multimethod matrix. *Psychological Bulletin,* 56, no. 2 (1959): 81–105.

31. Winett, R. A., King, A. C., and Altman, D. G. *Health Psychology and Public Health: An Integrative Approach.* New York: Pergamon Press, 1989.

32. Stokols, D. *The future of interdisciplinarity in the School of Social Ecology.* Available at www.drugabuse.gov/ttuc/Readings.html. Published 1998. Retrieved March 25, 2005.

33. Fuqua, J. *Transdisciplinary scientific collaboration: An exploration of the research process.* Doctoral dissertation (2002). School of Social Ecology, University of California, Irvine.

34. Hildebrand-Zanki, S., Cohen, L., Perkins, K., Prager, D. J., Stokols, D., and Turkkan, J. *Barriers to Transdisciplinary Research in Youth Tobacco Use Prevention. A Report from the Working Group to the Youth Tobacco Use Prevention Initiative.* Washington, D.C.: Center for the Advancement of Health and the Robert Wood Johnson Foundation, 1998.

35. Rhoten, D., and Parker, A. Risks and rewards of an interdisciplinary research path. *Science, 306* (2004): 2046.

36. Stokols, D., Fuqua, J., Gress, J., Harvey, R., Phillips, K., Baezconde-Garbanati, L., et al. Evaluating transdisciplinary science. *Nicotine Tobacco Research,* 5, Suppl 1 (2003): S21–39.

37. Stokols, D., Harvey, R., Gress, J., Fuqua, J., and Phillips, K. In vivo studies of transdisciplinary scientific collaboration: Lessons learned and implications for active living research. *American Journal of Preventive Medicine,* 28, no. 2S2 (2005): 202–213.

38. Shortliffe, E. H., Patel, V .L., Cimino, J. J., Barnett, G. O., and Greenes, R. A. A study of collaboration among medical informatics research laboratories. *Artificial Intelligence in Medicine,* 12(1998): 97–123.

39. Tuckman, B. W. Developmental sequence in small groups. *Psychology Bulletin,* 63, no. 6 (1965): 384–399.

40. Rosenberg, M. Cognitive structure and attitudinal affect. *Journal of Abnormal and Social Psychology,* 53 (1956): 367–372.

41. Abrams, D. B. Applying transdisciplinary research strategies to understanding and eliminating health disparities. *Health Education and Behavior,* 33, no. 4 (2006): 515–531.

42. Morgan, G., Kobus, K., Gerlach, K. K., Neighbors, C., Lerman, C., Abrams, D. B., et al. Facilitating transdisciplinary research: The experience of the transdisciplinary tobacco use research centers. *Nicotine & Tobacco Research,* 5, Suppl 1 (2003): S11–S19.

43. Lesser, E. L. Leveraging social capital in organizations. In E. L. Lesser, ed., *Knowledge and Social Capital: Foundations and Applications,* pp. 3–16. Boston: Butterworth-Heinemann, 2000.

44. Hall, K., Feng, A., Moser, R., Stokols, D., and Taylor, B. Moving the science of team science forward: Collaboration and creativity. *American Journal of Preventive Medicine,* 35, no. 2S (2008): 243–249.

45. Florin, P., and Wandersman, A. An introduction to citizen participation, voluntary organizations, and community development: Insights for empowerment through research. *American Journal of Community Psychology,* 18 (1990): 41–54.

46. Gray, B. Conditions facilitating interorganizational collaboration. *Human Relations,* 38 (1985): 911–936.

47. Schermerhorn, J. J. Determinants of interorganizational cooperation. *Academy of Management Journal, 18* (1975): 846–856.

48. Hall, K., Stokols, D., Moser, R., Taylor, B., Thornquist, M., Nebeling, L., et al. The collaboration readiness of transdisciplinary research teams and centers: Findings from the National Cancer Institute TREC baseline evaluation study. *American Journal of Preventive Medicine,* 35, no. 2S (2008): 161–172.

49. Buehler, R., Griffin, D., and Ross, M. Exploring the "Planning Fallacy": why people underestimate their task completion times. *Journal of Personality and Social Psychology,* 67 (1994): 366–381.

50. Kerner, J., Rimer, B., and Emmons, K. Introduction to the special section on dissemination: Dissemination research and research dissemination: How can we close the gap? *Health Psychology,* 24, no. 5 (2005): 443–446.

51. National Cancer Institute. *NCI-NIH Conference on the Science of Team Science: Assessing the Value of Transdisciplinary Research.* Available at http://videocast. nih.gov/Summary.asp?File=13474 and http://videocast.nih.gov/Summary. asp? File=13471. Published 2006. Retrieved February 17, 2008.

CHAPTER

9

HOW VULNERABILITIES AND CAPACITIES SHAPE POPULATION HEALTH AFTER DISASTERS

CRAIG HADLEY, SASHA RUDENSTINE, SANDRO GALEA

LEARNING OBJECTIVES

- Describe some of the ways that natural and human disasters affect the health of urban populations.

- Identify antecedent social, political, and environmental factors that can influence how a population responds to a disaster.

- Discuss the value and limits of epidemiological and anthropological insights into the consequences of disasters.

- Compare and contrast the health and social impact of Hurricane Katrina and the September 11 attack on the World Trade Center.

Several recent high-profile natural disasters (e.g., the southeast Asian tsunami of 2004 and the Gulf Coast hurricanes in the United States of 2005) and terrorist events (e.g., the September 11, 2001, terrorist attacks and the March 11, 2004, Madrid train bombings) have heightened awareness of disasters as important determinants of population health and have resulted in a concomitant increased interest in the consequences of disasters. Although the sporadic nature of lay and scientific reporting about high-profile disasters may suggest that these events are episodic and rare, general surveys of the U.S. population suggest that individual exposure to disasters is quite high and that approximately 10 percent of the U.S. population will experience a disaster during their lifetime.[1,2] Comparable international data suggest that since the mid-1980s, hundreds of millions of individuals worldwide have been affected by disasters, be it in the form of terrorism, famine, forced relocation, or political violence.[3] These figures suggest that although definitions of disasters and the approaches used to study them may be quite disparate,[4,5] disasters have been and remain a relatively common piece of the human experience.[6] Despite the mental and physical health burden that disasters exact,[7] academic and public health interest in disasters remains episodic at best and in many cases falls along disciplinary lines. Public health perspectives on disasters have typically centered on a medical model of disaster preparedness and generally less on the broader issues of why some populations appear to suffer greater health consequences of disasters than others.

Our objectives for this chapter are largely theoretical and conceptual. We suggest that greater attention to the social-ecological determinants of the postdisaster context may prove useful in understanding why some populations suffer more than others and that such an approach reveals unique insights for prevention and intervention. We also suggest that data collection and analysis methods that combine qualitative and quantitative methods and are informed by different disciplinary perspectives are critical in identifying factors that promote or undermine health in the postdisaster setting. We then outline a conceptual model that is useful for understanding the underlying determinants of population health in the postdisaster setting. The model calls attention to the underlying vulnerabilities and capacities that influence health and well-being, which we illustrate by drawing examples from the disaster literature and through three case studies. We conclude by examining the unique impact of disasters on the world's growing urban population.

SOCIAL AND ECONOMIC DETERMINANTS OF HEALTH AFTER DISASTERS

Socioecological perspectives on the determinants of population health suggest that factors at multiple levels of influence contribute to individual and population health.[8] These may include macrolevel historical and political factors, mesolevel factors such as social networks, and microlevel factors such as race/ethnicity.[9,10] Within this paradigm, it has been suggested that the determinants of population health may usefully be conceptualized as either vulnerabilities (e.g., poor aggregate socioeconomic status) or capacities (e.g., natural resources) and that population health reflects the interplay between underlying vulnerabilities and capacities and intermittent stressors (e.g., disasters) and protective factors (e.g., delivery of aid or other material resources).[11]

We suggest that social determinants at multiple levels of influence are also likely to influence health and well-being in the postdisaster context. This is a position close to that taken by geographers and anthropologists to explain why disasters occur; indeed, Hoffman and Oliver-Smith[4] explicitly define a disaster as "a process leading to an event that involves a combination of a potentially destructive agent from the natural or technological sphere and a population in a socially produced condition of vulnerability." Consistent with this approach and seemingly developed in parallel, public health practitioners have also identified a range of social-ecological factors that predict the severity of impact on health and well-being across disaster settings. This consilience of approaches is exemplified by the work of Blaikie et al.[12] whose comprehensive model of the factors leading to disaster builds off the work of Hewitt.[13] Briefly, Blaikie et al.'s model calls attention to multiple layers of influence, including history, class, resources, power, as well as aspects of the built environment and the interaction of these factors with a hazard. Hazards, or the physical agent of the disaster (e.g., flood, fire, etc.), are but one part of the equation producing disasters. Disasters are produced when a hazard intersects with existing vulnerabilities, which as stated earlier, are generated through a range of factors. This model can be usefully extended to include the health and well-being of populations in the postdisaster setting.

The social-ecological model can also be usefully extended to include not just vulnerabilities but also capacities, which are protective social and ecological features. Such a framework may be useful in the postdisaster context. This view encourages the researcher to identify underlying population-level factors that act as constants in promoting or eroding health and well-being in the pre- and postdisaster setting. A wide range of factors may be considered as underlying vulnerabilities, such as the paucity of material resources (e.g., low income) available to a given human population or the presence of a natural tectonic fault line that predisposes a population to earthquakes. Conversely, examples of underlying capacities may include social capital, abundant availability of natural resources, high levels of contributions to public goods, or a dispersed and effective informal safety net. However, the intermittent stressors that interact with existing vulnerabilities and capacities include the closure of a large employer or a hazard; these are inevitable events whose occurrence is neither frequent nor predictable. Protective events, such as the opening of a new school or an increase in group cohesiveness due to the success of a local sports team, also occur intermittently. Importantly, these intermittent influences, which interact with the underlying conditions, shape health at any particular moment in ways that are not necessarily amenable to standard epidemiological analyses.

Although this perspective is relatively new in our thinking about the consequences of disasters, the suggestion that we can understand population health as the outcome of trade-offs between population vulnerabilities and capacities is not novel. Nor is the idea that understanding the social and ecological conditions of the affected imperative to understanding how and why populations vary in their capacities and vulnerabilities. Diverse academic disciplines have long considered the factors that determine or covary with vulnerability.[14, 15] Still others have postulated that vulnerability can include genetic and biological vulnerability at the individual level[16] and social vulnerability at the group level.[17] In the study of disaster preparedness, it has long been recognized that certain populations are also more vulnerable to the effects of disasters than others,[18] and detailed case studies, often carried out by anthropologists,[4] have shown that multiple layers of history, ecology, and culture overlap to produce and augment existing group-level vulnerability.

Virchow, a physician-anthropologist, reports in his mid-nineteenth century writings an ethnomedical description of several Bavarian villages in which he makes precisely the same distinction between population-level vulnerabilities and capacities. He uses extensive ethnographic observation to understand population-level variability in these two factors. For instance, after a lengthy ethnographic account of the settlement and living conditions in several villages, he notes "the untoward conditions of social life in [these villages] are offset to a great extent by the beneficial influence of the elevation of the land and the formation of the soil, and that [as a result] this poverty-stricken . . . population, which faces death by starvation every single year of crop failure, shows a mortality rate almost as low as that prevailing in the best countries of the old world."[19] A high level of poverty, which acts as a population-level vulnerability, is countered by the ecological positioning of the area, a capacity that accounts for the low levels of mortality. Clearly, in many cases, vulnerabilities and capacities do not necessarily represent separate dimensions but rather ends of a spectrum, and in most cases, the lack of a specific capacity may represent a specific population-level vulnerability.

Although the full range of vulnerabilities and capacities that may influence population health after disasters is broad and locally specific, we have elsewhere made an attempt to delineate some of the general elements that might influence postdisaster consequences.[20] These elements include geography and history, demographic and political structures, community wealth and asset holdings, and aspects of the built environment and formal and informal social environments.

As underlying factors, geography and history contribute to outcomes of disasters in several ways. First and most obviously, some areas are naturally more at risk than are others. In these areas, the risk of recurrent disasters is virtually unavoidable, and the exigencies of geography then highlight the fact that there is likely no solution for the total elimination of these disasters. Geography also plays an important role in structuring the postdisaster response. News of a disaster event in isolated communities may take far longer to reach aid agencies or the media (as in the case of the Darfur famine of 2004–2005) than it might after disasters in more readily accessible locations. Similarly, the ability of agencies to provide aid may well be limited in geographically distant or difficult locales. For example, it took more than a week for domestic and international aid efforts to reach some victims of the devastating 2005 earthquakes in the Kashmir region that killed an estimated 80,000 people.[21]

Historical processes also influence the postdisaster outcome, particularly as related to historical-political relationships. As Olsen and colleagues[22] point out, many of the most disaster prone countries worldwide are in areas that are of little security interest to the United States or other developed countries and therefore receive minimal emergency funding. Colonial historical relations also influence responses and therefore postdisaster consequences. In an interesting recent example, the 7.5 magnitude earthquake that hit Mozambique in February 2006 was notably benign in part due to building codes imposed on the country by Portugal during the colonial period.[23] Political structures and systems of governance establish the parameters (e.g., taxation, federal-state relations) that shape many of the other contextual factors influencing health after disasters. For example, analyses of state failures such as those that have occurred in Liberia and Somalia and which often precede or predispose to disasters show that these events are far more likely to occur in partial as compared to fully democratic regimes.[24] Similarly, postdisaster response may be influenced by political structures and governance, as we describe in more detail later.

Even within areas that share geographic, historical, and political structures, the level of community wealth acts as a local vulnerability or a capacity. There is an abundance of research in public health demonstrating that aggregate community socioeconomic status is associated with health, independent of individual socioeconomic position. Community socioeconomic status encompasses multiple domains, including high rates of poverty and unemployment and lower education and income levels.[25] Empirically, low community socioecological status (frequently also referred to as community deprivation) is a determinant of health outcomes, including health-related behaviors, mental health, infant mortality rate, adult physical health, coronary heart disease, and mortality even after accounting for individual-level factors.[26] Low community socioeconomic status may affect residents' health through two primary mechanisms: (a) by limiting the availability of salutary resources that may be beneficial to residents' well-being and (b) through psychosocial stress accompanying a chronic shortage of essential resources.[27] These social mechanisms also explain how community socioeconomic status may influence health in the disaster context. After disasters, when both formal and informal resources are limited, societies with a priori fewer resources are less likely to have access to salutary resources such as health and social services or food reserves. Consistent with this line of reasoning, Norris et al.[28] showed that individuals who lived in developing countries and presumably had fewer protective resources were at far greater risk of experiencing poor health outcomes in the postdisaster setting than those living in the United States. They report in their meta-analysis that 78 percent of the samples from developing countries showed signs of postdisaster impairment compared with 25 percent of the samples from the United States.

The physical environment is perhaps one of the most obviously central features of context to postdisaster recovery. Structures like buildings, bridges, and other infrastructure may be vulnerable to natural or human-made disasters and may directly influence the postdisaster context and the severity of the disaster consequences. For example, features of the physical environment can be immediately linked to fatality rate after disasters as seen in the recent earthquakes of comparable magnitude in Kobe, Japan, in 1995 and Bam, Iran, in 2003 that were associated with 5,200 and 26,000 deaths, respectively.[21, 29] Much of this difference was attributed to the different quality of buildings; Japanese buildings had been reinforced to cope with earthquake tremors, but much of the Iranian city of Bam collapsed with the earthquake, killing thousands of residents.[30] Clearly, given that more than half of the global population is or very soon will be living in urban settings, this has important consequences for health and well-being in postdisaster settings.[28] This rapid urbanization creates tremendous challenges in part because many urban dwellers will be living in slums, which are likely loci of multiple physical vulnerabilities.[31]

Culture, which coexists with these elements, is likely to be an important element structuring postdisaster outcomes. Culture, defined as beliefs or rules of behavior that are passed on from one individual to another by some form of social learning,[32] may influence individual and community responses to disasters as well as the health consequences thereafter, such as health-seeking behavior, mental health experiences, and the provision of resources by dominant groups. Because members of groups often, by definition, share norms and beliefs, groups of people will likely experience, react, and respond in very different ways to the same disaster event. Among this set of beliefs, some researchers have suggested that differing and culturally specific norms related to fatalism may alter both pre- and postdisaster responses.[33] Some evidence to support this claim has been shown through interviews with survivors of Hurricane Andrew. There is also the possibility that expressions of posttraumatic stress disorder and other mental health morbidity may vary by ethnic or cultural group.[34] Despite culture's seemingly important role, few studies analyze the role of culture in the postdisaster milieu. These limitations reflect, in part, a lack of ethnography used in the immediate postdisaster context[35] and difficulties in measuring shared norms and beliefs. Additionally, cooperation and the capacity to mobilize or create informal political or social groups may be a critical resource in the postdisaster situation. For instance, in rural Tanzania, a local vigilante group was instrumental in enforcing a ban on intervillage trading to reduce the spread of cholera, and in another situation, they successfully cooperated to defend a large amount of rice left roadside after a rice-bearing truck crashed (B. Paciotti, personal communication, April 14, 2006). Such widespread cooperation, which varies quite dramatically between cultures and groups,[36, 37] could have a substantial impact in the postdisaster setting where many other salutary resources are limited.

The complexity of the determinants of population health after disasters suggests it is unlikely that any single disciplinary perspective or framework will afford us the tools to fully understand how the determinants of population health interrelate to shape the health of populations. An interdisciplinary approach that simultaneously capitalizes on epidemiological rigor and anthropology's "radically contextualizing" roots has the potential to draw on quantitative and qualitative methods that can be complementary and help us to understand the etiology of the health consequences of these events. For example, the social autopsy approach, which integrates multiple levels of causation, was used to explore the underlying causes of differential health outcomes following the Chicago heat wave. This approach could begin to assess whether vulnerabilities and capacities act in isolation or interact at the individual and community levels with cultural, socioeconomic, and global political and historical forces to produce specific health outcomes after a disaster. Thus, the epidemiologic focus on categorical health outcomes can be augmented by historical and ethnographic data that can link the consequences of disasters to declining tax revenues, poor and myopic government planning, racial discrimination, and high rates of individual- and community-level poverty.

We use here three relatively recent disasters as case studies to illustrate the roles of vulnerabilities and capacities acting and interacting across multiple levels as well as the value of adopting a historical, cross-cultural, social science perspective. First, we examine the social determinants in influencing health and well-being in two similar crises resulting from political rather than environmental events. Next, we explore the social determinants of outcomes following Hurricane Katrina and the events of September 11, 2001. In each case, we draw on various data sources to highlight underlying vulnerabilities and capacities and attempt to show how these influences produce and reproduce differential outcomes within and between populations.

HUMANITARIAN CRISES IN ANGOLA AND THE BALKANS

In the postconflict periods following the political crises in Angola[38] and the Balkans,[39, 40] health outcomes varied markedly between these two countries. In both cases, political instability led to large-scale population displacement and social unrest, and the displaced peoples were almost entirely reliant on food assistance. Despite these similarities, the prevalence of undernutrition in the Kosovar population (one of the many ethnic groups within the Balkans) remained at approximately 2 percent throughout the crisis, whereas the prevalence of undernutrition in Angola increased throughout the crisis from 2.3 percent to 15 to 21 percent. Why did the prevalence of undernutrition increase by nearly tenfold in the Angola case, whereas there was no detectable increase in the levels of undernutrition in the Balkans? In both cases, large numbers of people were affected by violent political instability that brought about disastrous consequences for the provision of government and social services, and both resulted in substantial opportunity costs. To the wage earner in the Balkans, the disaster brought with it lost wages. To the farmer in Angola, the disaster brought unplanted crops or harvests consumed by rebel forces or internally displaced people.[40]

At least three key differences in population vulnerabilities and capacities emerge, which likely account for the vastly different health consequences observed in these humanitarian disasters. In the case of Angola, humanitarian aid was in short supply. The UN's 2002 calls for humanitarian assistance repeatedly fell short of their mark, with only 30 percent of the appeal being funded during critical periods of the crisis.[41, 42] One report expressed surprise and dismay, noting that "it is alarming . . . that the UN Consolidated Inter-Agency Appeal (CAP) has so far met with a very poor response from the international donor community, despite the emergency having been branded as the worst crisis in the world at present."[43] Emergency aid that did appear often was unable to be efficiently transferred to those most in need, in large part because of the large number of land mines placed by the opposition UNITA forces. In the Balkans, international aid agencies were able to take preemptive action and to reach locations, and thus continue to deliver vital aid in the postcrisis period. The UN assessment was that "overall, the international community has been successful in preventing acute [nutritional] wasting, among the Kosovan refugees."[44]

At the community and individual level, these two populations differed considerably in overall wealth. In the Balkans, which lacked the extreme poverty found in Angola, this enabled wealth redistribution and therefore acted as a population-level capacity, whereas in Angola low levels of wealth disallowed redistribution, and social networks were powerless to assist those in need. Further, household food insecurity assessments identified critical shortfalls in food in Angola, but this was not necessarily the case in the Balkans. Subsequent assessment showed that a large number of Albanian households (another ethnic group within the Balkans) had family members living either abroad or outside the conflict area who were sending remittances that were critical for protecting households from food insecurity.[40] Yet, in the Angola case, because few households had family living outside the conflict area, few people received remittances, and lacking such safety nets, shocks to the households were not successfully buffered. These patterns suggest that variation in health outcomes in the postdisaster period are linked to global variation in international aid and perhaps to global migration patterns, which enable individuals to relocate and send remittances, thereby diminishing the negative impact of decline in social services during a conflict period.

To put this in the context of our conceptual model, privileged political positions and global migration patterns are likely underlying capacities to the extent that they facilitate emergency aid donations and the ability of individuals to redistribute resources through remittances. This later point may be particularly salient in light of the rapidly urbanizing global community and the hypothesized reduction in informal safety nets that are expected to accompany this shift. Some have hypothesized that formal safety networks will emerge to take over the functions of informal safety nets, but the available evidence from sub-Saharan Africa does not support any clear urban bias in the availability of formal safety nets.[45] As in the Angola example, urbanization may be associated with limited formal and informal safety nets, which in the post-postdisaster setting erodes health and well-being. Preexisting health conditions, in this case undernutrition, also contribute to a reduced capacity to effectively respond in the context of markedly increased stress. Thus, these cases illustrate how during and after a disaster, individual, community, and global forces interact to position populations along distinct tracks that lead some to stable or improved health and others to poor health outcomes.

HURRICANE KATRINA

Hurricane Katrina was a category 3 hurricane when it hit the Gulf Coast of the United States on August 29, 2005. Despite sufficient warning and officials at all levels being "acutely aware of Katrina and the risk it posed," the storm contributed to more than 1,800 deaths, billions of dollars of damage, and the displacement of between 700,000 and 1.2 million people.[46] Austin[47] provides an excellent overview that mixes historical reports with current ethnography to illustrate how power, resources, and geography created vulnerabilities in the region even before Hurricane Katrina hit. In addition to the preexisting geographic and power vulnerabilities, socioeconomic vulnerabilities already existed at both the state and individual level; the three states (Louisiana, Alabama, and Mississippi) that bore the burden of the storm were among the poorest in the United States,[48] a fact that has implications for the citizenry and the level of support available in crisis situations. Groups with preexisting vulnerabilities were predicted to be differentially affected by the storm, and media coverage and preliminary reports suggested poverty and race were key predictors of risk of damage to material and physical resources.

Two separate reports confirm this general assessment but offer a more nuanced perspective.[46, 49] An examination of census tract data reveals that the overall population living in areas considered damaged by Federal Emergency Management Agency (FEMA) criteria were disproportionably black (45.7 percent vs. 26 percent black in nondamaged areas). Damaged areas also had a higher proportion of individuals living in rental homes (45.7 percent vs. 30 percent in nondamaged areas) and greater percentages of people living below the poverty line (20.9 percent vs. 15.3 percent in nondamaged areas) and who were unemployed (7.6 percent vs. 6.0 percent in nondamaged areas). Death reports also show that elderly white individuals were at the highest risk of death. To be sure, there were also areas with considerable damage that disproportionally comprised individuals who were white and wealthy, yet the statistical patterns reveal deep social divides. These patterns of differential impact have significant implications for current and future health consequences.[50] More than 500,000 people are estimated to have an unmet need for mental health services when the number of medical professionals is near its nadir. In addition to the health impact of depression and other common mental disorders, depression is associated with hypertension, heart disease, and diabetes. Mental health outcomes are also expected to give rise to increased rates of substance use and abuse. Further, consistent with our model, the impact of these health outcomes is unlikely to fall equally on all. Some evidence, for instance, suggests that African Americans are less likely than other racial/ethnic groups to seek care for mental health morbidities such as posttraumatic stress disorder following disasters.[51] Higher rates of poverty and lower rates of health insurance, which will be amplified by the reduced availability of social services, may also undercut attempts to rebuild physical and mental health and economic well-being.[52]

Hurricane Katrina therefore exacerbated preexisting vulnerabilities. Although in many cases effective governance or formal safety networks can act as population-level capacities and serve to attenuate, protect, or eliminate negative health effects experienced as a result of population-level vulnerabilities, this was largely not the case with Hurricane Katrina. In the case of Katrina, the governmental response was described as "uncoordinated" and "hampered by ineptitude, lack of leadership and bureaucratic turf wars across all levels of government."[53] Consequently, despite being warned that the storm would be disastrous, the governmental response lagged, and the primary response did not occur until two days after Katrina landfall.[54] Part of this delay was due to confusion at multiple levels within the government. Local governments believed that the federal government would take primary responsibility and the lead, but the federal government believed that in disaster situations, "the role of the federal government is not and should not ever be that of a first responder."[54] Rather, FEMA believed "states have the primary responsibility for emergency preparedness and response in their jurisdictions,"[54] although planning exercises simulating a disaster of this magnitude led to the conclusion that an event of the magnitude of Katrina would require first-line federal response.

Others noted that FEMA was unable to actually carry out its job because of changes in the department's structure, and increasing amounts of energy focused on being prepared to deal with terrorist strikes. Part of the poor response also appears to have stemmed from a limited appraisal of how other similar humanitarian crises have unfolded in the other parts of the world, representing a Western-centric public health model. Thus, despite an awareness that large numbers of individuals would be evacuated (this assumption was built into simulation exercises), governmental responses seemed to contain little information on how to handle mass displacement of the population. There is a voluminous literature from foreign refugee crises that would have been helpful in planning such a response.[55] Nieburg et al. point out that one of the primary lessons from such foreign refugee crises is to have sufficient water and appropriate food on hand to feed large numbers of displaced individuals; this is a lesson that was apparently not learned on several prior occasions in which the Superdome was used as a shelter.[56]

Although in this case the formal response was delayed, informal safety nets quickly emerged. The notion that postdisaster behavior is marked by widespread deviance, including looting, panic, and extreme psychological dysfunction, is referred to as the disaster myth.[57] In contrast to the disaster myth, empirical research on population behavior in the postdisaster setting rarely conforms to that predicted by the disaster myth model. Rather, behavior is often highly prosocial, calm, and rational. In his ethnographic account of helping behavior during Katrina, Ethridge[58] describes the emergence of "leaderless" prosocial behavior in a group of individuals temporarily occupying a high school. Group consensus emerged over a range of behaviors and tasks, and many norms temporarily fell by the wayside. For instance, age hierarchies broke down, and youth played a critical role in fetching supplies, in part because older individuals were incapacitated by infections on their extremities (due to limited facilities for bathing). Again, this case study documents how multiple lines of evidence reveal multiple layers of vulnerabilities and capacities that interact to amplify the deleterious impact of disasters on vulnerable populations.

SEPTEMBER 11, 2001, TERRORIST ATTACKS ON NEW YORK CITY

The New York City (NYC) metropolitan area is the largest and most densely populated metropolitan area in the United States.[48] Although estimates of population size vary depending on the areas selected as boundaries of the metropolitan area, approximately 15 million people live in the vicinity of NYC in the tristate area of New York State, New Jersey, and Connecticut. Perhaps as a result of the preeminent role played by NYC in national discourse, the attacks on the World Trade Center (WTC) were perceived as an attack on the United States. The attacks themselves started on 8:46 A.M. on the morning of September 11, 2001, and consisted of two hijacked airplanes hitting the WTC towers, which eventually collapsed. Two other airplanes were also hijacked that day with one crashing into the Pentagon and the other into a field in Pennsylvania. During the day of September 11, "fog of war" rumors had many in the NYC metropolitan area afraid for their lives. Early rumors of more planes being hijacked and aimed for other NYC and national targets were rife. As round-the-clock, real-time television coverage of the attacks saturated the airwaves, millions in the area saw images first of people waving for help from the towers of the WTC and then of the towers falling. Meanwhile, countless residents of the tristate area knew someone or were related to someone who was working in the WTC. Disrupted communications systems meant that many were uncertain about the fate of family or friends for most of the day of September 11 and, in many cases, for days after the attacks.

In many respects, the aftermath of the terrorist attacks on New York City represented a model of community mobilization in response to a mass trauma. There was a highly visible and mostly effective mobilization of municipal and national resources to aid those affected by the attacks and a rapid engagement of resources to assist the population of the area both in the short term and in the relative long term. Approximately $20 billion in federal aid was routed to New York City in the aftermath of the attacks.[59] For example, Project Liberty was a free service established to provide counseling after the attacks.[60] It was established soon after the September 11 attacks and was fully functional until 2004, at which point several of the services it provided were reduced. All services were terminated in 2005. During its existence, Project Liberty provided services to approximately 750,000 persons in the NYC metropolitan area.[61] It made as a core part of its mission specific outreach efforts aimed at ensuring that all residents of New York City would avail themselves of services if needed. However, despite the outpouring of national attention after the attacks and the relatively effective functioning of official governmental resources in the aftermath of the attacks (particularly when compared with the response after Hurricane Katrina, as discussed earlier), the health consequences of the September 11, 2001, terrorist attacks clearly reflected underlying vulnerabilities that were largely predicated on socioeconomic circumstance.

Several studies have amply documented that the psychological and behavioral consequences of the September 11, 2001, terrorist attacks extended well beyond those who are typically considered victims of such disasters and into the general population.[35, 62–65] Persons who were more exposed to the disaster (e.g., persons who lived closer to the WTC complex, persons who had a friend or relative killed in the attacks) were more likely to have psychological symptoms and adverse health behavior than were those who were not directly exposed to the disaster. Overall, it has been estimated that persons directly affected by the attacks were 3.5 times more likely to have adverse mental health symptoms after the attacks than persons who were not directly affected.[66] However, once direct and immediate exposure to the attacks is taken into consideration, the extension of the consequences of these attacks to the general population provides several examples of the role of social vulnerabilities and capacities in shaping health after this disaster.

One of the more consistent observations that emerged from research carried out after the September 11, 2001 terrorist attack was the differential risk of psychopathology among different ethnic groups. Several studies showed that Hispanics had a higher prevalence of psychopathology than did other racial/ethnic groups[63, 67] and specific analyses showed that Hispanics of Dominican or Puerto Rican origin were more likely than other Hispanics and non-Hispanics to report symptoms consistent with posttraumatic stress disorder (PTSD) after the September 11 terrorist attacks.[63] In one study that attempted to understand the reason behind these differences, it was shown that Dominicans and Puerto Ricans were more likely than persons of other races/ethnicities to have lower incomes, to be younger, to have lower social support, to have had greater exposure to the September 11 attacks, and to have experienced an emotional reaction upon hearing of the September 11 attacks. These variables accounted for 60 to 74 percent of the observed higher prevalence of probable PTSD in these groups.[63]

The role of pre- and postdisaster income as determinants of postdisaster functioning and well-being was reinforced in other analyses after this event. For example, one analysis that focused on the longitudinal risk of PTSD after the September 11, 2001, attacks found that unemployment at any time after the attacks predicted PTSD persistence even when accounting for a range of other potentially confounding covariates. In addition, high levels of perceived work stress predicted PTSD persistence among persons employed after September 11, 2001, and this was associated with poor mental health.[68] Therefore, in the aftermath of the September 11 attacks, individual socioeconomic position and job status both contributed to differences in postdisaster mental health and may explain many of the other differences observed between racial/ethnic groups after this event.

A further illustration of this point has been recent work that showed empirically that properties of urban neighborhoods of residence were associated with the individual risk of psychopathology after the September 11, 2001 attack, even after accounting for individual vulnerabilities. Specifically, in this postdisaster context, neighborhood-level income inequality has been shown to be associated with depression among persons with lower income.[69] It has been hypothesized that persons with individual socioeconomic disadvantage may be more socially or economically marginalized and dependent on local resources and hence more vulnerable to the consequences of this particular disaster. Other work has shown that neighborhood poverty was associated with the risk of incident depression in the years after the attacks even when accounting for individual socioeconomic status.[70] Taken together, data pulled from studies on mental health outcomes following the September 11 attacks amply demonstrate the role of vulnerabilities and capacities and how these play out across individuals, groups, and communities. In addition, the events of September 11, 2001 illustrate how the uniquely urban characteristics of population density and diversity, complexity, and income inequality, described in Chapter One of this volume, influenced how this disaster affected health.

IMPLICATIONS FOR PREVENTION AND INTERVENTION

Underlying socioeconomic vulnerabilities—both individual and ecological—contributed to shaping health after the September 11, 2001 attack, much as they did after Hurricane Katrina and after the humanitarian crises in Angola and the Balkans. These events are clearly substantially different, and the mobilization of external resources in response to these events is dramatically different both in scope and effectiveness. However, social and ecological factors consistently influence health and well-being after all these events, further reinforcing the premise guiding this chapter that underlying conditions represent a spectrum of vulnerabilities and capacities that shape postdisaster health and functioning. In addition, postdisaster interventions, while potentially helpful as protective factors, cannot obviate the role played by baseline factors in shaping the outcomes of disasters.

Therefore, the conceptual model presented here suggests and the case studies illustrate how the production of population health in the aftermath of disasters reflects a combination of underlying vulnerabilities and capacities interacting with the disaster stressor itself and potentially mitigated by postdisaster protective factors. These case studies also call attention to the interrelations of global-, community-, and individual-level factors in shaping health after disasters. Our understanding of these processes is enhanced by the use of a combination of approaches from anthropology and epidemiology that consider how vulnerabilities and capacities operate in tandem and interact across levels of units of analysis. Thus, although we can understand the causes of morbidity and mortality outcomes in New Orleans from a biomedical or proximate perspective, clearly the ultimate or upstream causes lie in preexisting health and economic inequalities in the United States, in the interactions between the oil industry and the wetlands, and in the mismanaged governmental attempts to protect citizens of the affected areas. Similarly, we can see that appealing to family members living outside the affected area is a critical source of support in some situations, but this capacity is not universally shared and likely varies widely both within and between communities. The discussions of Hurricane Katrina and Angola show that, in some cases, regardless of the existence of individual-level capacities, governmental forces can act as barriers to action and, at worst, contribute to poor outcomes. The studies about the September 11, 2001 attack similarly highlight the interplay among individuals, groups, and communities. These case studies draw attention to the important role of context in shaping postdisaster outcomes.

We suggest that there are several implications of the observations drawn here for those concerned with public health promotion. The model of vulnerabilities and capacities presented here strongly suggests that traditional understandings of "disaster preparedness" might be substantially broadened to include elements that may have been seen as outside the purview of disaster preparedness and even public health. The model we propose seeks to include social inequalities, aspects of the built environment, and informal social support, for example, as key components that will influence or mitigate the postdisaster environment. It might reasonably be argued that affecting features of the social environment, such as those just mentioned, that influence postdisaster health is a challenge beyond the scope of most public health practitioners and is certainly outside the scope of disaster preparedness. However, we believe that the approach taken in this chapter strengthens arguments that propose structural changes because they will pay off in general public health and in the postdisaster setting. Further proof of this concept comes from Norris et al.[28] In their analyses, they report a consistent finding across studies that individuals who were more distressed before a disaster are likely to experience more distress after a disaster. In this chapter and more so elsewhere,[20] we have pointed out that disaster outcomes reflect and amplify preexisting vulnerabilities, which strengthens the case that these determinants should not be overlooked in the effort to mitigate disaster consequences.

There are multiple examples throughout history when public health has indeed acted on contextual factors that expand considerably beyond the realm of individual exposure or behavior. For example, it was public health efforts to improve sanitary conditions in cities that led to sentinel improvements in European cities' infrastructure and attendant reductions in morbidity and mortality throughout the nineteenth century.[71] Effecting structural changes requires sentinel shifts in policies that may influence underlying determinants. The current increased awareness of disasters and their potential consequences creates an opportunity for advocacy and action to improve underlying features of context that may influence the health of populations after disasters. Such advocacy and action constitute a valid task for public health professionals.

If aspects of the social environment indeed influence postdisaster outcomes and are amenable to intervention, then a second implication of this work is that capacities and vulnerabilities are locally and culturally specific and that the relevant tools are needed to identify these. Once identified, these local assets can be leveraged to reduce the impact of disasters through early warning systems, protect vulnerable members of the community, and improve responses in the postdisaster period. Furthermore, uncovering and leveraging local capacities are particularly relevant in resource-poor settings where higher level public health services may be absent or ineffective. Nevertheless, our understanding of these capacities and vulnerabilities is currently biased toward already known capacities and largely based on those spelled out in the nondisaster social epidemiological literature. We suspect that research methods such as ethnographic and community-based participatory research designs may provide vital insights about how individuals and communities function in the face of a disaster and that knowledge of these local resources may be particularly fruitful in mitigating the postdisaster response and explaining population health variation.

A final implication of our ideas here is that the world's population is now dominated by urban dwellers. Projections estimate that by 2030, 5 billion people will be living in urban areas throughout the world. Although urban living is associated with a range of beneficial features, there are also large numbers of poor individuals in these settings.[72] This is increasingly true in those areas that are witnessing the most rapid urban growth: Asia and Africa.[72] The perspective that we have put forward here (and others have advanced elsewhere[12]) suggests that poorer individuals moving to or growing up in these settings will not only have reduced access to material resources, but their political voices will be silenced, and their living conditions will likely expose them to pollutants and increase vulnerability to hazards. Dense housing and narrow roads coupled with a range of heating and cooking materials and a lack of publicly funded firefighters put urban dwellers at increased risk of hazards and disasters. The peripheral positioning of many slums also makes them likely to experience floods. These same conditions, along with material deprivation and food insecurity, also erode health and well-being in the predisaster setting. Unfortunately, cities do not appear to be proactively preparing for a disaster: Of 109 cities in Africa and Asia, 34 percent lacked building codes, 46 percent lacked hazard mapping, and 54 percent did not have hazard insurance available for public or private buildings.[72] We suggest that these pre-existing vulnerabilities set the stage for a tremendous burden in the event of disasters in urban areas worldwide.

SUMMARY

In this chapter, we have sought to extend public health perspectives on disasters from the typical approach—which uses a medical model of disaster preparedness—to the broader issue of why some populations appear to suffer greater health consequences of disasters than others. Our objectives were largely theoretical and conceptual. We suggested that greater attention to the socioecological determinants of the postdisaster context may help to reveal insights for prevention and intervention to reduce the disparate impact of disasters. We also suggested that data collection and analysis methods that combine qualitative and quantitative methods and are informed by different disciplinary perspectives are critical in identifying factors that promote or undermine health in the postdisaster setting. We presented a conceptual model that called attention to the underlying vulnerabilities and capacities that influence health and well-being, which we illustrated by drawing examples from the disaster literature and through three case studies. We concluded by examining the unique impact of disasters on the world's growing urban population.

DISCUSSION QUESTIONS

1. How did the social conditions in New Orleans prior to Hurricane Katrina affect how the storm influenced health?

2. The authors of this chapter argue that structural changes that reduce inequality and increase social support prior to disasters can help to mitigate the adverse impacts. What do they mean and do you agree or disagree?

3. The authors present several case histories of political and natural disasters to illustrate their points. How do these case studies illustrate—or contradict—the framework the authors present in this chapter? What are the strengths and weaknesses of a case study methodology?

4. What are the pathways by which urban disasters can affect mental health?

NOTES

1. Burke, Jr., F. M. Acute-phase mental health consequences of disasters: Implications for triage and emergency medical services. *Annals of Emergency Medicine,* 28 (1996): 119–128.

2. Kessler, R. C., Sonnega, A., Bromet, E., Hughes, M., and Nelson, C. B. Posttraumatic stress disorder in the national comorbidity survey. *Archives of General Psychiatry,* 52 (1995): 1048–1060.

3. Nates, J. L., and Moyer, V. A. Lessons from Hurricane Katrina, tsunamis, and other disasters. *Lancet,* 366, no. 9492 (2005): 1144–1146.

4. Hoffman, S., and Oliver-Smith, A., eds. *Catastrophe and Culture.* Santa Fe, N.M.: School of American Research, 2002.

5. Quarantelli, E. J. What is a disaster? Six views of the problem. *International Journal of Mass Emergencies and Disasters,* 13, no. 3 (1995): 221–229.

6. Prentice, A. Fires of life: The struggles of an ancient metabolism in a modern world. *Nutrition Bulletin,* 26 (2001): 13–27.

7. Noji, E. K. Disasters: Introduction and state of the art. *Epidemiology Review,* 27 (2005): 3–8.

8. Kaplan, G. A. What is the role of the social environment in understanding inequalities in health? *Annual Report New York Academy of Sciences,* 896 (1999): 116–119.

9. Krieger, N. Theories for social epidemiology in the 21st century: An ecosocial perspective. *International Journal of Epidemiology,* 30, no. 4 (2001): 668–677.

10. Winterhalder, B., and Smith, E. A. Analyzing adaptive strategies: Human behavioral ecology at twenty-five. *Evolutionary Anthropology,* 9, no. 2 (2000): 51–72.

11. Galea, S., Nandi, A., and Vlahov, D. The epidemiology of post-traumatic stress disorder after disasters. *Epidemiology Review,* 27 (2005): 78–91.

12. Blaikie, P., Cannon, T., Davis, I., and Wisner, B. *At Risk: Natural Hazards, People's Vulnerability, and Disasters.* London: Routledge, 1994.

13. Hewitt, K. *Interpretations of Calamity from the Viewpoint of Human Ecology.* Boston: Allen & Unwin, 1983.

14. Bankoff, G. Constructing vulnerability: The historical, natural and social generation of flooding in metropolitan Manila. *Disasters,* 27 (2003): 224–238.

15. Turner, II, B. L., Kasperson, R. E., Matson, P. A., et al. A framework for vulnerability analysis in sustainability science. *Proceedings of the National Academy of Sciences USA,* 100 (2003): 8074–8079.

16. Heath, A. C., and Nelson, E. C. Effects of the interaction between genotype and environment research into the genetic epidemiology of alcohol dependence. *Alcohol Research & Health,* 26 (2002): 193–201.

17. McKeehan, I. V. A multilevel city health profile of Moscow. *Social Science & Medicine,* 51 (2000): 1295–1312.

18. Oliver-Smith, A. Anthropological research on hazards and disasters. *Annual Review of Anthropology,* 25 (1996): 303–328.

19. Virchow, R. I. Report on the typhus epidemic in Upper Silesia. In L. T. Rather, ed., *Collected Essays on Public Health and Epidemiology,* Vol. 1, pp. 11–12. Canton, Mass.: Science History Publications, 1985

20. Galea, S., Hadley, C., and Rudenstine, S. Context and the consequences of disasters: A population health perspective. *American Journal Disaster Medicine,* 1 (2006): 37–47.

21. USAID. *Pakistan Quake Relief.* Washington, D.C, USAID. May 2006. www .usaid.gov/locations/asia_near_east/documents/south_asia_quake/pakistan_ quakerelief.pdf.

22. Olsen, G. R., Carstensen, N., and Høyen, K. Humanitarian crises: What determines the level of emergency assistance? Media coverage, donor interests and the aid business. *Disasters,* 27, no. 2 (2003): 109–126.

23. Goering, L. Colonial past aids Mozambique in surviving quake. *Chicago Tribune* (February 24, 2006).

24. Esty, D. C., and Ivanova, I., eds. *Global Environmental Governance: Options and Opportunities.* New Haven, Conn.: Yale School of Forestry and Environmental Studies, 2002.

25. Berkman, L., and Kawachi, I. *Social Epidemiology.* Oxford: Oxford University Press, 2001.

26. Pickett, K. E., and Pearl, M. Multilevel analyses of neighborhood socioecological context and health outcomes: A critical review. *Journal of Epidemiology and Community Health,* 55, no. 2 (2001): 111–122.

27. Williams, D. R., Lavizzo-Mourey, R., and Warren, R. C. The concept of race and health status in America. *Public Health Report,* 109 (1994): 26–41.

28. Norris, F. H., Friedman, M. J., and Watson, P. J. 60,000 disaster victims speak: Part II. Summary and implications of the disaster mental health research. *Psychiatry,* 65, no. 3 (2002): 240–260.

29. Daley, R. W., Brown, S., Archer, P., et al. Risk of tornado-related death and injury in Oklahoma, May 3, 1999. *American Journal of Epidemiology,* 161, no. 12 (2005): 1144–1150.

30. The Associated Press. Major earthquakes around the world over the past 80 years. *USA Today* (October 5, 2005).

31. UNFPA. State of the World Population 2007: Unleashing the Potential of Urban Growth. New York: United Nations Population Fund, 2007.

32. Richerson, B., and Boyd, R. *Not by Genes Alone: How Culture Transformed Human Evolution.* Chicago: University of Chicago Press, 2005.

33. Perilla, J. L., Norris, F. H., and Lavizzo, E. A. Ethnicity, culture and disaster response: Identifying and explaining ethnic differences in PTSD six months after Hurricane Andrew. *Journal of Social and Clinical Psychology,* 21 (2002): 20–45.

34. Marsella, A. J., Friedman, M. J., Gerrity, E. T., and Scurfield, R. M. *Ethnocultural Aspects of Posttraumatic Stress Disorder: Issues, Research, and Clinical Applications.* Washington, D.C.: American Psychological Association, 1996.

35. Galea, S., Ahern, J., Resnick, H., Kilpatrick, D., Bucuvalas, M., Gold, J., and Vlahov, D. Psychological sequelae of the September 11 attacks in Manhattan, New York City. *New England Journal of Medicine,* 346 (2002): 982–987.

36. Henrich, J., Boyd, R., Bowles, S., et al. "Economic man" in cross-cultural perspective: Behavioral experiments in 15 small-scale societies. *Behavioral and Brain Sciences,* 28, no. 6 (2005): 795–815; discussion 815–855.

37. Paciotti, B., Hadley, C., Holmes, C., and Borgerhoff Mulder, M. Grass-roots justice in Tanzania. *American Science,* 93 (January/February 2005): 58–63.

38. United Nations Sub-Committee on Nutrition. *Report on the Nutrition Situation of Refugees and Displaced Populations,* Report No. 26. Geneva: United Nations, 1999.

39. United Nations Sub-Committee on Nutrition. *Report on the Nutrition Situation of Refugees and Displaced Populations,* Report No. 30. Geneva: United Nations, 2000.

40. United Nations Administrative Committee on Coordination, Sub-Committee on Nutrition (ACC/SCN) in collaboration with International Food Policy Research Institute (IRPRI). *Fourth Report on the World Nutrition Situation: Nutrition Throughout the Life Cycle.* Geneva: United Nations, 2000.

41. United Nations Sub-Committee on Nutrition. *Report on the Nutrition Situation of Refugees and Displaced Populations.* Report No. 39–43. Geneva: United Nations, 2002.

42. United Nations Sub-Committee on Nutrition. *Report on the Nutrition Situation of Refugees and Displaced Populations.* Report No. 42. Geneva: United Nations, 2003.

43. United Nations Sub-Committee on Nutrition. *Report on the Nutrition Situation of Refugees and Displaced Populations.* Report No. 38. Geneva: United Nations, 2002.

44. United Nations Sub-Committee on Nutrition. *Report on the Nutrition Situation of Refugees and Displaced Populations.* Report No. 27. Geneva: United Nations, 1999.

45. Ruel, M. J., Haddad, L., Garrett, J. L, et al. Some urban facts of life: Implications for research and policy. *World Development,* 27, no. 3 (2000): 1917–1938.

46. Gabe, T., Falk, G., McCarty, M., and Mason, V. W. *Hurricane Katrina: Social-demographic characteristics of impacted areas.* Available at www.gnocdc.org/reports/crsrept.pdf. Washington, D.C.: Congressional Research Service. Published November 4, 2005. Accessed June 26, 2008.

47. Austin, D. Coastal exploitation, land loss, and hurricanes: A recipe for disaster. *American Anthropologist,* 108, no. 4 (2006): 671–691.

48. U.S. Census Bureau. GCT-P14. *Income and poverty in 1999: 2000.* Available at http://factfinder.census.gov/servlet/GCTTable?_bm=y&-geo_id=01000US&-_box_head_nbr=GCT-P14&-ds_name=DEC_2000_SF3_U&-format=US-9. Accessed June 26, 2008.

49. Logan, J. *The impact of Katrina: Race and class in storm-damaged neighborhoods.* Available at www.s4.brown.edu/Katrina/report.pdf. Published 2005. Accessed June 26, 2008.

50. Weisler, R. H., Barbee, J. G., and Townsend, M. H. Mental health and recovery in the Gulf Coast after Hurricanes Katrina and Rita. *JAMA,* 296, no. 5 (2006): 585–588.

51. Boscarino, J. A., Galea, S., Adams, R. E., Ahern, J., Resnick, H., and Vlahov, D. Mental health service and medication use in New York City after the September 11, 2001 terrorist attack. *Psychiatric Services,* 55, no. 3 (2004): 274–283.

52. Wittenauer, C. Baton Rouge mayor: Big problems still exist. *The Associated Press* (February 23, 2006).

53. Jakes L. Report: Government-wide Katrina failings rampant, government-wide failings to blame for Katrina response, House report finds. *The Associated Press* (February 12, 2006).

54. CQ Transcriptions. Former FEMA director testifies before Congress. Transcript of the House hearings today on the federal, state and local response to Hurricane Katrina. *CQ Transcriptions* (September 27, 2005).

55. Nieburg, P., Waldman, R. J., and Krumm, D. M. Hurricane Katrina. Evacuated populations—lessons from foreign refugee crises. *New England Journal of Medicine,* 353, no. 15 (2005): 1547–1549.

56. O'Brien, K., and Bender, B. Chronology of errors: How a disaster spreads. *Boston Globe* (September 11, 2005).

57. Fisher, H. *Response to Disaster: Fact Versus Fiction and Its Perpetuation.* Lanham, Md.: University Press of America, 1998.

58. Ethridge, R. Bearing witness: Assumptions, realities, and the otherizing of Katrina. *American Anthropologist,* 108, no. 4 (2006): 799–813.

59. United States General Accounting Office. *Disaster assistance: Federal aid to the New York City area following the attacks of September 11th and challenges confronting FEMA.* Available at www.gao.gov/new.items/d031174t.pdf. Published 2003. Accessed July 25, 2006.

60. Project Liberty. *Project liberty history.* New York State. Available at www.projectliberty.state.ny.us/whatwaspl-history.htm. Accessed July 25, 2006.

61. New York State Office of Mental Health. *2005–2009 statewide comprehensive plan for mental health service services. Appendix 5: Project Liberty service delivery.* New York State Office of Mental Health. Available at www.omh.state.ny.us/omhweb/statewideplan/2005/appendix5.htm. Accessed July 25, 2006.

62. Galea, S., Vlahov, D., Resnick, H., et al. Trends in probable post-traumatic stress disorder in New York City after the September 11 terrorist attacks. *American Journal of Epidemiology,* 158, no. 6 (2003): 514–524.

63. Galea, S., Vlahov, D., Tracy, M., Hoover, D., Resnick, H., and Kilpatrick, D. G. Hispanic ethnicity and post-traumatic stress disorder after a disaster: Evidence from a general population survey after September 11. *Annals of Epidemiology,* 14, no. 8 (2004): 520–531.

64. Vlahov, D., Galea, S., Resnick, H., et al. Increased consumption of cigarettes, alcohol, and marijuana among Manhattan residents after the September 11th terrorist attacks. *American Journal of Epidemiology,* 555 (2002): 988–996.

65. Vlahov, D., Galea, S., Ahern, J., Resnick, H., and Kilpatrick, D. Sustained increased consumption of cigarettes, alcohol and marijuana among Manhattan residents following the events of September 11, 2001. *American Journal of Public Health,* 94, no. 2 (2004): 253–254.

66. Galea, S., and Resnick, H. Posttraumatic stress disorder in the general population after mass terrorist incidents: Considerations about the nature of exposure. *CNS Spectrums,* 10, no. 2 (2005): 107–115.

67. Schlenger, W., Caddell, J., Ebert, L., et al. Psychological reactions to terrorist attacks: Findings from the National Study of Americans' Reactions to September 11. *JAMA,* 288, no. 5 (2002): 581–588.

68. Nandi, A., Galea, S., Tracy, M., et al. Job loss, work stress, job satisfaction and the persistence of posttraumatic stress disorder one year after the September 11 attacks. *Journal of Occupational and Environmental Medicine,* 46, no. 10 (2004): 1057–1064.

69. Ahern, J., and Galea, S. Social context and depression after a disaster: The role of income inequality. *Journal of Epidemiology Community Health,* 60 (2006): 766–770.

70. Galea, S., Ahern, J., Nandi, A., Tracy, M., Beard, J., and Vlahov, D. Urban neighborhood socioeconomic status and incidence of depression: Evidence from a population-based cohort study. *Annals of Epidemiology,* 17 (2007): 171–179.

71. Coleman, C. *Death Is a Social Disease: Public Health and Political Economy in Early Industrial France.* Madison: University of Wisconsin Press, 1982.

72. United Nations. *Challenge of the Slums.* Nairobi, Kenya. United Nations Settlement Programme, 2003.

CHAPTER

10

IMMIGRANTS AND URBAN AGING: TOWARD A POLICY FRAMEWORK

MARIANNE FAHS, ANAHÍ VILADRICH, NINA S. PARIKH

LEARNING OBJECTIVES

- Describe major trends in aging and immigration and discuss how these trends will affect the composition of urban populations.

- Identify common assumptions about aging and immigration and analyze the factual basis of these assumptions.

- Discuss the influence of municipal policies in transportation, housing, food, and other areas on the health of older immigrants.

- Describe policies that will support healthy aging among immigrants living in cities.

THE NEW URBAN DEMOGRAPHY: BABY BOOMERS AND IMMIGRANTS

The first "baby boomer" turns sixty-five in 2011, followed by 76 million others, representing an increase of 117 percent in the population of persons aged sixty-five years and older by 2030. Figure 10.1 presents the U.S. Census estimates of the average annual rates of growth for the population of older adults over time. Cities, where older people increasingly tend to concentrate, face enormous challenges. The implications for public health policy in U.S. cities, as well as cities across the globe, are complex, as the aging population is not only growing but also living longer. Indeed, this new demographic wave of baby boomers is predicted to have such a major impact on our urban economic and political landscape that some have coined the term "demographic tsunami." There is no doubt that the ramifications of this phenomenon for cities are unparalleled in history. The implications for public health in the United States, as well as globally, are enormous and complex.

Policymakers concerned with healthy urban aging will face not only a doubling in cities' older demographic but also an unprecedented increase in the percentage of elderly who are nonwhite. As shown in Figure 10.2, nonwhite elderly will increase from 16 percent of the total elderly population in 2000 to 36 percent by 2050.[1] This increase follows the most recent wave of immigration, which occurred after the 1965 Immigration Act, the largest wave ever experienced in U.S. history.[2] Thus, many of

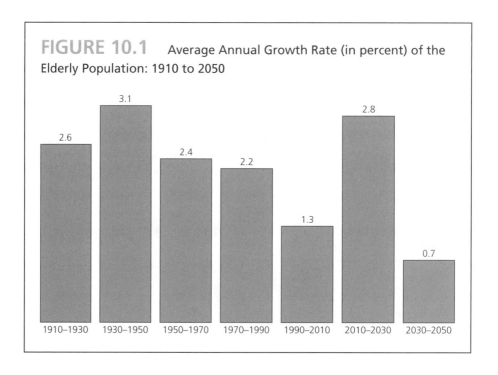

FIGURE 10.1   Average Annual Growth Rate (in percent) of the Elderly Population: 1910 to 2050

these more diverse older people will be immigrants aging in a foreign land. Older immigrants in the United States will not only become more numerous but also increasingly diverse in terms of gender, income, ethnicity, and language.

How cities respond to the public health challenges of healthy urban aging will make a critical contribution to the resolution of the current policy debate on aging. The debate centers on the controversy over the extent to which this new wave of older adults will pose an unsustainable economic "burden," requiring new cuts in Medicare or Social Security, as advocated by some policy analyses and leaders, or instead will bring new economic growth and prosperity, as many economists and others suggest is possible.[3] A reasoned analysis of the factors affecting healthy urban aging can help guide decision makers to make more informed choices.

This chapter examines key social, economic, and policy issues at the intersection of these demographic trends in our cities. Our intent is to contribute to new ways of thinking to help support the development of a new urban landscape promoting healthy

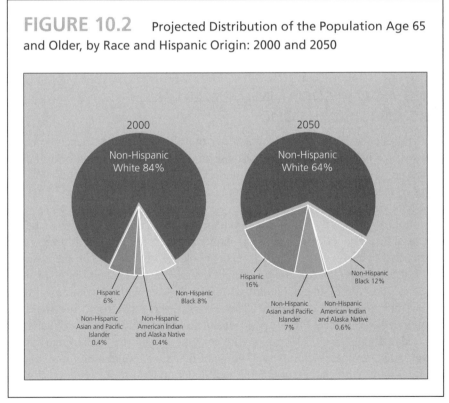

FIGURE 10.2 Projected Distribution of the Population Age 65 and Older, by Race and Hispanic Origin: 2000 and 2050

Note: Data are middle-series projections of the population. Hispanics may be of any race. These data refer to the resident population.

Source: U.S. Census Bureau, Population Projections.

aging for all. Recently, researchers have begun investigating multiple determinants of healthy aging, including neighborhood and environmental determinants. Yet there are no theoretical models to define and predict which factors are associated with successful aging in an urban environment.[4] The intent of this chapter is to develop a policy framework to contribute toward the identification of prominent features of urban policy and urban neighborhoods likely to have differential impacts on healthy urban aging among immigrants. Because many of these features are modifiable, identifying those aspects of neighborhood environments and policy having significant influence on healthy aging can provide insight to policymakers interested in addressing disparities in successful aging and improving healthy aging overall.[5]

In this chapter, we first provide a brief overview and critique of the economic and social debate influencing our current policies on health and aging. We then review several major studies that address the effects of the built and social environment on health and health trajectories of urban older adults, with a particular focus on immigrants and immigrant health. Finally, we present a multilevel conceptual framework for healthy urban aging, adapted from the fields of gerontology and urban public health, and discuss the need to extend and modify this model to focus on healthy aging among immigrants. Based on this framework, we suggest incremental steps toward a public health policy agenda for healthy urban aging.

ECONOMIC AND SOCIAL INFLUENCES ON AGING AND HEALTH POLICY

Policy and economics are closely linked. If the ultimate goal of a new conceptual framework for healthy urban aging among immigrants is to help inform and guide effective policy, it is first important to understand what economic undercurrents are shaping contemporary policy. Furthermore, it is critical for policy analysts to understand what evidence supports these underlying economic assumptions.

Economists generally agree that population aging, contrary to popular belief, is not a causal factor necessarily leading to an increased economic burden—for example, the rising cost of health care.[6, 7] In their recent book, *Aging Nation: The Economics and Politics of Growing Older in America,* Schulz and Binstock take issue with the dire forecasts of those predicting economic demise associated with population aging, calling them the "Merchants of Doom."[3] These doomsayers stoke the widely held belief that continued government financing of pensions and health care costs will lead to economic and political "crises" associated with an aging population.[8] Schulz and Binstock, however, point out that the future well-being of the whole population (of all ages) has "very little to do with 'population aging' and much to do with technological change, investments in people (education) and businesses . . . and many other non-aging factors that in large part determine the rate of economic growth. Simply equating population aging with economic demise is 'voodoo demographics.'"[3]

To build our framework for evidence-based urban aging policy, we begin by briefly reviewing the prevailing assumptions that influence the contemporary policy arena on aging and immigrants and the evidence behind these assumptions, which relies heavily on economic indicators. To better understand the contextual environment that shapes public health policies for older urban immigrants, we discuss five prevailing economic assumptions about aging and immigration.

Assumption 1: Older Adults Are a Drain on the Economy

The reality: The older (50+) population currently represents $2 trillion in consumer spending, an amount sure to increase as the population grows older.[9] This rising consumer demand will stimulate many industries. These industries include the high-tech industry, where breakthroughs in products using technology useful to older adults, such as robotics, will occur, as well as the more traditional "silver industries" associated with older adult consumers such as assisted living housing, pharmaceuticals, the banking system, the travel industry, and long-term care insurance.

Assumption 2: Older Adults Are a Drain on the Health Care System

The reality: The health care industry, one of the fastest growing employment sectors in the country and fueled by increasing demand among older adults, will be a powerful economic stimulus, particularly in large urban centers.[10] In the health care market, as in all others, expenses to consumers provide income to producers.[7] Thus, increased expenses associated with health care for a growing population of older adults lead to job growth and income for health care workers. A recent study by the Urban Institute finds health care to be the leading employer in twenty major U.S. cities, and the Department of Labor predicts tremendous job growth in health care over the next several decades.[11, 12]

But how high can health care expenditures grow before we start depriving other sectors of the economy, such as education or housing? The issue is not one of absolute growth but of relative growth compared to the economy as a whole. In fact, according to a recent study, health care costs can increase 1 percent faster than real per capita economic growth with no adverse consequences for the next seven decades; that is, we would not have to decrease spending in any other economic sector through 2075. A 2 percent differential still takes us through the next three decades with no other spending decreases.[13]

Assumption 3: Immigrants Are a Drain on the Economy and the Health Care System

The reality: Similar to older adults, prevailing assumptions concerning immigrants focus on the burden that immigrants represent to the U.S. economy and the health care system.[14] Yet consistent data show immigrants contribute substantially to tax revenues through productive labor.[14] Moreover, health expenditures appear to be substantially lower for immigrants than for U.S.-born groups.[15, 16]

Assumption 4: Preventive Medicine Is Not Cost Effective After Age Sixty-Five

The reality: Health economists have shown strikingly cost-effective results ever since preventive medicine for older people first began to be systematically examined twenty years ago.[17, 18] Actual cost savings have been documented in the literature for programs focusing on immigrant elderly.[19] In a recent study of the value of disease prevention among the elderly, Goldman and colleagues demonstrated prevention among the elderly could be very cost effective.[20] For instance, hypertension control could reduce health spending by $890 billion over the next twenty-five years, while adding 75 million disability-adjusted life years. Reducing obesity back to 1980s levels would save more than $1 trillion.[20]

Assumption 5: Increased Longevity Will Cause Large Health and Social Costs from Degenerative Disease, Disability, and Economic Decline

The reality: As stated at the beginning of this section, economic theory does not predict a causal association between longevity and economic decline. Instead, the available economic data show a positive association between increasing longevity and economic growth. A recent study of developing countries calculated a ten-year gain in life expectancy translated into nearly one additional percentage point of annual income growth.[21] This favorable economic finding could apply to urban neighborhoods as well. In New York City, for instance, as in other world economic capitals, people are now living longer than the national average.[22] It is possible to speculate further that decreasing disparities in longevity across neighborhoods would similarly lead to increased urban prosperity.

Economic wealth is defined by more than market value; it includes social value as well. A recent study estimated that increased longevity between 1970 and 2000 added more than $3 trillion per year to national wealth.[23] This is an enormous hidden increase in social value that is not considered by standard market analyses.

Moreover, older people are staying healthy longer. New data show old-age disability rates declined for all socioeconomic groups over the past two decades.[24] These findings provide new evidence in support of the "compression of morbidity" hypothesis.[25] This hypothesis suggests, as people live longer, age-related morbidity begins later in life; that is, morbidity is "compressed" into the later stages of life.

Finally, male and female immigrants have 3.4 and 2.5 years, respectively, longer life expectancy than those born in the United States.[26] In contrast to some studies that link the length of immigrants' stay in the United States with increasing unhealthy practices, other studies suggest that immigrants' healthy habits may provide a sort of "health insurance policy" against disease, particularly among impoverished elderly newcomers.[27, 28] In an ethnographic study of forty- to seventy-year-old Indian immigrants in Canada, Choudhry reported older women's strategies to continue a healthy lifestyle were based on maintaining a good diet, participating in physical activity, and practicing weight control, as well as having regular spiritual prayers and good relationships with others.[29] In a study of older women who had come to the United States from the former Soviet Union, researchers found that participants tended to decrease their risk for coronary heart disease as they followed a more "Americanized" way of life.[30]

This brief review of the conventional wisdom that informs current policy debates on aging, immigration, and health shows that many of these assumptions are patently false or subject to empirical challenge.

Alternative Conceptual Models

An understanding of the complex interactions of urban neighborhoods with the economic, social, environmental, and behavioral factors associated with healthy aging among older immigrants suggests that good public health policy can also be good economic policy. Contrary to prevailing assumptions on aging, the available economic data show a positive association among aging, longevity, and economic growth. Thus, public health policy can play a substantial role in promoting healthy aging among immigrants while simultaneously promoting urban economic vitality. There is a pressing need for more research to better understand how and where urban neighborhood environments and policy influence health and health trajectories among older immigrants and to identify modifiable neighborhood features that can improve the health and social well-being of older adult immigrants.

In the gerontology literature, models of productive and successful aging dispute deterministic age-related frailty as a biological inevitability; rather, they focus on understanding determinants of healthy aging—that is, the biological and social mechanisms causally linked to cognitive and functional performance. There are many terms for "healthy aging," including "successful aging" and "productive aging," two of the best known. According to Rowe and Kahn, *successful aging* is the combination of low probability of disease, high physical and mental functioning, and active engagement with life.[31] Their emphasis is on the interaction between biological and functional capacities. Butler introduced the concept of *productive aging* to emphasize the economic value associated with healthy aging.[32] Both of these concepts are useful to incorporate in a conceptual framework for healthy urban aging. Although a growing literature documents the effectiveness of individual-level evidence-based interventions for the promotion of physical activity, improved nutrition, chronic disease management, and prevention of cognitive decline and depression for older adults, the fundamental reality is that the factors that influence health are behavioral, social, and environmental.[33] To date, few interventions for older people or older immigrants adequately address these social and environmental determinants.

To develop a policy model for healthy aging in the context of urban environments, a conceptual framework for healthy urban aging must move beyond individual predictors of health and economic outcomes and incorporate the broader social, biological, and physical determinants of health for older adults. These include transportation, physical activity, social networks, access to health and social services, economic and social security, community involvement, and housing. In the next section, we explore these influences.

SOCIAL AND ENVIRONMENTAL CONSIDERATIONS

What Is a Neighborhood?

A rapidly growing body of literature explores the effects of social, institutional, and physical characteristics of neighborhoods on health behaviors[34, 35] and health outcomes.[36] Gerontologists have suggested that neighborhood environments might be particularly significant for the functional health and well-being of older adults. Yet no consensus has been reached on the most appropriate way to characterize the physical and social environments of neighborhoods or even how to define them. There does seem to be a growing agreement that "neighborhood" refers to a geographic unit, with relative homogeneity in housing type and population, as well as some level of social interaction and symbolic significance to residents.[37, 38] However, the subjectivity of neighborhood boundaries[39] is also widely accepted,[40] particularly in cities, where local travel is easy and frequent and neighborhood boundaries are likely to be malleable. Social connections, common use of public facilities (e.g., schools, post office, shopping areas), and physical barriers (e.g., railroad tracks) may lead to an overlap in residents' neighborhood definitions, but their perceptions are also affected by individual characteristics, such as gender, age, educational attainment, mobility, and daily activities.[37, 41]

We define neighborhood characteristics to include safety, density, socioeconomic status (SES), wealth disparity, access to public transport, access to retail and recreational facilities, and general aesthetic qualities. In addition to these general neighborhood features, housing factors such as size, home ownership, and condition and social factors such as measures of social cohesion, social capital, participation in social groups, and cultural norms are important components of a conceptual framework for successful urban aging.

Physical Environment and Health Status

Extensive evidence suggests that local physical environments affect a myriad of health-related outcomes, including self-rated health, mortality, depression, chronic conditions, and health behaviors.[35, 36, 42–47] Some recent work on the influence of the social environment suggests a positive association between the social resources of a community and health.[48–50] Although studies show that neighborhood characteristics significantly affect health among different subgroups of the adult population, researchers still know very little about how the local environment influences the health of older adults.[45, 51–53] Even less is known about the specific influence of neighborhoods on the well-being of older immigrants.

It is likely that neighborhood context plays a salient role in the quality of life of older adults, particularly among immigrants. Older residents rely on the proximate resources of the neighborhood, spend a majority of their time in a localized area, and have a strong commitment and emotional attachment to their community.[54] Several studies demonstrate that the health of older adults varies based on characteristics of the area, including neighborhood socioeconomic status (SES). Krause found that compared with those who lived in better off residential areas, older adults who lived in deteriorated neighborhoods were significantly more likely to report poorer health status.[45] Robert and colleagues used data from a nationally representative sample to show that neighborhood SES was associated with health status and comorbidity of older adults independent of individual-level SES.[53, 55, 56] In a 2002 study, Balfour and Kaplan used longitudinal data and found that older adults who reported living in neighborhoods with excessive noise, inadequate lighting, and heavy traffic experienced a greater risk of functional decline one year later compared with those residing in communities with fewer environmental problems.[51]

Of particular interest is a recent study that examined neighborhood effects and health status among older Mexican Americans. As expected, older adults who lived in adverse neighborhood environments, compared with those who resided in better environments, were more likely to report poorer health status. In addition to the association between neighborhood economic disadvantage and poor health status, Patel and colleagues found that older adults who lived in a neighborhood near the Mexico-U.S. border compared with those who did not were more likely to report poorer health status.[57] Furthermore, relative to older Mexican Americans who did not live in neighborhoods with other Latinos, those who did were more likely to report better health, demonstrating the importance of multiple contextual domains when assessing the association between neighborhood effects and health, in particular among immigrant groups.

Physical Activity

One health-related behavior that has been increasingly linked to the neighborhood environment is physical activity.[35, 58, 59] Certainly, the social and physical environment, including transportation policies and decisions, create opportunities that either facilitate or hinder the promotion of physical activity. Although there is strong evidence that a physically active lifestyle is important in the prevention of chronic disease and promotion of health and well-being, physical activity levels tend to progressively decline with increasing age.[60] Limited cross-sectional research in older adults suggests that lower levels of physical activity are associated with higher levels of psychological distress and with a lower health-related quality of life.[61] There is also evidence that physical activity is protective against incident depression and falls in older adults. However, predictors of exercise adherence that have been developed in younger adults are unreliable in this group.[62]

Notably, among older adults, regular physical activity improves mobility, coordination, and balance, as well as other health benefits that improve overall health and well-being.[63–66] As with most data on health behaviors, there is limited research on physical activity patterns that compare U.S.- and foreign-born residents. Few studies have suggested that immigrants compared with their U.S.-born counterparts are less likely to engage in physical activity.[67] Yet among older immigrants, with increased time in the United States and greater acculturation, participation in leisure-time physical activity increased after controlling for other demographic factors.[68, 69]

Recent evidence suggests that community characteristics, including street design, proximity of facilities, lighting, aesthetics (e.g., trees and greenery), and safety are the most important determinants of physical activity.[70, 71] A study in Houston, Texas, found that nearly 60 percent of disabled and elderly residents lacked sidewalks in their neighborhoods.[72] Clearly, fear of crime and a lack of accessible areas for walking create barriers to physical activity among older adults. Furthermore, a recent investigation examining the multilevel effects of the built environment on walking patterns of older adults revealed significant interneighborhood variability in walking activities among older residents. These differences were explained by such environmental characteristics as high employment density, high household density, greater areas of open and green spaces, and more street intersections.[73]

On the one hand, dispersed communities, problematic community design, and the lack of safe environments may make it difficult for many individuals, especially older adults, to walk in their own neighborhoods.[74, 75] Living in neighborhoods with high levels of noise, litter, crime, vandalism, graffiti, and abandoned buildings may result in persons being less likely to engage in physical activity out of fear of exercising in the neighborhood.[76]

On the other hand, several factors in the physical and social environment have been found to promote physical activity among older adults. Using data from the Behavioral Risk Factor Surveillance System (BRFSS), researchers found that other likely influences on physical activity included physician advice, proximity to facilities, social support, health literacy, and childhood practices.[62, 77, 78] Personal attributes of older people that have been associated with higher levels of activity include being male, younger age, ability to travel independently, better physical functioning, adequate fruit and vegetable intake, and perceptions of high self-efficacy[61, 77–80] Although individual behaviors and attitudes, including safety issues for older adults, are important factors in health-related outcomes, structural barriers, including social, economic, and political processes, have contributed to the creation and development of the physical and social environment and to the growing disparities in health by social class, race and ethnicity, age, and gender.[81]

These studies suggest that the characteristics and amenities of a neighborhood are important for the physical and mental health of older adults, including immigrant elders. As many older adults reside in their communities for decades, a phenomenon commonly referred to as "aging in place," it will become increasingly important to develop policies that can create and sustain supportive environments for older residents.

Isolation and Neighborhood Conditions: Effects on Immigrants' Mental Health

Depression is a major public health problem, particularly later in life. Among older adults, depression has been found to lead to declined role functioning, increased risk of physical disability, and other medical illnesses.[82–84] Prevalence of depression among community dwelling older adults is limited by small sample size, but reported rates of depression range from 1 to as high as 27 percent.[83, 85, 86] Older immigrants appear to be more vulnerable to and more affected by mental illness than other groups, particularly with regard to depression, memory loss, and mood alterations.[87, 88] Overall, older immigrants present more mental health problems than their younger counterparts, particularly among women from different ethnic groups.[30]

It has long been thought that certain characteristics of the urban environment, in particular, community disorganization, may influence population mental health. Yet, empirical evidence linking neighborhood characteristics and health is primarily focused on physical health. Recent studies examining the relationship between neighborhood context and mental health have found that neighborhood deprivation and disorganization are associated with depression, even after accounting for individual income and education status.[89–94] The implication of this research is that there are characteristics of economically deprived neighborhoods that influence mental health beyond the effect of economic deprivation itself. The ongoing identification of these characteristics would provide the opportunity to model structural interventions that might influence an individual's risk of developing a mental illness regardless of socioeconomic status. Although there is no research focused specifically on older adults in this regard, such a hypothesis is supported by a recent randomized controlled trial that moved families from high-poverty neighborhoods to nonpoor neighborhoods. The results showed that both parents and children who moved reported fewer psychological distress symptoms than did control families who did not move, despite no other changes in their economic situation.[95]

Robert and colleagues examined data from the Alameda County Study to assess the theoretical proposition that neighborhood conditions, either stressful or supportive, would increase or decrease the risk of poor mental health. Study results revealed neighborhood characteristics to be associated with depression.[96] In another recent study with older Mexican Americans, results showed that low neighborhood SES was associated with higher levels of depressive symptomatology, and higher levels of concentration of older Latinos in a neighborhood was associated with lower levels of mental health problems.[97] Similar results were found in a study conducted by Kubzansky and colleagues assessing neighborhood context and depression. Findings suggest that individuals who lived in economically disadvantaged neighborhoods compared with those who resided in better off communities were more likely to report higher levels of depression.[92]

Social Capital

Recent studies on the effect of social capital report differential access to social resources (e.g., belonging to community organizations and community services), differences mediated in part by immigrant household composition (i.e., single-mother families vs. elderly units) and migratory age (i.e., young-at-arrival elderly vs. old-at-arrival elderly).[98]

Even though there is no definitive consensus on the relationship between the built environment and social capital, several studies have demonstrated that walkable neighborhoods and mixed land use in communities are associated with an improved sense of community among residents.[99, 100] The built environment can also have negative consequences. For example, geographic isolation; little social contact with neighbors, friends, or community members; and increased use of computers and television can encourage isolation.[101, 102]

The creation of supportive neighborhood or community networks could lead to higher levels of social capital, which in turn have been shown to be associated with lower levels of morbidity and mortality and self-rated health.[48, 103] Moreover, establishing and maintaining supportive social networks and having accessible transportation options are particularly important for older adults as they protect from social isolation and create healthy and productive communities. Whether the dense social networks associated with ethnic enclaves promote social integration of older immigrants warrants further study.

Transportation: Mobilizing Social Networks

Recent research has focused on the connection between transportation and health. Transportation decisions have the potential to either promote or obstruct the development and maintenance of healthy communities and neighborhoods. Specifically, transportation is closely associated with social isolation.[104] Travel for great distances or lack of transport options prevents individuals from developing meaningful social networks that provide valuable support and assistance on a regular basis and contribute to individuals' quality of life and well-being. For older adults, the connection between transportation policy and health is critical. Without adequate, affordable, and readily accessible transportation options, older adults are limited in participating in physical activities, getting to health and other social service organizations, and establishing supportive networks.[104, 105] Furthermore, as the distance traveled for social and health services, work, or leisure activities increases, and mass transit is not available, there is an elevated risk of vehicular accidents as well as pedestrian injuries and fatalities.[106, 107] Of note, pedestrian injuries and deaths are highest among children and older adults.[108] As more immigrants move from inner cities to suburbs, their access to public transportation may decline.

Living Alone: The Pervasive Impact of Loneliness and Isolation

Living arrangements and frail or absent social networks appear to be omnipresent risk factors for mental health illnesses among elderly immigrants in the United States.[109] Living alone and having fewer financial resources are indeed among the most common predictors of depression among aging immigrants.[110] Isolated individuals are more numerous at the top of the age pyramid, particularly among those who have experienced the loss of significant others (e.g., in the case of widowers), have undergone emotional loneliness (lack of intimate attachment), or are removed from supportive kin.[111] Loneliness is considered a public health problem among immigrants, both in itself and as it relates to other mental health ailments.[112] Although, as noted by Klinenberg, there are differences between the objective and subjective indicators of isolation and loneliness—isolation being an objective marker and loneliness a more subjective feeling—both have an impact on elderly physical and emotional health.[113] This concurs with current strong evidence that links social interactions with positive health outcomes.[114–116]

Studies of Koreans in the United States have led to a better understanding of the relationship between social integration and mental health outcomes as well as of immigrants' coping strategies against chronic disease. Kim's research on predictors of loneliness among elderly Korean immigrants found that women reported higher levels of feeling lonely than previously found in the literature. Of note, women's dissatisfaction with their perceived social support was the greatest predictor of loneliness, despite their marital status.[111] In a study aimed at determining the relationship of Korean immigrants' alienation to place of residence, Moon concluded that foreign-born residents may minimize their adjustment problems either by living in ethnic enclaves or by socializing with members of their own ethnic group.[117] Studies of postmigration effects on mental health outcomes show that mental health issues did not appear until after migration to the United States.[118] In a study of immigrants' living arrangements and depression, Wilmoth and Chen found that depressive symptoms were more prevalent among those living alone, a finding that calls attention to the relationship between social integration (measured on the basis of counting on social networks and perception of social support) and mental health outcomes.[110]

A study of social integration and health status among Asian Indian immigrants (fifty years and older) found an association between poor health status and older age, being female, and longer residence in the United States.[69] Diwan and colleagues also found that satisfaction with friendships was a predictor of positive affect, suggesting the need for interventions leading to immigrants' social integration.[119] Miller et al. reported that Russian female immigrants who were older, had lived fewer years in the United States, and took antidepressants reported more symptoms of depressive mood.[30] These findings support the results of a study on gender differences in distress among immigrants from the former Soviet Union.[120] The authors found that older age and less time in the United States predicted higher levels of stress among both male and female immigrants. Women reported more distress than men, a finding that correlates with having lower educational attainment and lacking sponsoring agents (i.e., friends and family) and supportive organizations (e.g., religious groups) in the United States.

Wilmoth and Chen also found that immigrant status and living arrangements interact in predicting depressive symptoms.[110] Studies examining the prevalence of mental disorders among Mexican immigrants and U.S.-born Mexican Americans show that Mexican immigrants present healthier mental health profiles than their U.S.-born ethnic kin in spite of their lower socioeconomic status. The authors partially attribute these results to the protective effect of traditional family networks that are more prevalent among first-generation migrants compared with successive generations.[121] In the next section, we further explore the impact of the social and physical environment on immigrants' health status with a focus on the effect of social isolation on elderly mental health conditions. The need to promote social integration at different levels (e.g., family, neighborhood, community) and the importance of ecological approaches that address the obstacles to immigrant social incorporation are pivotal in promoting healthy aging indicators among the foreign-born population in the United States.

Dynamic Social Networks and Changing Filial Expectations

Immigrants' health status assessment must take into account the impact of family transitions and household mobility.[122] Generally, different immigrant groups in the United States have different intergenerational family living arrangements. Significantly, individuals who migrated to the United States after the age of fifty appear to be more dependent on their families than those who emigrated earlier,[123] particularly when they become ill.[124] Parents who had immigrated recently, especially Asians and those from Central and South America, were more likely to live with their children, who typically provided most of the household income, a trend that decreases over time.[125] Long-term incorporation, which is usually correlated with membership in groups and English proficiency, appears to be related to higher degrees of healthy independence and autonomy at older age. For example, lifetime migration patterns and ethnic involvement were significant predictors of nursing home placement among a sample of elderly European Americans who migrated to Florida after retirement.[126] Immigrant grandparents' participation in raising their children's offspring in the United States has become one of the most widespread family strategies to deal with stressors and crises and to address national shortages in affordable child care.[127] This suggests the emergence of new risks for aging immigrants in the United States as they become caregivers for troubled families and children with behavioral disorders.

As immigrants grow older, their children also face emerging difficulties in developing coping strategies that seek to balance cultural traditions, filial values and obligations, along with changing personal expectations. According to Jones et al., Asian American immigrant women involved in filial caregiving are at special risk of encountering health problems due to the conflicting demands they face while mobilizing family and personal resources.[128] Lan studied the transformation of caring modalities for elderly, middle-class Taiwanese and Hong Kong immigrant families in California and found a rise in the commoditization of care (e.g., via third parties in institutional and ambulatory settings), with the family as the main agency arranging for older adults' caring networks.[129] By recruiting home care practitioners, immigrant families help re-create "fictive kin" through which elderly parents and their adult children try to adjust to (and negotiate with) cultural norms of filial care. Similar results were found in a study on the impact of children's emigration on nonimmigrant Asian Indian elderly parents.

Miltiades reports that parents substitute for their children's help by relying on hired assistants, a solution that provides both groups with higher independence but may not counteract the feelings of depression and loneliness experienced by older adults left behind.[130] In addition, Lee and Farran found depressive symptoms among Koreans and Korean Americans, mostly females, who were caregivers of older relatives suffering from dementia.[131] In a study on mother-daughter conflicts in caregiving practices, Usita and Du Bois reveal the clashes emerging from contrasting needs between elderly immigrants' claims for care and attention vis-à-vis their daughters' complaints of their mothers' control and endless demands.[132]

In a study of elderly Koreans in the United States, Sung and Kim noted that contrary to the belief that Asian elders and their children keep the traditional custom of coresidence, elderly Koreans tended to live independently from their children as they grew older in the United States, primarily due to the availability of welfare programs.[133] In the same vein, Kim and Lauderdale, who studied the living arrangements of elderly Koreans in the United States, found that the likelihood of independent arrangements correlated with the availability of subsidized housing near Korean ethnic communities.[134] Similar results were reported by Burr and Mutchler in a study on older Mexican immigrants' living conditions, which revealed that moving to areas with higher concentration of Latinos increased the likelihood of living alone, particularly among older Mexican immigrants.[135] A study of elderly Chinese Americans found a switch from traditional expectations of family obligations and filial liaisons to more dependence on friends and neighbors as a central support system.[136] Furthermore, when examining the patterns of morbidity and mortality of elderly Mexican Americans living in high- and low-density Mexican American neighborhoods, Eschbach et al. found that the sociocultural advantages of living in *el barrio* (high-density Mexican area) outweighed the neighborhood's poverty.[137]

The foregoing studies suggest that ethnic vicinity provides additional incentives and support for independent living arrangements. Conceptualizations of older immigrant support networks should distinguish between older adults living alone in ethnically homogeneous communities and those in heterogeneous communities. To counteract the increasing constraints in physical and mental health that aging immigrants face in terms of physical and mental well-being, many seek diverse support networks as they approach retirement age.[138]

Roles for Public Health Researchers and Practitioners

In advancing a public health policy agenda for an aging immigrant population in the United States, health professionals and public health advocates have an important role to play in advancing accurate information on the contributions and needs of aging immigrants, while countering false assumptions concerning economic productivity and social service utilization.[139] Life-course perspectives can be pivotal in providing a better understanding, particularly taking into account that healthy aging must be understood within the context of an immigrant's life cycle.[140] For example, preretirement years are particularly crucial to immigrant patterns of physical and emotional health later in life.[138]

We have highlighted the need for multilevel and interdisciplinary approaches to yield a better understanding of the determinants of healthy aging among immigrants in the United States. A growing literature, summarized earlier, documents a complex multilevel interaction in older adults among functional and mental health, social connections, the physical environment, and physical activity. Healthy aging is both a predictor and an outcome of higher levels of physical activity and better mental health. All of these relationships take place in and interact with the physical and social environment. Only within this complex context can we begin to define the specific characteristics and circumstances of older immigrants. Acknowledgment of immigrant differences is vital but should not keep us from recognizing central common influences on health such as gender, socioeconomic status, municipal policies, and neighborhood environments. At the same time, researchers need to respect the unique role of religion, national traditions, and cultural values among different immigrant groups.[141, 142]

TOWARD A CONCEPTUAL FRAMEWORK

The body of literature reviewed in the previous section initiates a theoretical and empirical foundation for an integrated conceptual framework for healthy urban aging among immigrants. Clearly, the determinants of healthy aging among immigrants are multilevel. Yet despite a new and growing body of research demonstrating that characteristics of urban neighborhoods affect healthy aging, much of this phenomenon remains unexplored and unspecified, particularly among vulnerable older immigrants.

To investigate central scientific questions about the interaction of urban environment factors and health behavior interventions and to assist urban neighborhoods to better use social, economic, and built environmental factors to support efforts to promote healthy aging among older immigrants, it is useful to conceptualize the complex phenomena as multilayered. Figure 10.3 presents a multilevel characterization of the determinants of healthy urban aging. Public policies and socioeconomic conditions form the structure for healthy aging and include national and local public policies, particularly those affecting immigrants, such as immigration policy, Medicare and Medicaid eligibility, welfare policies, housing conditions, options for long-term care, availability, quality, and affordability of education/training, and access to transportation.

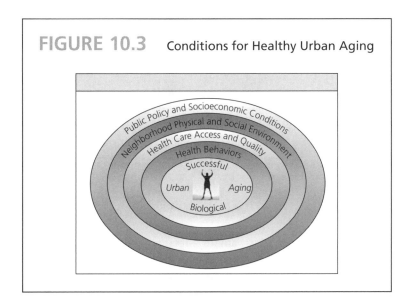

FIGURE 10.3   Conditions for Healthy Urban Aging

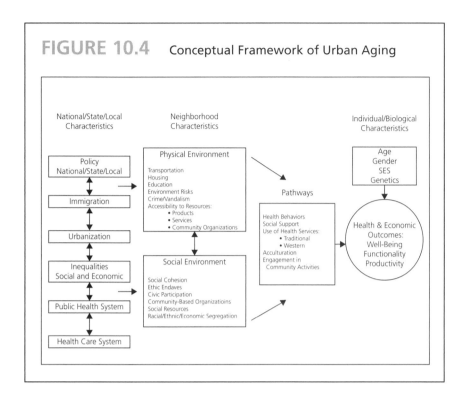

FIGURE 10.4 Conceptual Framework of Urban Aging

These characteristics interact with the social and physical characteristics of neighborhoods, such as food availability, living conditions, and public parks, as well as with the availability of quality and accessible health care programs and services, to influence personal health behaviors, such as diet, activity, smoking, alcohol consumption, and drug use. These are likewise influenced at the individual level by social, psychological, and biological characteristics.

The conceptual framework of urban aging shown in Figure 10.4 presents possible pathways to study how the effects of public policies interact with specific physical and social neighborhood characteristics to influence health outcomes. As we have seen, research to date has addressed only selected determinants. If we are to create an evidence base for the effectiveness of specific policies and programs to improve healthy aging among immigrants, future research must address the multilayered complexity found in the interaction between policy and urban neighborhood characteristics as these interactions influence the familiar pathways to health found at the individual level.

A PUBLIC HEALTH RESEARCH AND POLICY AGENDA

Policies to improve health and economic outcomes for older immigrants must address societal and community characteristics, including public safety, affordable housing, accessible transportation, and opportunities for involvement in the community. Resources are required to develop "age-friendly" or "active living" communities.[91, 143, 144] In 2005, the World Health Organization (WHO) launched the Global Age-Friendly Cities Project to engage cities to become age friendlier—that is, to encourage active aging by "optimizing opportunities for health, participation and security in order to enhance quality of life as people age" and "to tap the potential that older people represent for humanity."[145] With focus groups from thirty-three cities around the world, the WHO project defined eight areas of urban living of particular concern to older people: outdoor spaces and buildings; transportation; housing; social participation; respect and social inclusion; civic participation and employment; communication and information; and community support and health services. The project provides a useful checklist of core age-friendly city features for each of the eight areas and thus can serve as a guide for the development of specific urban public health policy goals.

Unfortunately, the WHO guide is somewhat limited in its applicability to the United States with Portland, Oregon, being the sole U.S. city represented in the development of the guide. Specific challenges in terms of health insurance availability and health care access for older immigrants in the United States are not addressed. However, as the WHO guide emphasizes, interventions solely geared to expanding health service access are not fully suitable to the needs of vulnerable older adults. For example, Freidenberg reports in her study of elder Puerto Ricans living in *El Barrio* (East Harlem, NYC) that despite the increasing allocation of resources to health care facilities, a serious unmet need experienced by older Puerto Ricans is difficulty in remaining independent at home.[140]

Many aspects concerning the supply, organization, and financing of health and social services are decided by the state or national government rather than the city, of course. To adequately respond to older adults' needs, it will be necessary to prompt policymakers with local research focused on specific aspects of the environmental context that influence healthy aging among some of the most vulnerable older members of society. However, an urban public health agenda for healthy aging can advance policy through the development of an evidence base for effective demonstrations and interventions at the local level. Population-specific plans must be able to capture local risk factors across and within immigrant groups.[140] By acknowledging older immigrants' subdifferences within ecological-defined areas, it will be possible to better allocate scarce resources. The policy relevance of such research often can be enhanced by including economic outcomes and by using techniques such as cost-effectiveness analysis, cost-benefit analysis, and impact analysis.[146, 147] Thus, an important area for further research is to better understand, describe, and quantify the economic benefits to urban neighborhoods and society that are associated with improvements in health outcomes for older adults.

Policy Recommendations

1. *Reducing disparities in income and education.* Policies to improve income and educational opportunities will improve health and increase longevity.[148]An interesting

model developed and implemented in Baltimore called the Experience Corps involved disadvantaged older adults in the support of early childhood reading. It demonstrated successful health outcomes as well as cost effectiveness.[149] Similar models, targeted to immigrant communities, should be developed and rigorously assessed to inform policy and program development within urban immigrant neighborhoods.

2. *Investing in the built environment.* Optimal physical infrastructure is conducive to improved health indicators at both the community and the individual levels. Given the large amount of time that older adults spend in localized areas,[54] policies targeting neighborhoods' physical and social capital are crucial, including those based on improving service infrastructure, transportation, and community resources, such as recreational facilities and active senior citizen centers.[45, 144] The consideration of spatial and social change (e.g., improvement or deterioration of infrastructure) is also important, particularly in the case of neighborhoods experiencing rapid gentrification. The built environment is a proximate determinant of physical activity and thus contributes to overall health status particularly related to older adults' quality of life.[70, 71, 73] Policies focused on improving the physical environment include investing in well-kept sidewalks, green areas, street design and intersections, access to public transportation, lighting, and aesthetics.

3. *Increasing neighborhoods' safety indicators.* Fear of crime affects older adults' ability to cope with simple and essential tasks, including shopping for basic food, cashing checks, and even socializing with neighbors.[113] As Freidenberg observes in the case of older adults in a Puerto Rican population, in spite of the fact that crime reported by older adults is low, fear of crime is high.[140] Hence, policy solutions to promote neighborhood safety programs should aim to provide companionship and support to vulnerable elders, including chaperone services and transportation to places of entertainment and social integration (e.g., senior citizens centers, cultural programs outside the neighborhood, and churches).

4. *Overcoming social isolation and improving mental health indicators.* The strengthening of community networks can lead to higher levels of social capital, which in turn is related to lower levels of mortality and better self-rated health.[48, 103] Policy recommendations include providing access to formal and informal supportive networks and webs through outreach efforts aimed at connecting older immigrants with voluntary organizations, ethnic-related groups, peer-support programs, and supportive housing. In addition, support for community programs not only would help improve health outcomes but would also prevent social reclusion and depression among isolated immigrant elders. As previously reported in this chapter, policy programs aimed at improving mental health indicators should address formal services (e.g., community health clinics) as well as informal counseling services, such as the ones provided by faith organizations,[141] which together may contribute to counter the stigma related to mental health conditions.

5. *Considering household composition (stable and transient).* Improving income variables based on personal indicators may ignore the ways by which scarce resources

are distributed through informal webs to satisfy population-based needs. For example, elderly minorities often spend large amounts of their income on feeding network members who may not formally live in the same household; consequently, reducing out-of-pocket expenses via food cooperatives could be a viable solution.[140] Housing assets differ between those living with others and those living alone with limited access to social webs. Policy solutions aimed at providing affordable housing should prioritize services for those reclusive and without relatives.[113]

In conclusion, healthy aging will result in longer, more productive lives, with the potential of increased economic capacity at the neighborhood level.[32] Policymakers who move precipitously to correct invented dual economic threats of a growing aging and immigrant population may instead exacerbate unintended negative economic and health consequences. A better approach is to support the development of new knowledge and evidence to better understand how to catalyze and support the social and economic advances possible with successful and productive aging. The existence of a prosperous, well-educated, and healthy older immigrant population can be an important asset to society through both its market and its participation in voluntary programs, such as after-school programs for children.[150] As a result, policies stressing "elder power"—that is, older adults' active engagement in productive activities—will lead not only to a greater sense of fulfillment, social recognition, and self-efficacy in late life but may also enhance older adults' and their families' social and economic contributions to society. The challenges are great, but the opportunities are exciting for well-designed multilevel urban research to contribute to improved policies that will support both healthy aging among immigrants and improved economic productivity in our urban neighborhoods.

SUMMARY

In this chapter, we examined key social, economic, and policy issues at the intersection of two demographic trends that are shaping cities in the United States and elsewhere: the aging of the population and growing rates of immigration. We provided a brief overview and critique of the economic and social debate influencing our current policies on health and aging. The chapter encouraged new ways of thinking to help support the development of an urban social and physical environment that promotes healthy aging for all. We examined the differential impact of these environments on older immigrant and nonimmigrant urban populations. We then proposed a policy framework that can contribute to the identification of prominent and modifiable features of urban policy and urban neighborhoods that define and predict which factors are associated with successful aging in urban settings. Our findings can provide insight to policymakers interested in addressing disparities in successful aging and improving healthy aging overall.

DISCUSSION QUESTIONS

1. What are different levels of influence on the health of older immigrants? Which levels do you think are the most important influences on the mental health of older immigrants?

2. Some people believe that older people and immigrants are drains on the economy, whereas others argue that these groups make important contributions to our society and economy. What is the evidence for these contradictory positions? What is your opinion on this question?

3. What policy changes might make cities friendlier and healthier places for older immigrants?

4. What are some ways that municipal policies interact with the culture of different immigrant groups to influence their health?

ACKNOWLEDGEMENT

An earlier version of this chapter was presented as a working paper in the Franklin & Eleanor Roosevelt Faculty Seminar on Urban Public Policy, Hunter College, 2006.

NOTES

1. Bullato, R. A., and Anderson, N. B. *Understanding Racial and Ethnic Differences in Health in Late Life: A Research Agenda.* National Research Council. Washington, D.C.: National Academies Press, 2004.

2. Kandula, N. R., Kersey, M., and Lurie, N. Assuring the health of immigrants: What the leading health indicators tell us. *Annual Review of Public Health,* 25 (2004): 357–376.

3. Schulz, J. H., and Binstock, R. H. *Aging Nation: The Economics and Politics of Growing Older in America.* Westport, Conn.: Praeger, 2006.

4. Longino, C. F., Jr. Exploring the connections: Theory and research. *Journal of Gerontology B: Psychological Sciences and Social Sciences,* 60B (2005): S172.

5. Lynch, J., and Smith, G. D. A life course approach to chronic disease epidemiology. *Annual Review of Public Health,* 26 (2005): 1–35.

6. Cutler, D. M. The potential for cost savings in Medicare's future. *Health Affairs,* 24 (2005): R77–R80.

7. Reinhardt, U. E. Does the aging of the population really drive the demand for health care? *Health Affairs,* 22 (2003): 27–39.

8. Bipartisan Commission on Entitlement and Tax Reform. *Commission Findings.* Washington, D.C.: U.S. Government Printing Office, 1994.

9. Moody, H. R. Silver industries and the new aging enterprise. *Generations,* 28 (2004): 75–78.

10. Lowenstein, R. The health sector's role in New York's regional economy. *Current Issues in Economics and Finance,* 1 (1995): 1–6.

11. Rogers, D., Toder, E., and Jones, L. *Economic Consequences of an Aging Population* (Occasional paper no. 6. The Retirement Project). Washington, D.C.: The Urban Institute, 2000.

12. U.S. Department of Labor, Bureau of Labor Statistics (BLS). *Tomorrow's jobs.* Available at www.bls.gov/oco/oco2003.htm. Published 2007. Accessed June 23, 2008.

13. Chernew, M. E., Hirth, R. A., and Cutler, D. M. Increased spending on health care: How much can the United States afford? *Health Affairs,* 22 (2003): 15–25.

14. Berk, M. L., Schur, C. L., Chavez, L. R., and Frankel, M. Health care use among undocumented Latino immigrants: Is free health care the main reason why Latinos come to the United States? A unique look at the facts. *Health Affairs,* 19 (2000): 51–64.

15. Mohanty, S. A., Woolhandler, S., Himmelstein, D. U., Pati, S., Carrasquillo, O., and Bor, D. H. Health care expenditures of immigrants in the United States: A nationally representative analysis. *American Journal of Public Health,* 95 (2005): 1431–1438.

16. Muennig, P., and Fahs, M. C. Health status and hospital utilization of recent immigrants to New York City. *Preventative Medicine,* 35 (2002): 225–231.

17. Fahs, M. C., Mandelblatt, J., Schechter, C., and Muller, C. The cost-effectiveness of cervical cancer screening for the elderly. *Annals of Internal Medicine,* 177 (1992): 520–527.

18. Mandelblatt, J., and Fahs, M. C. The cost-effectiveness of screening for cervical cancer among elderly low-income women. *JAMA,* 259 (1988): 2409–2413.

19. Cantor, S. B., Fahs, M. C., Mandelblatt, J. S., Myers, E. R., and Sanders, G. D. Decision science and cervical cancer. *Cancer,* S98 (2003): 2003–2008.

20. Goldman, D. P., Cutler, D. M., Shang, B., and Joyce, G. F. The value of elderly disease prevention. *Forum for Health Economics & Policy*, 9 (Biomedical Research and the Economy), Article 1. Available at www.bepress.com/fhep/biomedical_research/1. Published 2006. Accessed June 23, 2008.

21. Bloom, D. E., and Canning, D. The health and wealth of nations. *Science,* 287 (2000): 1207–1209.

22. NYC Department of Health and Mental Hygiene (NYCDOHMH). *Summary of New York City vital statistics, 2001.* Available at www.nyc.gov/html/doh/downloads/pdf/vs/2001sum.pdf. Accessed June 23, 2008.

23. Murphy, K. M, and Topel, R. H. The value of health and longevity. *Journal of Political Economy,* 114 (2006): 871–904.

24. Schoni, R. F., Freedman, V. A., and Martin, L. G. Why is late-life disability declining? *Milbank Quarterly,* 86 (2008): 47–89.

25. Manton, K. G., Stallard, E., and Corder, L. Changes in morbidity and chronic disability in the U.S. elderly population: Evidence from the 1982, 1984, and 1989 National Long Term Care Surveys. *Journal of Gerontology B: Psychological Sciences and Social Sciences,* 50 (1995): S194–204.

26. Singh, G. K., and Miller, B. A. Health, life expectancy, and mortality patterns among immigrant populations in the United States. *Canadian Journal of Public Health,* 95 (2004): I14–I21.

27. Viladrich, A. Tango immigrants in New York City: The value of social reciprocities. *Journal of Contemporary Ethnography,* 34 (2005): 533–559.

28. Viladrich, A. *Social careers, social capital and access barriers to health care: The case of the Argentine minority in New York City.* Doctoral dissertation. Graduate School of Arts and Sciences, Columbia University, 2003.

29. Choudhry, U. K. Health promotion among immigrant women from India living in Canada. *Image- the Journal of Nursing Scholarship,* 30 (1998): 269–274.

30. Miller, A. M., Sorokin, O., Wilbur, J., and Chandler, P. J. Demographic characteristics, menopausal status, and depression in midlife immigrant women. *Women's Health Issues,* 14 (2004): 227–234.

31. Rowe, J. W., and Kahn, R. L. Successful aging. *Gerontologist,* 37 (1997): 433–440.

32. Butler, R. N. The study of productive aging. *Journal of Gerontology B: Psychological Sciences and Social Sciences,* 57 (2002): S323.

33. McGinnis, J. M., and Foege, W. H. Actual causes of death in the United States. *JAMA,* 270 (1993): 2207–2212.

34. Duncan, C., Jones, K., and Moon, G. Smoking and deprivation: Are there neighborhood effects? *Social Science & Medicine,* 48 (1999): 497–505.

35. Yen, I. H., and Kaplan, G. A. Poverty area residence and changes in physical activity level: Evidence from the Alameda County Study. *American Journal of Public Health,* 88 (1998): 1709–1712.

36. Kawachi, I., and Berkman, L. F. *Neighborhoods and Health.* New York: Oxford University Press, 2003.

37. Chaskin, R. Perspectives on neighborhood and community: A review of the literature. *Social Service Review,* 7 (1997): 521–547.

38. Gephart, M. A. Neighborhoods and communities as contexts for development. J. Brooks-Gunn, G. J. Duncan, and L. J. Aber, eds., *Neighborhood Poverty: Context and Consequences for Children,* Vol. 1, pp. 1–43. New York: Russell Sage Foundation, 1997.

39. Gould, P., and White, R. *Mental Maps.* London: Routledge, 2002.

40. Furstenberg, F., and Hughes, M. The influence of neighborhoods on children's development: A theoretical perspective and a research agenda. In J. Brooks-Gunn, G. J. Duncan, and L. J. Aber, eds., *Neighborhood Poverty: Policy Implications in Studying Neighborhoods,* Vol. 2, pp. 23–47. New York: Russell Sage Foundation, 1997.

41. Burton, L., Price-Spratlen, T., and Spencer, M. B. On ways of thinking about measuring neighborhoods: Implications for studying context and developmental outcomes for children. In J. Brooks-Gunn, G. J. Duncan, and L. J. Aber, eds., *Neighborhood Poverty: Policy Implications in Studying Neighborhoods,* Vol. 2, pp. 132–144. New York: Russell Sage Foundation, 1997.

42. Anderson, R. T., Sorlie, P., Backlund, E., Johnson, N., and Kaplan, G. A. Mortality effects of community socioeconomic status. *Epidemiology,* 8 (1997): 42–47.

43. Cagney, K. A., Browning, C. R., and Wen, M. Racial disparities in self-rated health at older ages: What difference does the neighborhood make? *Journal of Gerontology B: Psychological Sciences and Social Sciences,* 60B (2005): S181–S190.

44. Diez-Roux, A. V., Nieto, F. J., Muntaner, C., et al. Neighborhood environments and coronary heart disease: A multilevel analysis. *American Journal of Epidemiology,* 146 (1997): 48–63.

45. Krause, N. Neighborhood deterioration and self-rated health in later life. *Psychology and Aging,* 11 (1996): 342–352.

46. LeClere, F. B., Rogers, R. G., and Peters, K. D. Ethnicity and mortality in the United States: Individual and community correlates. *Social Forces,* 76 (1997): 169–198.

47. Yen, I. H., and Kaplan, G. A. Poverty area residence and changes in depression and perceived health status: Evidence from the Alameda County Study. *International Journal of Epidemiology,* 28 (1999): 90–94.

48. Kawachi, I., Kennedy, B. P., and Glass, R. Social capital and self-rated health: A contextual analysis. *American Journal of Public Health,* 89 (1999): 1189–1193.

49. Veenstra, G. Social capital and health (plus wealth, income inequality and regional health governance). *Social Science & Medicine,* 54 (2002): 849–868.

50. Wen, M., Browning, C. R., and Cagney, K. A. Poverty affluence and income inequality: Neighborhood economic structure and its implication for self-rated health. *Social Science & Medicine,* 57 (2003): 843–860.

51. Balfour, J. L., and Kaplan, G. A. Neighborhood environment and loss of physical function in older adults: Evidence from the Alameda County Study. *American Journal of Epidemiology,* 155 (2002): 507–515.

52. Diez-Roux, A. V. Invited commentary: Places, people and health. *American Journal of Epidemiology,* 155 (2002): 516–519.

53. Robert, S. A., and Li, L. Age variation in the relationship between neighborhood socioeconomic context and adult health. *Research on Aging,* 23 (2001): 233–258.

54. Wen, M., Cagney, K. A., and Christakis, N. A. Effect of specific aspects of community social environment on the mortality of individuals diagnosed with serious illness. *Social Science & Medicine,* 61 (2005): 1119–1134.

55. Robert, S. A. Community-level socioeconomic status effects on health. *Journal of Health and Social Behavior,* 39 (1998): 18–37.

56. Robert, S., and House, J. S. SES differentials in health by age and alternative indicators of SES. *Journal of Aging and Health,* 8 (1996): 359–388.

57. Patel, K. V., Eschbach, K., Rudkin, L. L., Peek, M. K., and Markides, K. S. Neighborhood context and self-rated health in older Mexican Americans. *Annals of Epidemiology,* 13 (2003): 620–628.

58. Booth, K. M., Pinkston, M. M., and Poston, W. S. Obesity and the built environment. *Journal of American Diet Association,* 105 (2005): S110–117.

59. Frank, L. D., Schmid, T. L., Sallis, J. F., et al. Linking objectively measured physical activity with objectively measured urban form: Findings from SMARTRAQ. *American Journal of Preventative Medicine,* 28 (2005): 117–125.

60. U.S. Department of Health and Human Services. *Physical Activity and Health: A Report of the Surgeon General.* Atlanta, Ga.: Centers for Disease Control and Prevention, National Center for Chronic Disease Prevention and Health Promotion, 1996.

61. Lim, K., and Taylor, L. Factors associated with physical activity among older people: A population-based study. *Preventative Medicine,* 40 (2005): 33–40.

62. Schutzer, K. A., and Graves, B. S. Barriers and motivations to exercise in older adults [Review]. *Preventative Medicine,* 39 (2004): 1056–1061.

63. Aranceta, J., Perez-Rodrigo, C., Gondra, J., and Orduna, J. Community-based program to promote physical activity among elderly people: The Gerobilbo study. *Journal of Nutrition, Health and Aging,* 5 (2001): 238–242.

64. Dannenberg, A. L., Jackson, R. J., Frumkin, H., Schieber, R. A., Pratt, M., Kochtitzky, C., and Tilson, H. H. The impact of community design and land-use choices on public health: A scientific research agenda. *American Journal of Public Health,* 93 (2003): 1500–1508.

65. Fillit, H. M., Butler, R. N., O'Connell, A. W., et al. Achieving and maintaining cognitive vitality with aging. *Mayo Clinic Proceedings,* 77 (2002): 681–696.

66. Houde, S. C., and Melillo, K. D. Cardiovascular health and physical activity in older adults: An integrative review of research methodology and results. *Journal of Advanced Nursing,* 8 (2002): 219–234.

67. Jacobs, D. H., Tovar, J. M., Hung, O. L., Kim, M., Ye, P., Chiang, W. K., and Goldfrank, L. R. Behavioral risk factor and preventive health care practice survey of immigrants in the emergency department. *Academic Emergency Medicine,* 9 (2005): 599–608.

68. Crespo, C., Smit, E., Carter-Pokras, O., and Anderson, R. Acculturation and leisure-time physical inactivity in Mexican American adults: Results from the NHANES III, 1988–1994. *Americal Journal Public Health,* 91 (2001): 1254–1257.

69. Jonnalagadda, S. S., and Diwan, S. Health behaviors, chronic disease prevalence and self-rated health of older Asian Indian immigrants in the U.S. *Journal of Immigrant Health,* 7 (2005): 75–83.

70. Giles-Corti, B., and Donovan, R. The relative influence of individual, social, and physical environment determinants of physical activity. *Social Science & Medicine,* 54 (2002): 1793–1812.

71. King, A. C., Castro, C., Wilcox, S., et al. Personal and environmental factors associated with physical inactivity among different racial-ethnic groups of U.S. middle-aged and older-aged women. *Journal of Health Psychology,* 19 (2000): 354–364.

72. Markham, J. P., and Gilderbloom, J. I. Housing quality among the elderly: A decade of changes. *International Journal of Aging and Human Development,* 46 (1998): 71–90.

73. Li, F., Fisher, J., Brownson, R. C., and Bosworth, M. Multilevel modeling of built environment characteristics related to neighborhood walking activity in older adults. *Journal of Epidemiology Community Health,* 59 (2005): 558–564.

74. Pate, R. R., Pratt, M., Blair, S. N., Haskell, W. L., Macera, C. A., Bouchard, D., et al. Physical activity and public health: A recommendation from the Centers for Disease Control and Prevention and the American College of Sports Medicine. *JAMA,* 273 (1995): 402–407.

75. Pollard, T. Policy prescriptions for healthier communities. *American Journal of Health Promotion,* 18 (2003): 109–113.

76. Ferraro, K. F., and LeGrange, R. L. Are older people most afraid of crime? Reconsidering age differences in fear of victimization. *Journal of Gerontology B: Psychological Sciences and Social Sciences,* 47 (1992): S233–S244.

77. Booth, M. L., Owen, N., Bauman, A., et al. Social-cognitive and perceived environment influences associated with physical activity in older Australians. *Preventative Medicine,* 31 (2000): 15–22.

78. Wilcox, S., Bopp, M., Oberrecht, L., et al. Psychosocial and perceived environmental correlates of physical activity in rural and older African American and white women. *Journal of Gerontology B: Psychological Sciences and Social Sciences,* 58 (2003): 329–337.

79. King, W. C., Belle, S. H., Brach, J. S., et al. Objective measures of neighborhood environment and physical activity in older women. *American Journal of Preventative Medicine,* 28 (2005): 461–469.

80. Woo, J., Goggins, W., Sham, A., et al. Social determinants of frailty. *Gerontology,* 5 (2005): 402–408.

81. Northridge, M. E., and Sclar, E. A joint urban planning and public health framework: Contributions to health impact assessment. *American Journal of Public Health,* 93 (2003): 118–121.

82. Abrams, R. C., Lachs, M., McAvay, G., Keohane, D. J., and Bruce, M. L. Predictors of self-neglect in community-dwelling elders. *American Journal of Psychiatry,* 159 (2002): 1724–1730.

83. Lebowitz, B. D., Pearson, J. J., Schneider, L. S., et al. Diagnosis and treatment of depression in late life: Consensus statement update. *JAMA,* 278 (1997): 1186–1190.

84. Penninx, B. W., Leveille, S., Ferrucci, L., van Eijk, J. T., and Guralnik, J. M. Exploring the effect of depression on physical disability: Longitudinal evidence from the established populations for epidemiologic studies of the elderly. *American Journal of Public Health,* 89 (1999): 1346–1352.

85. Robins, L. N., and Regier, D. A. *Psychiatric disorders in America: The Epidemiological Catchment Area Study.* New York: Free Press, 1991.

86. Steffens, D. C., Skoog, I., Norton, M. C., Hart, A. D., Tschanz, J. T., Plassman, B. L., Wyse, B. W., Welsh-Bohmer, K. A., and Breitner, J. C. Prevalence of depression and its treatment in an elderly population: The Cache County Study. *Archives of General Psychiatry,* 57 (2000): 601–607.

87. Marwaha, S., and Livingston, G. Stigma, racism or choice: Why do depressed ethnic elders avoid psychiatrists? *Journal of Affective Disorders,* 72 (2002): 257–265.

88. Suen, L.J.W. U.S. predictive model of memory for the elderly Taiwanese immigrants. *Dissertation Abstracts International. Section B: The Sciences and Engineering,* 62, no. 2-B (2001): 787.

89. Silver, E., Mulvey, E. P., and Swanson, J. W. Neighborhood structural characteristics and mental disorder: Faris and Dunham revisited. *Social Science & Medicine,* 55 (2002): 1457–1470.

90. Latkin, C. A., and Curry, A. D. Stressful neighborhoods and depression: A prospective study of the impact of neighborhood disorder. *Journal of Health and Social Behavior,* 44 (2003): 34–44.

91. Galea, S., and Vlahov, D. Urban health: Evidence, challenges, and directions. *Annual Review of Public Health,* 26 (2005): 341–365.

92. Kubzansky, L. D., Subramanian, S. V., Kawachi. I., et al. Neighborhood contextual influences on depressive symptoms in the elderly. *American Journal of Epidemiology,* 162 (2005): 253–260.

93. Ross, C. E., and Mirowsky, J. Neighborhood disadvantage, disorder, and health. *Journal of Health and Social Behavior,* 42 (2001): 258–276.

94. Ross, C. E., and Jang, S. J. Neighborhood disorder, fear, and mistrust: The buffering role of social ties with neighbors. *American Journal of Community Psychology,* 28 (2000): 401–420.

95. Leventhal, T., and Brooks-Gunn. J. Moving to opportunity: An experimental study of neighborhood effects on mental health. *American Journal of Public Health,* 93 (2003): 1576–1582.

96. Robert, R. E., Kaplan, G. A., Shema, S. J., and Strawbridge, W. J. Prevalence and correlates of depression in an aging cohort: The Alameda County Cohort Study. *Journal of Gerontology B: Psychological Sciences and Social Sciences,* 52B (1997): S252–S258.

97. Ostir, G. V., Eschbach, K., Markides, K. S., et al. Neighborhood composition and depressive symptoms among older Mexican Americans. *Journal of Epidemiology and* 57 (2003): 987–992.

98. Hao, L., and Kawano, Y. Immigrants' welfare use and opportunity for contact with co-ethnics. *Demography,* 38 (2001): 375–389.

99. Glynn, T. Psychological sense of community: Measurement and application. *Human Relation,* 34 (1981): 789–818.

100. Nasar, J., and Julian, D. The psychological sense of community in the neighborhood. *Journal of American Planning Association,* 61 (1995): 178–184.

101. Goran, M. I., and Treuth, M. S. Energy expenditure, physical activity, and obesity in children. *Pediatric Clinics of North America,* 48 (2001): 931–953.

102. Bashir, S. A. Home is where the harm is: Inadequate housing as a public health crisis. *American Journal of Public Health,* 92 (2002): 733–738.

103. Kawachi, I., Kennedy, B. P., Lochner, K., and Prothrow-Stith, D. Social capital, income inequality, and mortality. *American Journal of Public Health,* 87 (1997): 1491–1498.

104. Gorman, D., Douglas, M. J., Conway, L., Noble, P., and Hanlon, P. Transport policy and health inequalities: A health impact assessment of Edinburgh's transport policy. *Public Health,* 117 (2003): 15–24.

105. Jackson, R. J., and Kochtitzky, C. *Creating a Healthy Environment: The Impact of the Built Environment on Public Health.* Sprawl Watch Clearinghouse Monograph Series. Atlanta, Ga.: Centers for Disease Control and Prevention, U.S. Department of Health and Human Services, 2005.

106. Ewing, R., Pendall, R., and Chen, D. Measuring sprawl and its impact. *Smart Growth America.* Available at www.smartgrowthamerica.org/sprawlindex/sprawlindex.html. Published 2002. Accessed October 20, 2005.

107. Frumkin, H. Urban sprawl and public health. *Public Health Reports,* 117 (2002): 201–217.

108. McCarthy, M. Transport and health. In M. M. Wilkinson, ed., *Social Determinants of Health,* pp. 132–154. Oxford: Oxford University Press, 1999.

109. Plawecki, H. M. The elderly immigrant: An isolated experience. *Journal of Gerontology and Nursing,* 26 (2000): 6–7.

110. Wilmoth, J. M., and Chen, P. C. Immigrant status, living arrangements, and depressive symptoms among middle-aged and older adults. *Journal of Gerontology B: Psychological Sciences and Social Sciences,* 58 (2003): S305–313.

111. Kim, O. Predictors of loneliness in elderly Korean immigrant women living in the United States of America. *Journal of Advanced Nursing,* 29 (1999): 1082–1088.

112. Ponizovsky, A. M., and Ritsner, M. S. Patterns of loneliness in an immigrant population. *Comprehensive Psychiatry,* 45 (2004): 408–414.

113. Klinenberg, E. *Heat Wave: A Social Autopsy of Disaster in Chicago.* Chicago: University of Chicago Press, 2002.

114. Berkman, L. F. Assessing the physical health effects of social networks and social support. *Annual Review of Public Health,* 5 (1984): 413–432.

115. Berkman, L. F., Glass, T., Brissette, I., and Seeman, T. E. From social integration to health: Durkheim in the new millennium. *Social Science & Medicine,* 51 (2000): 843–857.

116. House, J. S., Landis, K. R., and Umberson, D. Social relationships and health. *Science,* 241 (1988): 540–544.

117. Moon, J. Alienation of elderly Korean American immigrants as related to place of residence, gender, age, years of education, time in the U.S., living with or without children, and living with or without a spouse. *International Journal of Aging and Human Development,* 32 (1991): 115–124.

118. Ahmad, F., Shik, A., Vanza, R., Cheung, A. M., George, U., and Stewart, D. E. Voices of South Asian women: Immigration and mental health. *Women's Health,* 40 (2004): 113–130.

119. Diwan, S., Jonnalagadda, S. S., and Balaswamy, S. Resources predicting positive and negative affect during the experience of stress: A study of older Asian Indian immigrants in the United States. *Gerontologist,* 44 (2004): 605–614.

120. Aroian, K. J., and Norris, A. Assessing risk for depression among immigrants at two-year follow-up. *Archives of Psychiatric Nursing,* 16 (2002): 245–253.

121. Escobar, J. I., Hoyos, N. C., and Gara, M. A. Immigration and mental health: Mexican Americans in the United States. *Harvard Review of Psychiatry,* 8 (2000): 64–72.

122. Lin, G. Elderly migration: Household versus individual approaches. *Papers in Regional Science,* 76 (1997): 285–300.

123. Angel, R. J., Angel, J. L., Lee, G. Y., and Markides, K. S. Age at migration and family dependency among older Mexican immigrants: Recent evidence from the Mexican American EPESE. *Gerontologist,* 39 (1999): 59–65.

124. Angel, J. L., Angel, R. J., and Markides, K. S. Late-life immigration: Changes in living arrangements and headship status among older Mexican-origin individuals. *Social Science Quarterly,* 81 (2001): 389–403.

125. Glick, J. E., and Van Hook, J. Parents' co-residence with adult children: Can immigration explain racial and ethnic variation. *Journal of Marriage & Family,* 64 (2002): 240–253.

126. Stoller, E. P., and Pezynski, A. T. The impact of ethnic involvement and migration patterns on long-term care plans among retired sunbelt migrants: Plans for nursing home placement. *Journal of Gerontology B: Psychological Sciences and Social Sciences,* 58 (2003): S369–376.

127. Goodman, C. C., and Silverstein, M. Latina grandmothers raising grandchildren: Acculturation and psychological well-being. *International Journal of Aging and Human Development,* 60 (2005): 305–316.

128. Jones, P. S., Zhang, X. E., and Meleis, A. I. Transforming vulnerability. *Western Journal of Nursing Research,* 25 (2003): 835–853.

129. Lan, P. Subcontracting filial piety: Elder care in ethnic Chinese immigrant families in California. *Journal of Family Issues,* 23 (2002): 812–835.

130. Miltiades, H. B. The social and psychological effect of an adult child's emigration on non-immigrant Asian Indian elderly parents. *Journal of Cross-Cultural Gerontology,* 17 (2002): 33–55.

131. Lee, E. E., and Farran, C. J. Depression among Korean, Korean American, and Caucasian American family caregivers. *Journal of Transcultural Nursing,* 15 (2004): 18–25.

132. Usita, P. M., and Du Bois, B. C. Conflict sources and responses in mother–daughter relationships: Perspectives of adult daughters of aging immigrant women. *Journal of Women & Aging,* 17 (2005): 151–165.

133. Sung, K. T., and Kim, M. H. The effects of the U.S. public welfare system upon elderly Korean immigrants' independent living arrangements. *Journal of Poverty,* 6 (2002): 83–94.

134. Kim, J., and Lauderdale, D. S. The role of community context in immigrant elderly living arrangements: Korean American elderly. *Research on Aging,* 24 (2002): 630–653.

135. Burr, J. A., and Mutchler, J. E. English language skills, ethnic concentration, and household composition: Older Mexican immigrants. *Journal of Gerontology B: Psychological Sciences and Social Sciences,* 58 (2003): S83–92.

136. Pang, E. C., Jordan-Marsh, M., Silverstein, M., and Cody, M. Health-seeking behaviors of elderly Chinese Americans: Shifts in expectations. *Gerontologist,* 43 (2003): 864–874.

137. Eschbach, K., Ostir, G. V., Patel, K. V., Markides, K. S., and Goodwin, J. S. Neighborhood context and mortality among older Mexican Americans: Is there a barrio advantage? *American Journal of Public Health,* 94 (2004): 1807–1812.

138. Buckley, C., Angel, J. L., and Donahue, D. Nativity and older women's health: Constructed reliance in the health and retirement study. *Journal of Women & Aging,* 12 (2000): 21–37.

139. Yoo, G. Shaping public perceptions of elderly immigrants on welfare: The role of editorial pages of major U.S. newspapers. *International Journal of Sociology and Social,* 21 (2001): 47–62.

140. Freidenberg, J. N. *Growing Old in El Barrio.* New York: New York University Press, 2000.

141. Gomberg, E. S. Treatment for alcohol-related problems: Special populations: Research opportunities. *Recent Developments in Alcoholism,* 16 (2003): 313–333.

142. Stanford, E. P., and Torres-Gil, F. M. Diversity and beyond: A commentary. *Generations,* 4 (1991): 5–6.

143. Ory, M., Hoffman, M. K., Hawkins, M., Sanner, B., and Mockenhaupt, R. Challenging aging stereotypes: Strategies for creating a more active society. *American Journal of Preventive Medicine,* 25, Suppl 2 (2003): 164–171.

144. Richie, B., Freudenberg, N., and Page, J. Reintegrating women leaving jail into urban communities: A description of a model program. *Journal of Urban Health,* 78 (2001): 290–303.

145. WHO. *Global Age Friendly Cities: A Guide.* Paris: World Health Organization, 2007.

146. Gold, M. R., Siegel, J. E., Russell, L. B., and Weinstein, M. C., eds. *Cost-Effectiveness in Health and Medicine.* New York: Oxford University Press, 1996.

147. Mauskopf, J. A., Sullivan, S. D., Annemans, L., Caro, J., Mullins, C. D., Nuijten, M., Orlewska, E., Watkins, J., and Trueman, P. Principles of good practice for budget impact analysis: Report of the ISPOR Task Force on good research practices—budget impact analysis. *Value Health,* 10 (2007): 324–325.

148. Meara, E. H., Richards, S., and Cutler, D. M. The gap gets bigger: Changes in mortality and life expectancy, by education, 1981–2000. *Health Affairs,* 27 (2008): 350–360.

149. Frick, K. D., Carlson, M. C., Glass, T. A., McGill, S., Rebok, G. W., Simpson, C., and Fried, L. P. Modeled cost-effectiveness of the Experience Corps Baltimore based on a pilot randomized trial. *Journal of Urban Health,* 81 (2004): 106–117.

150. Martinez, I. L., Frick, K. D., Glass, T. A., Carlson, M. C., Tanner, E., Ricks, M., and Fried, L. P. Engaging older adults in high impact volunteering that enhances health: Recruitment and retention in the Experience Corps Baltimore. *Journal of Urban Health,* 83 (2006): 941–953.

CHAPTER

11

REVERSING THE TIDE OF TYPE 2 DIABETES AMONG AFRICAN AMERICANS THROUGH INTERDISCIPLINARY RESEARCH

HOLLIE JONES, LEANDRIS C. LIBURD

LEARNING OBJECTIVES

- Describe the disproportionate burden of diabetes on African Americans and the pathways by which these disparities are produced.

- Compare the specific contributions that social psychology and critical medical anthropology can make to the study of type 2 diabetes among African Americans.

■ Analyze the pathways by which racial discrimination can influence health.

■ Discuss the value and limits of interdisciplinary approaches to the study of diabetes.

According to the Centers for Disease Control and Prevention, two of five African Americans born in 2000 have a lifetime risk of developing diabetes. Currently, 3.2 million, or 13.3 percent of African Americans aged twenty years or older have diabetes, making them 1.8 times more likely to have the disease than their white counterparts.[1] In the United States, an estimated 20.8 million people have diabetes, and of this number, 6.2 million—almost 30 percent—do not know it.[1] The risk for stroke is two to four times higher for people with diabetes, and adults with diabetes have heart disease death rates two to four times higher than adults without diabetes. Additionally, diabetes is the leading cause of kidney failure and, among adults aged twenty to seventy-four years, the leading cause of new cases of blindness.

Although the literature examining the complex pathophysiology of diabetes is expanding, we know that diabetes mellitus is a group of diseases characterized by high levels of blood glucose resulting from defects in insulin production, insulin action, or both. Type 2 diabetes, which accounts for 90 percent to 95 percent of all diagnosed cases of diabetes, usually begins as insulin resistance, a disorder in which cells do not use insulin properly. As the need for insulin increases, the pancreas gradually loses the ability to produce insulin.

In the epidemiological context, type 2 diabetes is associated with older age, obesity, family history of diabetes, history of gestational diabetes, impaired glucose metabolism, physical inactivity, and race and ethnicity.[1] African Americans, Hispanic/ Latino Americans, American Indians, and some Asian Americans and Native Hawaiians or Other Pacific Islanders are at particularly high risk for type 2 diabetes. Type 2 diabetes is also increasingly being diagnosed in children and adolescents.[1] Although the burden of diabetes in the United States is well documented, how the social-ecological context acts on population groups and on the body to increase risk for type 2 diabetes is not well understood.[2]

Epidemiology, clinical medicine, and biomedical research that locate risk within the physical sphere of the body portray risk as individual and not socially or historically determined. This thinking is problematic because the risk for developing diabetes is intimately intertwined with social, political, economic, and cultural environments. Increasingly, researchers are addressing the environmental factors that influence the higher prevalence of diabetes in communities of color, but much work remains to be done.[3–7] The need for interdisciplinary psychosocial and cultural research among African Americans with type 2 diabetes creates an ideal space to bring together psychology and medical anthropology. Together, these disciplines can expand our understanding of how best to reduce racial/ethnic disparities in diabetes beyond the traditional recommendations based on biomedical and epidemiological research.

In this chapter, we focus on critical social psychology and critical medical anthropology as tools for an interdisciplinary research agenda to reduce diabetes among

African Americans. Critical social psychology and critical medical anthropology research forefront race and ethnicity, ethnic identity, inequality and discrimination, and structural hindrances in the health care system as factors in the development of diabetes and in diabetes management. We discuss how ethnic identity and health care disparities undermine diabetes management. We review psychological and medical anthropological research methods and argue for a mixed-method approach. Finally, we propose research questions that integrate critical social psychology and critical medical anthropology perspectives, increase understanding of the experience of type 2 diabetes among urban African Africans, and inform the development of strategies to reduce the prevalence of diabetes in this community.

A DIALOGUE BETWEEN TWO DISCIPLINES: PSYCHOLOGY AND MEDICAL ANTHROPOLOGY

Although not easily isolated, psychological and cultural factors weigh heavily in the burden of diabetes among African Americans and other populations. Merging the fields of psychology and medical anthropology in urban health research allows researchers to consider the psychological and cultural factors that increase risk for diabetes and its complications, not to infer causation but to elaborate upon African American urban experiences that establish and perpetuate the risk for developing type 2 diabetes. Research that utilizes psychology and medical anthropology allows for more robust diabetes prevention and management interventions for African Americans at the individual, family, community, and policy levels. Our interdisciplinary theoretical approach recognizes that structural factors such as discrimination, segregation, inequality in schools and employment settings, and the unequal distribution of resources that facilitate health contribute to the diabetes disparities among African Americans.[8]

Psychology

Broadly, psychology examines the ways in which attitudes, behaviors, beliefs, personal characteristics, group dynamics, and experience influence individual behavior. Social psychology emphasizes intergroup dynamics, social identity, attitudes, discrimination, and prejudice and therefore lends itself to the study of diabetes disparities. The traditional social psychological approach, however, may not be enough to untangle the web of contextual factors that contributes to diabetes disparities.

Critical social psychology examines behavior in social contexts, particularly socioeconomic, historical, and political contexts.[9] For example, whereas population-based interventions focus on policy and population-level variables, critical social psychology focuses on the individual, while recognizing that the individual is nested within historical and social contexts and experiences structural factors that may hinder diabetes prevention and successful management. Psychological variables that may contribute to further understanding and alleviating the burden of diabetes in the African American community include perceptions of and experiences with racial discrimination, prejudice, ethnic identity, and cultural beliefs about health and disease. It is important to begin considering the relevance of these factors, given the complex individual behaviors required to prevent or manage type 2 diabetes effectively.

Critical social psychology recognizes race and ethnicity as social constructs, and a critical social psychological approach to diabetes disparities highlights historical context and avoids conceptual confounding by distinguishing between race and ethnicity.[10, 11] According to Jones,[10] race implies a genetic marker whereas ethnicity is thought to be mutable, controllable, and involve greater choice. Additionally, individuals grouped together on the basis of cultural similarities are ethnic groups, whereas a racial group is composed of people from various ethnicities. Research at the population level focuses on racial categories without recognizing the importance of ethnic identity as an independent construct.[12]

Although type 2 diabetes is strongly influenced by lifestyle, researchers need to consider how biological and social factors intersect to create a higher diabetes burden among African Americans. One area for future exploration is ethnic identity. Ethnic identity is a dynamic process that develops throughout the life span. It is important to note that ethnic identity is based in the group's self-definition as well as others' definition (public regard) of that particular ethnic group.[13] In this way, according to Nagel,[14] ethnicity is a dialectical process that arises out of interactions between individuals and audiences. One strategy would be to examine the extent to which ethnic identity is constructed outside the group and then adapted by the group in ways that may or may not be health promoting. Another potential strategy is to examine how awareness of being a member of a devalued racial/ethnic group can be a stressor with negative health effects.[15]

Inequality or Discrimination and Health   Racial and ethnic group membership is associated with differing degrees of inequality and discrimination. The legacy of inequality often leads to stress, which can negatively affect health.[16] Also, differences in health status, disease prevalence, and the distribution of resources and power can be partially attributed to social mechanisms that foster inequality.[17] Critical social psychology conceptualizes and examines the health impact of a society with a legacy of discrimination, including racial discrimination, which is defined as negative behavior toward a person based on negative attitudes toward the group to which that person belongs. Racial discrimination occurs at individual, institutional, and cultural levels and involves behavioral, cultural, psychological, and structural dynamics.[10]

In many ways, the experience of racial discrimination is subjective. Perceived discrimination is a person's perception of unfair treatment due to race or ethnic group membership.[10, 18, 19] In health care settings, the legacy of racial discrimination (e.g., the Tuskegee Syphilis Study) may influence levels of trust in physicians or in the medical system as a whole. This can have direct bearing on health-seeking behaviors, and for persons with diabetes, having confidence in the health care system is essential.

The connection between racial discrimination and health is based on the premise that encounters of this kind are chronic and stressful for African Americans and that the effects are cumulative over time.[20] People who experience racial discrimination often experience negative mental and physical health consequences as a result. In addition, the more discrimination a person experiences, the more at risk the person is for negative psychological and physical health outcomes.[21] Research among African Americans has shown that these experiences have deleterious consequences for physical and psychological health as well as for health behaviors.[16, 17, 21, 22] Research also suggests that, among African Americans with type 2 diabetes, more perceived racial discrimination is associated with higher depressive symptoms.[23] In sum, racial discrimination and related stressors may contribute to lower quality of life among African Americans with type 2 diabetes;[24] therefore, understanding racial discrimination is especially relevant when designing interventions for those who may have experienced discrimination.

Medical Anthropology

Medical anthropology is a subspecialty of cultural anthropology and includes academic medical anthropology, applied medical anthropology, biocultural medical anthropology, and critical medical anthropology. Medical anthropology maintains the cultural anthropology tradition of conducting cross-cultural analyses to examine how diverse cultures understand and respond to sickness and give "voice" to suffering populations, though not always with an action or applied orientation or agenda.[25] Distinctions between the categories of medical anthropology are mutable, and students are encouraged to engage the categories in dialogue and debate and to think across and between the categories to inform public health research.

According to Snow[26] and Pelto,[27] researchers in the category of applied medical anthropology ask questions such as these: What do people believe about illnesses, their causes, and treatments? What behaviors increase or decrease risk for selected diseases? What characteristics of health services encourage treatment-seeking behaviors? What changes in knowledge, behaviors, or disease-causing conditions can improve people's health? Applied medical anthropology examines how an understanding of culture in the patient-provider encounter can promote inclusion, create understanding of the sociocultural and material context of the patient, and eliminate disparities in the provision of health care. Also, academic and applied medical anthropology posit theoretical explanations of sickness that support, challenge, and reframe clinical efforts to improve patient adherence to biomedical regimens.[28, 29]

On the whole, medical anthropology is "concerned with the interrelationship of biological, social, and cultural factors in health and illness."[30] According to Lock and Scheper-Hughes,[31] "medical anthropology becomes the way in which all knowledge relating to the body, health, and illness is culturally constructed, negotiated, and renegotiated in a dynamic process through time and space." They add, "it is medical anthropology's engagement with the body in context that represents this subdiscipline's unique vision as distinct from classical social anthropology (where the body was largely absent) and from physical anthropology and the biomedical sciences (where the body is made into a universal object)." This focus on problematizing and understanding the body within a historical, political, and social frame aligns medical anthropology with critical social psychology.

Medical anthropology also posits cultural explanatory models of sickness and pathways to health, illness, and disease.[32] Although cultural and social anthropology have dominated discourse on culture throughout the twentieth century, examining culture and health and disease in the new millennium is challenging because "culture is increasingly hard to define, much less apply, to understanding social practices."[33] In urban centers worldwide, "the transnational flows of people and ideas that are part and parcel of globalization, the legacies of colonialism and, in consequence, a need to take power into account, have rendered older ideas of culture—as a relatively homogeneous set of understandings shared among a group of socially interacting people—conceptually obsolete."[32] Therefore, contemporary urban health research offers an opportunity to articulate new definitions of culture and the relationships between culture and health. Capturing the complexity of the historical and social construction of an urban cultural environment requires a systematic process of inquiry. Although such a task is daunting, intersections between medical anthropology and psychology can elaborate how individuals' social and physical environments and various cultural milieus interact to affect health.

Culture in research then must be defined such that "the essential links from the cultural, to the individual, to the biological" are made conceptually and empirically.[34] Janes[33] argues that in addition to a more precise definition of culture and "how it manages to get into the body," we must address "the role culture plays in human social life; understand how the 'stuff' of culture—ideas, symbols, meanings, shared understandings, morals, values, beliefs—are distributed within and among social groups within larger, complex social systems; and develop the conceptual tools and research methods to apprehend the links between culture as a shared experience on the world and individual experience." Rather than abandon culture as a viable domain for analysis, medical anthropology seeks to articulate more carefully cultural models as determinants of health, which invites epistemological refinements from other disciplines. Overall, medical anthropology research is important for contemporary urban areas in the United States and for those at risk for or diagnosed with type 2 diabetes. Knowing how people understand the disease and its prevention and management helps health care providers to undo misinformation and facilitate successful prevention and control.

Critical Medical Anthropology   A more recent theoretical framework within medical anthropology is critical medical anthropology, which incorporates political, economic, biocultural, feminist, phenomenological, and cultural-constructivists approaches. Like critical social psychology, critical medical anthropology examines the power relations in Western medicine to challenge the aims of Western medicine and to point out the ways that the nation-state imposes its economic and political agendas on the bodies of the population. The goals of critical medical anthropology include critiquing the materialist premises of biomedicine and challenging the economic and power relations of medical encounters.[35]

Baer et al.[36] argue that "a key component of health is struggle," and health is understood as "access to and control over the basic material and non-material resources that sustain and promote life at a high level of satisfaction." Questions that critical medical anthropologists consider about health are: Who has power over the agencies of biomedicine? How and in what form is this power delegated? What are the economic, sociopolitical, and ideological ends and consequences of these power relations? How is power expressed in the social relations within the health care delivery system? What are the principal contradictions of biomedicine and the arenas of struggle in the medical system? According to Hans Baer, one of the early framers of critical medical anthropology,

Critical medical anthropologists along with other critical medical social scientists maintain that bourgeois medicine by virtue of its integration in capitalist societies functions as (1) a mechanism for promoting the functional health of workers involved in the productive process; (2) an arena for profit-making; (3) a mechanism for maintaining and reproducing the working class; (4) an arena of social control and the reproduction of class, racial, ethnic, and gender relations; and (5) a mechanism of imperialist expansion and bourgeois cultural hegemony.[36]

In this context, "health" is an endpoint needed to support the economy rather than a resource for a full and satisfying life.

Bach et al.[37] conducted an analysis of more than 150,000 African American and white Medicare beneficiaries to establish empirically some of the underlying causes of health care disparities between African American and white patients aged sixty-five years and older. They interviewed more than 5,000 primary care physicians about the quality of health care they provided to their African American and white patients. In summary, Bach et al. found that "physicians working for plans in which African American patients were heavily enrolled provided primary care of a lower quality to all patients in the plan than did physicians working for plans in which fewer African American patients were enrolled."

Bach et al.[37] also found that physicians who treated a higher proportion of minority patients were less knowledgeable about preventive care practices and were less likely to be board certified in their primary specialty than physicians treating white patients. African American patients were more likely to visit African American physicians, and physicians with a large African American patient pool provided more charity care, derived a higher percentage of their incomes from Medicaid, and practiced more often in low-income neighborhoods. In addition, physicians who primarily treated African American patients reported facing considerable obstacles in gaining access to specialty referrals and high-quality diagnostic imaging services, which resulted in fewer screenings for diseases and more diagnoses when diseases were at relatively advanced stages. Bach et al. found that African American communities had fewer primary care physicians than white communities. In the United States, the distribution of physicians dictates quality care more than patients' choice. Undoing these structural inequalities is one of the aims of critical medical anthropology.

Critical medical anthropology, like critical social psychology, provides an opportunity to address race and racism, class, gender identity and health, and power within the health care system "as a key social-structural factor in health and in societal responses to illness."[38] Currently, medical anthropology and psychology in general are wanting in studies on the impact of race on health status and disparities in urban communities of color.[39, 40] More specifically, there is a lack of studies of how corporate practices and health care culture help shape disease risk. For example, corporate practices, by design, flood urban African American communities with food options that increase diabetes risk. Organizational culture and service delivery ideologies of the U.S. medical care system are established by health care administrators, physicians, and other allied health resources and industries. The privileging of a profit-driven system of care contributes to a health care culture that perpetuates inequality in clinical settings. This cultural dynamic contributes to diabetes disparities among African Americans by the rationing of access to specialty care, discouraging early diagnosis and treatment, and decreasing the likelihood that access to education about prevention will be provided from these same health care providers. Furthermore, health care administrators may be more interested in services that are reimbursable costs, as well as cost containment and minimization (e.g., Medicaid). Thus, health care administrators may implement policies that de-emphasize preventive treatment and services. These practices leave African Americans vulnerable to not having access to the level of expertise required to prevent diabetes and its complications.

In summary, the goals of medical anthropology are as varied as its theoretical and methodological perspectives but include understanding African Americans' conceptualizations of sickness to enhance communication between health care providers and consumers of health care[7, 41] and influencing public policy by fostering understanding of the sociocultural complexities of health issues.[30] Another goal is to integrate biological and cultural approaches to identify and eliminate risks to health by examining the ecological dimension of disease causation that "explicitly sets health, illness and disease within a system of mutually interacting organic, inorganic and cultural environments."[42]

ETHNIC IDENTITY AND THE EXPERIENCE OF BEING AFRICAN AMERICAN WITH TYPE 2 DIABETES

Ethnic Identity and Diabetes

Living in the context of inequality has an impact on health, and ethnic identity may influence the relationship between systems of inequality and health. Ethnic identity is an individual's sense of identification with a particular ethnic group and its beliefs, values, norms, and history.[43] A degree of choice is involved in ethnic identity. For example, although a person may appear to be African American, that person may not self-identify as African American for ideological reasons or because of membership in another ethnic group. How one self-identifies implies assumptions about health-related behaviors such as dietary preferences, a key component in diabetes self-management.

Ethnic identity, as conceptualized in social psychology, is created in external space and may develop in response to discriminatory practices or in opposition to other ethnic groups. In understanding African American ethnic identity, critical social psychologists highlight the social and historical conditions of African Americans in the United States and view ethnic identity formation as a complex phenomenon that embodies responses to centuries of oppression.

Although external influences on ethnic identity are important, it is equally important to note that ethnic identity exists in the absence of discrimination. For example, African American ethnicity is characterized by certain traditions (e.g., musical, religious expression, culinary preferences), many of which are defined from within the culture.[43] The more accurate interpretation then of ethnic identity acknowledges external structuring and internal agency in the formation and maintenance of ethnic identity[44, 45] as well as sociopolitical and cultural influences.

Similarly, health and health disparities are externally and internally structured. For example, urban communities with high concentrations of racial and ethnic minority populations often have more fast-food restaurants, low-quality convenience foods, tobacco products, and liquor stores. In African American communities, there are more fast-food restaurants and vendors of alcoholic beverages per capita than in white communities, and the consumption of the same is arguably higher among African Americans as well,[46] which is not unrelated to the aggressive marketing of these products to African American consumers. There is a paucity of research that has specifically addressed the role of corporate practices and policy on diabetes risk in ethnic minority urban communities. Additionally, high rates of crime and violence and a lack of green space or other options for recreational physical activity become disincentives for regular physical activity.[47]

Given the close association between obesity and type 2 diabetes, we can make some assumptions about the role of these factors on African Americans' diabetes burden. As Mechanic observed,

> The complex, dynamic (ever changing), and interactive nature of socio-ecologic conditions increase the risk for obesity and overweight in communities of color which confounds and undermines most public health interventions that have tended to isolate selected behaviors—namely nutrition and physical activity, and delivered interventions that are often de-contextualized, ahistorical, and overly dependent on theories of individual behavior change. Higher status as measured by social class or other indicators of social dominance, for example, allow people with more resources such as money, knowledge, social networks or power to be better positioned to take advantage of opportunities to protect their health relative to those in less favored socioeconomic positions.[48]

Some questions that researchers can address in future research are: To what extent do people's perceptions of social and physical environment structure their health behaviors and beliefs? Does changing the social and physical environment to one that invites good health choices inspire health-promoting behaviors? To what extent are sustained systems of social support tied to maladaptive health behaviors, including excessive alcohol consumption or preference for high fat, high sodium meals?

Ethnic Identity, Health Behavior, and Perceptions

Regardless of its origin, ethnic identity influences our perceptions, health behaviors, and relationships with others and the way we navigate through the world.[49] Ethnic identity can influence a person's health care choices, including preferences for doctors from specific ethnic backgrounds or ways of coping with chronic illness. Additionally, ethnic identity can influence levels of perceived discrimination in health care settings. One explanation for variability in perceptions of discrimination is that the significance of an event depends on the salience of the identity domain in which the event occurs.[50] In other words, a person with a stronger sense of ethnic identity may be more likely to notice cues that suggest discrimination and may find the event more relevant and stressful than those who are less strongly identified with an ethnic group. In this way, ethnic identity can act as a moderator for perceptions.

Recognizing the relevance of ethnic identity in the health care setting can be especially important in issues of trust and patient satisfaction so that interventions can be tailored to specific worldviews, cultural practices, community realities, and experiences.[7] Regarding trust, diabetes self-management may be partially contingent upon the patient-provider relationship. Several studies demonstrate a relationship between high levels of patient trust in providers and a patient's ability to complete diabetes care activities.[51] Poor patient-provider relations may further contribute to a sense of mistrust among African Americans of doctors, nurses, and the health care system.[52]

In terms of patient satisfaction, a study by Garroutte, Kunovich, Jacobsen, and Goldberg[12] among American Indians found that strong ethnic identity was associated with reduced satisfaction with the social skills and attentiveness of health care providers. This suggests that ethnic identity is a cultural factor that may influence patient evaluations of health care, their help-seeking behaviors, and attitudes toward health care providers. However, more research in this area is needed, particularly among African Americans.

Ethnic Identity as Coping

Ethnic identity among African Americans can be viewed as a protective factor, which may positively influence disease survival rates. Psychological literature suggests that protection exists at three levels: individual, familial, and societal,[53] and all three levels are evident in African American history and in ethnic identity theory. Although a major role of African American identity is to provide a sense of group affiliation, another is "to protect a person from psychological insults, and, where possible, to warn of impending psychological attacks that stem from having to live in a racist society."[54] Cross[55] suggests that a fully developed African American ethnic identity helps defend a person from negative psychological stress in societies that use behavioral strategies to enforce discrimination and racism.

Many who are diagnosed with diabetes are at increased risk for depression,[56,57] and their mental health needs often remain unmet. Negative treatment on the basis of race or ethnicity can cause depression and low life satisfaction among African Americans.[20,22,58] Given these race-related stressors, African Americans with type 2 diabetes may be at increased risk for depression. However, a person with a stronger African American ethnic identity may be able to protect self-esteem and maintain a "sense of perspective and personal worth in the face of racism."[44] These buffering effects may also extend to hypertension and depression in general.[20]

Ethnic Identity and Spirituality

For many African Americans, ethnic identity includes a sense of spirituality, or religion and religiosity.[55,59] Mattis and Jagers[60] differentiate between the two: religion is a system of beliefs about God shared by a specific community, whereas religiosity is the degree of adherence to an organized religion or belief system. Polzer[59] found that among African Americans spirituality impacts diabetes self-management because African Americans may turn to God, or "turn it over to God," to cope with diabetes. Mullings and Wali[61] found that African American women turned to faith institutions in times of crisis to discuss explicitly personal stressors and receive advice on ways to cope with stress. In addition to lending emotional support, many African American churches provide tangible support in the form of clothing, food donations, and housing resources.

Perhaps most important, African American churches provide social support through a sense of familial connection, which helps buffer stressors and helps people protect themselves from and cope with those stressors. But more research is needed to determine how interventions related to type 2 diabetes can be translated to churches or other spiritual meeting places. Additionally, given that spirituality can enhance preventive behavior and diabetes self-management, health care providers and those developing interventions for this population can address spirituality via culturally relevant care.

INTERDISCIPLINARY RESEARCH METHODS

Qualitative and quantitative research methods are used in medical anthropology and psychology. Multiple qualitative methods, such as interviews, participant observation, focus groups, and document analysis can be used to address specific research questions and test assumptions.[62] One useful qualitative approach in anthropology and psychology is ethnography.[62–64] Hammersley and Atkinson[64] describe ethnography as "the ethnographer participating, overtly or covertly, in people's daily lives for an extended period of time, watching what happens, listening to what is said, asking questions—in fact, collecting whatever data are available to throw light on the issues that are the focus of the research." Neuman[62] describes meaning-giving in ethnography, in that "displays of behavior do not give meaning; rather meaning is inferred, or someone figures out meaning. Moving from what is heard or observed to what is actually meant is at the center of ethnography."

The inductive nature of qualitative research allows significant topics and patterns to emerge as data are collected. Theory is built in the process. Ultimately, qualitative research can be used to better understand a group's perceptions and experiences with health and disease to develop or refine theory. Strengths of qualitative research include

- Its open-ended nature and flexibility. Researchers can probe with respondents for greater detail and clarity in answering questions. Additionally, based on information gained from the respondents, researchers can modify or add questions.

- The opportunity to pursue a research problem in multiple ways, such as using observational fieldwork data, interviews, focus groups, and relevant documents (library sources, newspapers and other archival data, diaries, field notes, photographs, videotapes, recorded oral histories, etc.).

- The perspective that all responses interest a researcher and not just the most frequently given responses.

- The option to return to respondents if there are gaps in the data or to ask additional questions. Furthermore, respondents can participate in interpreting and reporting data.

- Achieving greater validity in the findings than in quantitative methods.

Potential weaknesses of qualitative research include

- The labor and resources necessary, given its open-ended, unstandardized approach.

- The lack of standardization in data analysis. According to Bernard,[65] "most methods for quantitative analysis—things like factor analysis, cluster analysis, regression analysis, and so on—are really methods for data *processing* and for finding patterns in data." Computer programs such as Epi Info and SPSS analyze (i.e., process but do not interpret) data for the researcher. In qualitative research, existing computer programs manage data, and analysis is performed by the research team. Gaining consensus, or high intercoder reliability, is achievable but is labor and time intensive.

- Being vulnerable to critiques of data being subjective or anecdotal in a scientific community that prefers experimental design that utilizes standardized, statistically significant research. Although qualitative research is not standardized, it is systematic, and depth of information is achieved in that respondents can understand questions as intended and answer in their own words.

Ethnography, like other qualitative methods, is largely an interpretive social science, and the principal instrument of data collection, analysis, interpretation, and reporting is the researcher. However, the sociocultural position of the researcher affects research, choice of methods, and interpretation of findings; therefore, questions and challenges often associated with conducting qualitative research are: How do researchers minimize the impact of their intrusion into the social life cycle of the people studied? Does a "native" anthropologist fare better or worse than an anthropologist from another culture? What input should members of the community, typically referred to as informants, have in "signing off" on what is reported about them? How do we create a better balance between understanding culturally specific perspectives and experiences (the emic approach) and understanding general health-related perspectives and experiences across all groups (the etic approach) and the construction of meaning?

Researchers often combine qualitative and quantitative research techniques to increase confidence in research findings.[62, 65] This mixed methodology involves the "collection or analysis of both quantitative and qualitative data in a single study in which the data are collected concurrently or sequentially, are given a priority, and involve the integration of the data at one or more stages in the process of research."[66] The use of mixed methods has become more popular in the field of psychology and anthropology. When designing interventions to prevent diabetes or to minimize diabetes complications among African Americans, a mixed method approach might include quantitative methods such as survey or checklist methodologies or monitoring of glycemic control over time, while qualitative methods might include structured and unstructured interviews, focus groups, thematic analysis of intervention-related notes and observations, policy analysis, or ethnography.

Using mixed methods allows researchers to identify and explore issues facing African Americans that may not be captured using a single methodology and may help interventionists gain a more exact understanding of an intervention's effectiveness and enhance validity.[67] In such studies, the methodologies can be complementary and integrative:[68] quantitative data help determine the effectiveness of an intervention, and qualitative data help lend meaning to the intervention. For instance, supplementing HbA1c outcome data with qualitative data from focus groups can reveal greater detail about the intervention's effectiveness or flaws.[69] In this case, quantitative data help researchers determine effectiveness in lowering HbA1c among a target population, and the focus groups provide data on the aspects of the intervention that participants found challenging or useful.

Mixed methods can also be used to develop diabetes interventions for African Americans. Before designing an intervention, researchers could conduct in-depth interviews with African American women diagnosed with diabetes to understand their experiences with diabetes self-management and health care and its meaning to their lives.[70, 71] Conducting focus groups, interviews, and meetings with community members before implementing an intervention allows members to convey their needs and concerns and to identify possible barriers to the successful implementation of an intervention. The information then can be used to design a more effective intervention, which is key for communities with marginalized or underrepresented groups who may strongly mistrust medical research.

Mixed methods have several strengths. Data from a mixed methods intervention can be used to improve replication of an intervention. Mixed methods can help researchers further understand the phenomenon under study and improve upon intervention design in the future.[67] To address public health concerns such as diabetes, interdisciplinary research approaches using both quantitative and qualitative methodologies and more complex study designs will be required. Reversing the tide of diabetes among African Americans will require research approaches that focus on the person diagnosed with diabetes; that person's social, economic, cultural, and political environments; and the health care system in which that person is involved. These approaches can also be facilitated by a better understanding of the role of ethnic identity in diabetes-related behaviors and of barriers across the political-economic spectrum.

INTEGRATING SOCIAL PSYCHOLOGY AND MEDICAL ANTHROPOLOGY TO REDUCE THE BURDEN OF DIABETES

In this chapter, we attempted to fuse aspects of critical social psychology and medical anthropology to address type 2 diabetes among African Americans. Given the rise of new cases of diabetes and the risk of serious diabetes-related complications in the African American community, we can no longer rely solely on current approaches. Instead, innovative multidisciplinary approaches and research designs are required. Combining theoretical perspectives and research methodologies from multiple disciplines can help address this burden and provide a richer inquiry into the problem of type 2 diabetes for this population. Diabetes risk and management are highly influenced by a person's engagement with the social service and health care systems. Engagement with the health care system includes issues of access, trust, cultural competence, quality of care, perceptions of discrimination, and communication between patients and providers. Diabetes risk and management are also influenced by a variety of historical, social, cultural, structural, and psychological factors.

The contribution of critical social psychology is its theoretical and empirical understanding of ethnic identity and its focus on socioecological and historical contexts and the negative effects of racial discrimination on behavior. African American ethnic identity is protective and develops, at least partially, in response to hostile social experiences. Ethnic identity influences health-related behaviors, perceptions of discrimination in the health care system, trust of health care providers, and willingness to engage in preventive and management-related behaviors. Ethnic identity also influences dietary preferences, physical activity, and beliefs about disease. Many of these behaviors can lead to developing diabetes and related complications. This path can be redirected if family members, researchers, policymakers, educators, and health care providers are aware of the cultural, social, psychological, and historical dynamics that contribute to the rise of new cases of diabetes and diabetes-related complications.

Critical medical anthropology explores the dialectical relationship between biological, social, and cultural factors in health, illness, and disease management. Critical medical anthropology's principal contribution is to expose and critique the health care system for the characteristics that make it structurally unwelcoming to people of color and to critique power relations inherent in medical encounters. The goal is to create awareness and correct the problem. This theoretical orientation, in conjunction with critical social psychology and mixed method research methodologies, is a powerful strategy for addressing the diabetes crisis at a deeper level.

Questions Raised by an Interdisciplinary Approach

Integrating perspectives from critical social psychology and critical medical anthropology will increase our understanding of the experience of African Americans with type 2 diabetes. We must examine how culture, beliefs, and practices influence diabetes management and help-seeking behavior and how social and institutional inequality affects individual perceptions and health-related behaviors. For example, how might structural inequality in the health care system be dismantled so that the health outcomes and management behaviors for African Americans with type 2 diabetes are improved? What structural changes are needed in the health care system to ensure equitable, respectful, and high-quality care for African Americans and other ethnic groups? Structural inequalities include exposure to environmental toxins, poor quality housing[15] and community services, as well as lack of access to healthy, affordable foods, green space, and quality health care with providers familiar with African American culture.

Depending on social context, African Americans may interpret health messages and approach disease prevention in a manner consistent with their ethnic identity. One question to consider is what are the nuances of these interpretations and how can they be turned to a health-promoting direction? People bring their ethnic identity into the health care system, including their beliefs about disease and attitudes toward health care providers.[72] How might providers gain greater sensitivity to the nuances of ethnic identity and how it plays out in health behaviors? Those interested in intervening with this particular population must be aware of how cultural beliefs and experiences shape willingness to engage in health-promoting behaviors.

In conclusion, interdisciplinary approaches are needed because the literature is currently dominated by models that focus on individual-level patient education but do not measure meaning, the legacy of distrust of the health care system, the dehumanizing orientation of clinical care, or how social environments can alter psychological states[8] to facilitate or undermine a person's ability to act on a provider's recommendation. Medical anthropology has only recently become interested in African Americans with diabetes, and critical social psychology has just begun to tackle the interaction between social inequality and specific health-related behaviors. Combining theoretical and methodological approaches is an innovative and crucial strategy for reversing the tide of diabetes in the African American community.

SUMMARY

In this chapter, we used critical social psychology and critical medical anthropology as tools to suggest an interdisciplinary research agenda to reduce diabetes among African Americans. We examined how race and ethnicity, ethnic identity, inequality and discrimination, and structural barriers in the health care system influence the development of diabetes. We discussed how ethnic identity and health care disparities can undermine diabetes management. We described the legacy of distrust of the health care system, the dehumanizing orientation of clinical care, and the pathways by which social environments can alter psychological states to facilitate or undermine a person's ability to act on a provider's recommendation. Finally, we proposed research questions that integrate critical social psychology and critical medical anthropology perspectives, increase understanding of the experience of type 2 diabetes among urban African Africans, and inform the development of strategies to reduce the prevalence of diabetes in this community.

DISCUSSION QUESTIONS

1. What are some of the reasons that African Americans in the United States have higher rates of type 2 diabetes than Whites?

2. What research methods have been used to study disparities in diabetes, and what are the specific insights that each method can contribute?

3. What are some assets of African American communities that could be enlisted in efforts to reverse the epidemics of obesity and type 2 diabetes?

4. Now that you have studied this chapter, what advice would you give to public health planners designing interventions to reduce type 2 diabetes in African American communities?

NOTES

1. Centers for Disease Control and Prevention. *National diabetes fact sheet: General information and national estimates on diabetes in the United States, 2005.* Atlanta, Ga.: U.S. Department of Health and Human Services. Published 2005. Available at www.cdc.gov/diabetes/pubs/pdf/ndfs_2005.pdf.

2. Brown, A., Ang, A., and Pebley, A. The relationship between neighborhood characteristics and self-rated health for adults with chronic conditions. *American Journal of Public Health,* 95, no. 5 (2007): 926–932.

3. Schootman, M., Andresen, E. M., Wolinsky, F. D., et al. The effect of adverse housing and neighborhood conditions on the development of diabetes mellitus among middle-aged African Americans. *American Journal of Epidemiology,* 166 (2007): 379–387.

4. Jack. L., Jr., et al. Influence of the environmental context on diabetes self-management: A rationale for developing a new research paradigm in diabetes education. *Diabetes Educator,* 25, no. 5 (1999): 775–790.

5. Brody, G. H., Jack, L., Jr., Murry, V. M., Lander-Potts, M., and Liburd, L. Heuristic model linking contextual processes to self-management in African-American adults with type 2 diabetes. *Diabetes Educator,* 27 (2001): 685–693.

6. Liburd, L., Jack, L., Jr., Williams, S., and Tucker, P. Intervening on the social determinants of cardiovascular disease and diabetes. *American Journal of Preventative Medicine,* 29, no. 5S1 (2005): 18–24.

7. Liburd, L., and Vinicor, F. Rethinking diabetes prevention and control in racial and ethnic communities. *Journal of Public Health Management & Practice,* Suppl (November 2003): S74–S79.

8. Gelhert, S., Sohmer, D., Sacks, T., Mininger, C., McClintock, M., and Olufunmilayo, O. Targeting health disparities: A model linking upstream determinants to downstream interventions. *Health Affairs,* 27, no. 2 (2008): 339–349.

9. Fox, D., and Prilleltensky, I. *Critical Psychology: An Introduction.* London: Sage, 1996.

10. Jones, J. M. *Prejudice and Racism.* New York: McGraw-Hill, 1997.

11. Feiring, C., Coates, D. L., and Taska, L. Ethnic status, stigmatization, support and symptom development following sexual abuse. *Journal of Interpersonal Violence,* 16 (2001): 1307–1329.

12. Garroutte, E. M., Kunovich, R. M., Jacobsen, C., and Goldberg, J. Patient satisfaction and ethnic identity among American Indian older adults. *Social Science & Medicine,* 59, no. 11 (2004): 2233–2244.

13. Sellers, R. M., Smith, M. A., Shelton, J. N., Rowley, S. J., and Chavous, T. M. Multidimensional model of racial identity: A reconceptualization of African American identity. *Pers Soc Psychol Rev,* 2 (1998): 18–39.

14. Nagel, J. Ethnicity and sexuality. *Annual Review of Sociology,* 26 (2000): 107–133.

15. Braveman, P. Racial disparities at birth: The puzzle persists. *Issues in Science and Technology* (2008): 27–30.

16. Krieger, N. Does racism harm health? Did child abuse exist before 1962? On explicit questions, critical science, and current controversies: An ecosocial perspective. *American Journal of Public Health,* 93 (2003): 194–199.

17. Williams, D. R. Race, SES, and health: The added effects of racism and discrimination. In N. E. Adler, M. Marmot, B. S. McEwen, and J. Stewart, eds., *Socioeconomic Status and Health in Industrial Nations: Social, Psychological and Biological Pathways,* p. 896. New York: Annals of the New York Academy of Sciences, 1999.

18. Brody, G. H., Chen, Y., Kogan, S. M., Murry, V. M., Logan, P., and Luo, Z. Linking perceived discrimination to longitudinal changes in African American mothers' parenting practices. *Journal of Marriage & Family,* 70, no. 2 (2008): 319–331.

19. Brody, G. H., Chen, Y., Murry, V. M., McBride, V., et al. Perceived discrimination and the adjustment of African American youths: A five-year longitudinal analysis with contextual moderation effects. *Child Development,* 77, no. 5 (2006): 1170–1189.

20. Clark, R., Anderson, N. B., Clark, V. R., and Williams, D. R. Racism as a stressor for African Americans: A biopsychosocial model. *American Psychology,* 54, no. 10 (1999): 805–816.

21. Jones, H. L., Cross, W. E., and Defour, D. Race-related stress, racial identity, and mental health among black women. *Journal of Black Psychology,* 33, no. 2 (2007): 208–231.

22. Landrine, H., and Klonoff, E. A. The schedule of racist events: A measure of racial discrimination and a study of its negative physical and mental health consequences. *Journal of Black Psychology,* 22, no. 2 (1996): 144–168.

23. Wagner, J., and Abbott, G. Depression and depression care in diabetes; relationship to perceived discrimination in African Americans. *Diabetes Care,* 3 (2007): 362.

24. Hill-Briggs, F., Gary, T. L., Hill, M. N., Bone, L. R., and Brancati, F. L. Health-related quality of life in urban African Americans with type 2 diabetes. *Journal of General Internal Medicine,* 17, no. 6 (2002): 412–419.

25. Finkler, K. *Women in Pain: Gender and Morbidity in Mexico.* Philadelphia: University of Pennsylvania Press, 1994.

26. Snow, L. F. *Walkin' over Medicine.* Boulder, Col.: Westview Press, 1993.

27. Pelto, H. G., Goodman, A. H., Dufour, D. L., and Gretel, H. *Nutritional Anthropology: Biocultural Perspectives on Food and Nutrition.* New York: McGraw-Hill, 2000.

28. Kleinman, A. *The Illness Narratives: Suffering, Healing and the Human Condition.* New York: Basic Books, 1988.

29. Liburd, L., Namageyo-Funa, A., Jack, L., and Gregg, E. Views from within and beyond: Illness narratives of African American men with type 2 diabetes. *Diabetes Spectrum,* 17, no. 4 (2004): 219–224.

30. Mullings, L. *On Our Own Terms: Race, Class, and Gender in the Lives of African American Women.* New York: Routledge, 1996.

31. Lock, M., and Scheper-Hughes, N. A. Critical-interpretive approach in medical anthropology: Rituals and routines of discipline and dissent. In C. F. Sargent and T. M. Johnson, eds., *Medical Anthropology: Contemporary Theory and Method,* pp. 41–70. Westport, Conn.: Praeger, 1996.

32. Wilkinson, R. G. *Mind the Gap: Hierarchies, Health and Human Evolution.* New Haven, Conn.: Yale University Press, 2000.

33. Janes, C. R. Commentary: "Culture," cultural explanations, and causality. *International Journal of Epidemiology,* 35 (2006): 261–263.

34. Dressler, W. W. Commentary: Taking culture seriously in health research. *International Journal of Epidemiology,* 35 (2006): 258–259.

35. Scheper-Hughes, N. Three propositions for a critically applied medical anthropology. *Social Science & Medicine,* 30, no. 2 (1990): 189–197.

36. Baer, H. A., Singer, M., and Johnsen, J. H. Toward a critical medical anthropology. *Social Science & Medicine,* 23, no. 2 (1986): 95–98.

37. Bach, P. B., Pham, H. H., Schrag, D., Tate, R. C., and Hargraves, J. L. Primary care physicians who treat blacks and whites. *New England Journal of Medicine,* 351 (2004): 575–584.

38. Baer, H., Singer, M., and Susser, I. *Medical Anthropology and the World System: A Critical Perspective.* Westport, Conn.: Bergin & Garvey, 1997.

39. Bailey, E. J. *Anthropology and African American Health.* Westport, Conn.: Bergin & Garvey, 2000.

40. Dressler, W. W. Health in the African American community: Accounting for health inequalities. *Medical Anthropology Quarterly,* 7 (1993): 325–345.

41. Kleinman, A. *The Illness Narratives: Suffering, Healing and the Human Condition.* New York: Basic Books, 1998.

42. Armelagos, G. J., Leatherman, T., Ryan, M., and Sibley, L. Biocultural synthesis in medical anthropology. *Medical Anthropology Quarterly,* 14 (1992): 35–52.

43. Cokley, K. Racial(ized) identity, ethnic identity, and Afrocentric values: Conceptual and methodological challenges in understanding African American identity. *Journal of Counseling Psychology,* 52 (2005): 517–526.

44. Cross, W. E. The everyday functions of African American identity. In J. Swim and C. Stangor, eds., *Prejudice: The Target's Perspective,* pp. 267–279. New York: Academic Press, 1998.

45. Nazroo, J. Y., and Karlsen, S. Patterns of identity among ethnic minority people: Diversity and commonality. *Ethnic and Racial Studies,* 26, no. 5 (2003): 902–930.

46. Williams, D. R. African American health: The role of the social environment. *Journal of Urban Health,* 75 (1998): 300–321.

47. Cubbin, C., and Winkleby, M. A. Food availability, personal constraints, and community resources. *Journal of Epidemiology and Community Health,* 61 (2007): 932.

48. Mechanic, D. Who shall lead: Is there a future for population health? *Journal of Health Politics, Policy and Law*, 28, no. 2–3 (2003): 421–442.

49. Oyserman, D., Fryberg, S. A., and Yoder, N. Identity-based motivation and health. *Journal of Personality and Social Psychology*, 93, no. 6 (2007): 1011–1027.

50. Thompson, V. L. Variables affecting racial-identity salience among African Americans. *Journal of Social Psychology*, 139, no. 6 (1999): 748–761.

51. Bonds, D. E., Camacho, F., Bell, R. A., Duren-Winfield, V., Anderson, R. T., and Goff, D. C. The association of patient trust and self-care among patients with diabetes mellitus. *BMC Family Practice*, 5 (2004): 26.

52. Stark Casagrande, S., Gary, T. L., LaVeist, T. A., Gaskin, D. J., and Coppoer, L. A. Perceived discrimination and adherence to medical care in a racially integrated community. *Journal of General Internal Medicine*, 22 (2007): 389–395.

53. Arthur, M. W., Hawkins, J. D., Pollard, J. A., Catalano, R. F., and Baglioni, A. J. Measuring risk and protective factors for substance use, delinquency, and other adolescent problem behaviors. *Evaluation Review*, 26, no. 6 (2002): 575–601.

54. Cross, W. E., Parham, T. A., and Helms, I. E. The stages of black identity development: Nigrescence models. In R. L. Jones, ed., *Black Psychology*, 3rd ed., pp. 319–338. Berkeley, Cal.: Cobb & Henry, 1991.

55. Cross, W. E. Oppositional identity and African American youth: Issues and prospects. In W. D. Hawley, ed., *Toward a Common Destiny*, pp. 185–204. San Francisco: Jossey-Bass, 1995.

56. Goldney, R. D., Phillips, P. J., Fisher, L. J., and Wilson, D. H. Diabetes, depression, and quality of life. *Diabetes Care*, 27, no. 5 (2004): 1066–1070.

57. Lustman, P. J., and Clouse. R. E. Treatment of depression in diabetes: Impact on mood and medical outcome. *Journal of Psychosomatic Research*, 53, no. 4 (2002): 917–925.

58. Williams, D. R., and Williams-Morris, R. Racism and mental health: The African American experience. *Ethnicity & Health*, 5, no. 3–4 (2000): 243–268.

59. Polzer, R., and Shandor, M. M. Spirituality and self-management of diabetes in African Americans. *Journal of Holistic Nursing*, 23, no. 2 (2005): 230–250.

60. Mattis, J. S., and Jagers, R. J. A relational framework for the study of religiosity and spirituality in the lives of African Americans. *Journal of Community Psychology*, 29, no. 5 (2001): 519–539.

61. Mullings, L., and Wali, A. *Stress and Resilience: The Social Context of Reproduction in Central Harlem*. New York: Plenum Press, 2000.

62. Neuman, W. L. *Social Research Methods: Qualitative and Quantitative Approaches*. Boston: Allyn & Bacon, 2003.

63. Crane, J. G., and Angrosino, M. V. *Field Projects in Anthropology.* Prospect Heights, Ill.: Waveland Press, 1992.

64. Hammersley, M., and Atkinson, P. *Ethnography: Principles in Practice.* London: Routledge, 1995.

65. Bernard, H. R. *Research Methods in Anthropology.* Walnut Creek, Cal.: AltaMira, 2002.

66. Creswell, J. W., Plana Clark, V. L., Gutmann, M. L., and Hanson, W. E. Advanced mixed methods research designs. In A. Tashakkori and C. Teddlie, eds., *Handbook of Mixed Methods in Social and Behavioral Research,* pp. 209–240. Thousand Oaks, Cal.: Sage, 2003.

67. Creswell, J. W. *Research Design: Qualitative, Quantitative, and Mixed Methods Approaches.* Thousand Oaks, Cal.: Sage, 2003.

68. Creswell, J. W., Fetters, M. D., and Ivankova, N. V. Designing a mixed methods study in primary care. *Annals of Family Medicine,* 2, no. 1 (2004): 7–12.

69. Sarkisian, C. A., Brusuelas, R. J., Steers, W. N., et al. Using focus groups of older African Americans and Latinos with diabetes to modify a self-care empowerment intervention. *Ethnic Discussion,* 15 (2005): 203–291.

70. Seidman, I. *Interviewing as Qualitative Research: A Guide for Researchers in Education and the Social Sciences.* New York: Teachers College Press, 1998.

71. Trochim, W. M. K. *The Research Methods Knowledge Base,* 2nd ed. Cincinnati, Oh.: Atomic Dog Publishing, 2001.

72. Baptiste-Roberts, K., Gary, T. L., Bone, L. R., Hill, M. N., and Brancati, F. L. Perceived body image among African Americans with type 2 diabetes. *Patient Education and Counseling,* 60 (2006): 194–200.

PART

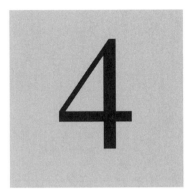

4

PUTTING INTERDISCIPLINARY APPROACHES INTO PRACTICE

12

USING INTERDISCIPLINARY APPROACHES TO STRENGTHEN URBAN HEALTH RESEARCH AND PRACTICE

**NICHOLAS FREUDENBERG, SUSAN KLITZMAN,
SUSAN SAEGERT**

LEARNING OBJECTIVES

- Describe the rationale for using interdisciplinary research approaches to study urban health problems.

- Discuss the stages of the interdisciplinary research process (defining the problem, creating and implementing a process, choosing partners, influencing policy and practice, and evaluating impact) and describe the key tasks in each stage.

- Analyze the unique challenges that face evaluators of interdisciplinary interventions to improve urban health.

- Identify specific ways that you can use interdisciplinary research approaches in your professional practice.

DOING INTERDISCIPLINARY RESEARCH AND PRACTICE

In the previous chapters of this volume, researchers from a variety of disciplines, professions, and specialization areas—including American studies, anthropology, economics, environmental health sciences, epidemiology, geography, health education, medicine, nutrition, political science, psychology, public health, social ecology, sociology, and urban planning—considered a range of urban health and social issues—including aging, air pollution, asthma, child development and poverty, diabetes, disasters, homelessness, housing foreclosures, hunger, immigration, obesity, racism, and tobacco use. The stories that emerge from these dizzying lists of disciplines and problems illustrate the complex challenges that face those seeking to improve the well-being of urban populations and the need for urban health researchers and practitioners to be able to cross traditional academic and professional boundaries if they are to be effective.

In this final chapter, we consider some of the central themes that run through this volume. Our focus is on *doing* interdisciplinary research and practice in urban health. In the last decade, a lively scholarly debate on the meaning, value, and tensions within inter- and transdisciplinary research has emerged.[1,2,3,4] However, our aim here is more practical: We seek to help readers move from an appreciation of interdisciplinary research to a capacity to do it—to apply the principles, concepts, and skills described in the previous chapters and developed elsewhere in recent years to their roles as urban health professionals and researchers.

We examine what we have learned about the practical application of the approaches, methods, and frameworks the authors describe and how our readers can apply these lessons in their work settings. Our sources for this discussion are the prior chapters, our own research and practice, described briefly in Chapter One, and our understanding of the recent literature on interdisciplinary research and practice. In the last several years, some new volumes and special journal issues on interdisciplinary research have been produced. These are described briefly in Table 12.1, and we encourage interested readers to consult these sources for a deeper understanding or for guidance on selected issues. Although much of the new attention to interdisciplinary research has emerged in the United States and Europe, it has also attracted researchers in Africa, Latin America, and Asia, suggesting its relevance in both the developed and developing world.[5,6,7]

In Figure 12.1, we present a schematic of the stages involved in doing interdisciplinary work on urban health. We conceptualize the process as a cycle—shown as a circle—in which researchers begin by defining the problem and then create a process for addressing the problem and implementing the research. Once the team of researchers

TABLE 12.1.   **Selected Recent Works on Interdisciplinary Research**

Title and authors	Publisher and publication date	Brief description
Creating Interdisciplinarity: Interdisciplinary Research and Teaching Among College and University Faculty. Lattuca, L.	Vanderbilt University Press, 2001	Analyzes the processes by which faculty from different disciplines pursue interdisciplinarity in their teaching and research across departments, disciplines, and institutions.
Expanding the Boundaries of Health and Social Science: Case Studies in Innovation. Kessel, F., Rosenfield, P. L., and Anderson, N. B., editors	Oxford University Press, 2003	Case studies of application of interdisciplinary methods on topics from brain science to HIV and human resilience. Prepared by Social Science Research Council and Office of Behavioral and Social Science Research at National Institute of Health.
Facilitating Interdisciplinary Research. Committee on Facilitating Interdisciplinary Research	National Academies Press, 2005	A review of interdisciplinary research with a focus on the organizational and institutional factors that facilitate or block this approach. Sponsored by the National Academies of Sciences and Engineering and the Institute of Medicine.
Handbook of Transdisciplinary Research. Hirsh-Hadorn, G., Hoffman-Riem, H., Biber-Klemm, S. et al., editors	Springer, 2008	Provides an overview of transdisciplinary research as applied to problems at the interface of science, society, and politics; most contributors are European researchers. Prepared by the Swiss Academies of Arts and Sciences.
Special Issue of *American Journal of Preventive Medicine*, "The Science of Team Science." Stokols, D., Hall, K. L., Taylor, B. K., Moser, R. B., and Syme, S. L.	Volume 35, Special Supplement, August 2008	Twenty articles on "team science" with sections on origins, theoretical perspectives, methodological contributions, the role of systems thinking, and future directions for the "science of team science."

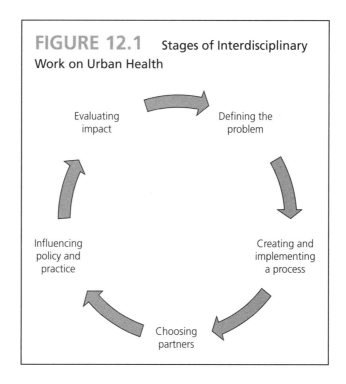

FIGURE 12.1 Stages of Interdisciplinary Work on Urban Health

is assembled, they will usually need to find other partners to help them understand the problem and carry out the research. Next the investigators look for ways to use their findings to influence policy and practice. Finally, the team evaluates the impact of their work to guide the next steps. Although the diagram shows the stages proceeding in a clockwise direction, in fact, research teams may on occasion return to previous stages. For example, after bringing in new partners, a team may choose to redefine the problem. In Chapter Seven, for example, it was only after talking to individuals who had experienced foreclosure that Saegert and her colleagues grasped its impact on health, thus modifying their research questions. Figure 12.1 also focuses on the research process itself rather than calling attention to the dynamic context in which the problem is unfolding. Again using the chapter on foreclosure and health as an example, as the research progressed, the media, political, and economic context moved from widespread denial of the foreclosure crisis to active engagement. This change affected the ways in which the research can lead to policy change and interventions.

Thus, we see interdisciplinary research as a dynamic and iterative process in which investigators move between steps in both directions as one set of problems is solved and new issues emerge. In the following pages, we discuss some of the issues that research teams face at each stage of the process, using examples from the previous chapters.

DEFINING THE PROBLEM

Only when a problem is clearly articulated can researchers decide whether or not it warrants interdisciplinary rather than disciplinary investigation. First, let's consider how to determine whether or not a problem meets the criteria for interdisciplinary research, and then let's take a step back and ask how best to frame a problem so as to define a researchable question.

Not every problem—not even every urban health problem—requires interdisciplinary research or intervention to solve. But in many of the case studies presented in this volume, the impetus for using an interdisciplinary approach to research or intervention was not an ideological commitment to interdisciplinarity but rather a consequence of the nature of the problem itself. What are some of the indications for an interdisciplinary rather than a disciplinary approach? And what kinds of problems are more suited to this approach?

First, investigators need to ask whether the problem's causes or consequences cross levels of organization. If they do, it may be that a single discipline will be insufficient. Second, if the investigators seek to solve as well as describe the problem they are studying—a basic premise of public health—then they need to ask whether their discipline has all or most of the tools needed for solution. If not, a broader team may be needed. Another way of saying this is to posit that if researchers want to move from basic or etiological research to applied work, from laboratory to bedside to population, a process recently labeled as translational science,[8] they probably need an interdisciplinary team. Third, if the problem is embedded in a complex social and physical environment or if it cuts across multiple sectors, more than one discipline may be needed to understand the influences of these external factors. Fourth, if researchers seek to address fundamental as well as proximate causes of a health problem, they may need to include researchers who can travel both upstream and downstream to understand these different levels of causes and the pathways by which they influence health. Finally, the research team needs to consider the scope of its mandate. If researchers are charged by larger social institutions with answering a narrow and specific question, a single discipline may suffice, whereas if the directive is to fix the problem, more complex investigations will be needed. For example, if researchers want to bring their findings into policy and practice arenas, they may need to find colleagues in other disciplines.

To illustrate, let's take the example of childhood asthma, a problem considered in Chapter Two. If the question is whether a particular medical treatment is effective in reducing asthma symptoms among children, a research team of one or two disciplines could probably design and carry out a study to answer it. If, however, the question is how to get an effective drug to the children who need it, how to help parents ensure their asthmatic children take the medicine properly, how to make sure that local health providers use the medicine effectively, or how to combine medical treatment with household or neighborhood environmental modification to further reduce symptoms, then the research team will need a much wider cast of characters. In sum, both the scope of the health problem under investigation and the types of questions that need to be answered dictate whether or not to use interdisciplinary research.

Framing the Problem

In every research endeavor, framing the problem is a key starting task. Interpreting the framing of social problems has recently emerged as a popular strategy in communications, social science, and public health research.[9, 10] "Frames" have been described as tools for defining a problem, diagnosing its cause, justifying solutions, and predicting its likely effects.[10]

In many complex questions that bring together multiple actors and stakeholders and draw on expertise of multiple disciplines, building in a reflection and possible reframing moment early in the process is wise.

Researchers and public health professionals always have choices in how to frame a problem. The decisions they make structure their opportunities for posing research questions and designing studies or interventions. How to frame a problem is both a scientific question and a political question—scientific in that it requires evidence and hypotheses on the more and less important causal factors and consequences and political in that any solution requires understanding who has power to solve the problem and what will move them to act. Although some researchers seek to avoid the second question, it is our belief that the public health ethic requires considering both simultaneously because the imperative is to improve population health, not simply to describe or analyze it.

To aid in our understanding of how framing a problem influences decisions about interdisciplinary research, we use the example of diabetes, a problem considered in Chapter Eleven. Diabetes can be considered from several different perspectives—for example, as a metabolic problem requiring adjustments in glucose metabolism, as a medical problem requiring effective medical management to prevent complications and treat symptoms, as a public health problem requiring control programs that reduce social and environmental risk factors and incidence in the population as a whole, as a social justice problem requiring efforts to shrink the growing disparities in morbidity and mortality among different socioeconomic and racial/ethnic groups, or as an economic problem imposing a growing burden on our work force, economy, and health care system. Each of these frames suggests a different solution and requires a different team of investigators to find answers. In Chapter Eleven, Jones and Liburd suggest that cultural and sociopolitical factors play a key role in shaping the differential impact diabetes has on different populations; they suggest that effective interventions may need to involve and be tailored to specific subpopulations.

No frame is by itself right or wrong, but the challenge is to match the frame of the problem with the expertise and mandate that researchers have to understand and address it. The case we make here and in the volume as a whole is that if the mandate is for researchers to improve the health of urban populations, then a broad, multilevel, and intersectoral framing of the problem is often more likely to lead to effective solutions than a narrower one. In the first chapter, we described the characteristics of cities that justified such an approach—population density and diverse, complex systems, a multiple array of human and social resources, and high levels of inequality. Health problems that are embedded in this context often require more comprehensive and holistic interventions than those that play out in a simpler environment.

To return to the example of diabetes, the rapid rate of increase of diabetes in U.S. cities;[11] its multifactoral roots in food systems,[12] urban design,[13] and health care organization; its driving role in fostering urban health disparities; and the substantial burden it is imposing on municipal economies[14] all suggest the value of framing the problem broadly and therefore initiating interdisciplinary investigation. These same characteristics of the diabetes problem also encourage the development of a process to include multiple constituencies and stakeholders in the task of framing the research questions to be answered.

Constructing Conceptual Models, Theories, or Frameworks

One of the greatest challenges facing interdisciplinary researchers is to isolate the variables of interest for study. On the one hand, the imperatives of interdisciplinary investigations are to consider multiple levels, domains, and constructs, often leading to a list of variables of interest longer than a New York City telephone directory. On the other hand, traditional research guidelines—and traditional funding agencies— often want researchers to identify a small number of variables, correctly noting that too many can lead to conceptual muddiness and analytic difficulties. To resolve this conundrum, some researchers find it helpful to construct conceptual models or frameworks, a simplification of the theories that explain the causes or consequences of the problem under study, and specify a limited number of variables of particular interest. For interdisciplinary researchers, these models often illustrate how forces operate or interact across levels of organization. In this volume, the authors of Chapter Four (Figures 4.1, 4.2, and 4.3) and Chapter Ten (Figure 10.3) and elsewhere have presented conceptual models to show relationships among their variables of interest.[15, 16]

Another tool that can help to frame a problem in a way that contributes to workable solutions is to use "systems science" to understand the problem within its broader dimensions. Green has noted that systems science or systems thinking can help "to unravel the complexity of causal forces in our varied populations, and the ecologically layered community and societal circumstances of public health practice."[17] Systems thinking provides quantitative and qualitative tools for analyzing complex systems, for understanding the dynamic interactions among variables of interest, and for identifying promising opportunities for intervention.[18, 19]

To give an example, one of us has analyzed the multiple systems that determine the health problems and needs of people leaving jails to identify opportunities for intervention at various levels.[20] Based on this analysis, a multilevel program was developed and tested.[21] Similarly, in Chapter Ten, Fahs and colleagues use systems thinking to assess the multiple influences on older urban immigrants and suggest policies and programs that can promote healthy aging for this population.

Often, the greatest contribution of interdisciplinary research is to create new more adequate conceptual frameworks for a problem based on ideas that arose in grappling with multiple disciplines' literatures. For example, in Chapter Six, Geronimus, a health scientist, and Thompson, a political scientist, first critically examine concepts of "normal development," drawing primarily on developmental psychology and normative sociological theories of the family. They then critique the underlying assumptions of most economic analyses enunciated in classical economic theory. In their third critique, they return more closely to the second author's core discipline. Throughout, their critical perspective is informed by a broad and interdisciplinary literature in cultural studies and critical race theory.

Even when interdisciplinary researchers adopt a less original conceptual framework, they often must read deeply in unfamiliar disciplines to understand the assumptions behind the theoretical and policy frames applied in the relevant literature. To meaningfully address the foreclosure issue and its relationship to health in Chapter Seven, the authors found that much of the relevant work and policy formulations on foreclosure derived from economic theory. In addition, research and thinking on the relationships among health, debt, foreclosure, and vulnerable populations ranged across disciplines from various subfields in psychology, through geography, public health, medicine, and sociology, as well as the interdisciplinary arenas of urban and policy studies.

CREATING A PROCESS FOR INTERDISCIPLINARY WORK

Once investigators have defined a problem and determined that an interdisciplinary approach may be warranted, the next task is to create the processes for carrying out the work. The steps include assembling a team, defining the processes and structures needed to build a supportive environment for collaboration, and selecting the methodologies and analytic strategies to be employed.

Assembling a Team

In this section, we discuss how to select members of an interdisciplinary research team; later, we discuss the task of developing collaborative relationships with external organizations. In practice, the distinction between these two levels may be arbitrary, but we think of the research team as comprising the individuals, whether trained researchers or community residents, who design, monitor, and carry out the research; external partners play a more limited role and usually are not involved in making operational decisions about the study.

Selecting members for an interdisciplinary research team requires paying attention both to individual and group characteristics. In our experience, attributes of good team members include a shared passion for understanding and reducing the problem under study, a willingness to listen to and consider different points of view, an openness toward broadening one's knowledge, experience working across traditional boundaries (whether disciplinary, sectoral, or level), confidence and good skills in their own home discipline, and a pragmatic rather than an ideological approach to questions of research design and methods. In many cases, interdisciplinary teams include individuals who have worked together before and already have experience in sorting through the relationship problems that inevitably arise in team research.

At the group level, effective teams establish and enforce group norms that support collaboration, value the contributions of each member, use problem-solving and conflict-resolution strategies to address problems that arise, and find ways to define and articulate a specific mission that drives their shared work.

Recently, a body of academic work studying team science has emerged. Stokols and his colleagues describe team science as initiatives "designed to promote collaborative—and often cross-disciplinary—approaches to analyzing research questions about particular phenomenon."[22] They distinguish team science from the "science-of-team-science," defined as "a branch of science studies concerned especially with understanding and managing circumstances that facilitate the effectiveness of team science initiatives."[22] By studying how teams make decisions and work together, researchers can identify successful strategies for teamwork.

How do interdisciplinary researchers decide who to invite to join their team? One logical starting point is the problem under study. What disciplines, skills, and experience are needed to answer the research question? Developing and evaluating an intervention to prevent diabetes in an African American community, the subject of Chapter Eleven, may require a health services researcher, a nutritionist, a physical activity researcher, an anthropologist, and an evaluator. By mapping the knowledge base on which a study rests, researchers can identify the expertise they need and then invite selected colleagues to join. In other cases, interdisciplinary collaboration can have a more serendipitous start. When two of the authors of Chapter Nine—Galea, a social epidemiologist, and Hadley, an anthropologist—discussed their common interests in the health consequences of disasters, each recognized that the other discipline could bring new insights into their research.

Urban health researchers often worry about when and how to bring community residents onto their research teams. Some begin with a philosophical commitment to community-based participatory research (CBPR) and would not begin a new study without bringing community residents into the planning process.[23] Others choose to bring in community residents on an as-needed basis, defining specific research questions that would benefit from community input. Two recent books provide guidance on the use of CBPR in health research.[24, 25]

In Chapters Two, Three, Five, Seven, and Eight, the authors show the value of participatory research, describing how having community residents, organizations, or others affected by the problem under study participate in the research process deepened the team's understanding. In our view, most interdisciplinary research on urban health would benefit from participation by a broader group of stakeholders, and perhaps defining a role for communities should be the default option, dispensed with only if there were strong contraindications.

We do, however, firmly believe that if researchers invite community residents, advocates, or others to join the research team, they should have an explicit rationale for such inclusion in the particular study and should have a clear negotiation on roles and responsibilities. To invite community residents to join a research team as window dressing is a disservice to both researchers and residents. In Chapter Eight, Fuqua et al. describe some of the problems that can emerge if community participants are not aware of their roles and stake in the research process. In the section on external partnerships below, we discuss other ways to engage community residents short of inviting them to serve as full members of the research team.

Interdisciplinary research teams may require a different style of leadership than a more traditional research group. Because no single discipline can claim theoretical supremacy or complete understanding and no single individual has the requisite knowledge for making decisions, a more collective leadership may lead to better processes. Defining scopes of responsibility within a team may help to allocate who decides what.

Is there an ideal size for an interdisciplinary research team? Several studies suggest that more effective teams have five to ten individuals, representing no more than four or five disciplines. Other factors associated with success include having a high proportion of tenured faculty members and external funding.[26]

Selecting Methods and Analytic Strategies

On the one hand, the selection and use of methods and analytic strategies in interdisciplinary research are no different from in disciplinary research. Researchers strive for reliability, validity, and generalizability and apply the same standards for assessing these constructs. On the other hand, because integration of findings is the ultimate goal of interdisciplinary research, investigators face an additional challenge: piecing together findings derived from different methods and analytic strategies into a coherent whole. Thus, an interdisciplinary team must consider in advance not only what methods to use to collect data on variables of interest but also how to combine findings from these different sources. Some useful starting points for this task are to agree on operational definitions of variables of interest; to construct, as described earlier, conceptual models or frameworks that show the relationships and interactions among variables at different levels of organization; and to develop integrative theories that might explain the question under study.

On a more interpersonal level, team members need to appreciate and value the insights from disciplines, methods, and analytic strategies other than their own. Those still caught in tired binary debates, for example, about the relative superiority of quantitative versus qualitative methods, individual- versus neighborhood-level phenomena, and the primacy of social versus natural science theory may not be suited for interdisciplinary research that draws from multiple methods, theories, and levels of research.

Building a Supportive Environment

As we have described, university-based interdisciplinary researchers face the usual stresses of academia: getting research funded, winning tenure and promotion, publishing the results of their research, and balancing the demands of research, teaching, and service as well as family, friends, and outside social and political commitments. In addition, interdisciplinary researchers face the particular challenges of learning new disciplines and methods, finding the extended time often needed to complete their research, developing relationships with colleagues and external partners in other disciplines and sectors, and having their work accepted by colleagues who may be skeptical of the value of interdisciplinary approaches. To cope with these stressors or to mitigate them, interdisciplinary researchers need to find ways to create environments that support their work.

At City University of New York, we developed several strategies to create supportive environments for interdisciplinary work in urban health. In 2002, several faculty members (including the editors of this volume) created the CUNY Urban Health Collaborative, an informal network of faculty, students, and staff working in some area of urban health. Over time, about 30 or 40 participants attended meetings regularly and more than 350 joined a list serve. The collaborative was too large and broad to serve as a research partnership, but it did create a space where faculty interested in finding colleagues or mentors in other disciplines could meet and seek partners, learn about funding opportunities, and discuss new methods and approaches to the study of specific urban health problems. A part-time graduate student research assistant helped to convene meetings, publicize events and funding opportunities, and organize faculty seminars. This low-cost, low-intensity network served as an incubator for more formal research partnerships that then developed specific research projects and applied for funding.[27]

In Chapter Five, Maantay and colleagues describe some of the ways that the South Bronx Environmental Justice Partnership created an organizational environment that could support the diverse participants in their study of childhood asthma. They describe the importance of having a safe space where individuals representing organizations with different missions and types of power could freely exchange ideas and solve problems, while acknowledging the fact that some outside factors were beyond their control.

CHOOSING INSTITUTIONAL AND COMMUNITY PARTNERS

Successful action-oriented, interdisciplinary urban health research requires multilevel and multisectoral partnerships. As noted by Fuqua, Stokols, and colleagues in Chapter Eight, transdisciplinary (TD) action research "comprises at least three kinds or phases of collaboration: (a) *scientific collaborations* among research investigators, (b) *community problem-solving coalitions* in which researchers work with community members to translate scientific knowledge into community problem-solving strategies, and (c) *intersectoral partnerships* involving representatives of organizations situated at local, state, national, and international levels, who work together to improve environmental, social, and health problems."

Several key elements of effective partnerships emerge from the case studies analyzed in this volume and elsewhere, including (a) recognition of each partner's unique knowledge and perspectives; (b) finding common elements in their respective institutional missions, goals, or agendas; (c) ensuring programmatic and institutional longevity; and (d) developing processes for resolving differences, conflict, and competition.

A few examples illustrate some of these principles in action. In the partnership between academic nursing and public health departments and a local health department's wellness program described by Zenk et al. in Chapter Three, the partners shared a commitment to understanding how the urban food retail system influences diet and health in low-income urban communities. In Chapter Five, Maantay and her colleagues described a partnership among a community organization, a large clinical system, a minority-serving educational institution, and a research-oriented medical school. Although the institutions represented seemingly diverse sectors (i.e., community advocacy, medical care, public higher education, and academic medicine), they were able to find common ground around improving the health and well-being of community residents and workers. In this case, the partnership worked to secure grant funding for the community-based organization so that it could hire full-time staff and maintain a meaningful and active presence.

In Chapter Eight, Fuqua and her colleagues describe the Tobacco Policy Consortium's development, in which over the course of several years, researchers' and community members' perspectives on tobacco control priorities became more similar as a result of repeated brainstorming sessions and collective discussions of the TPC's priorities. They began to share views on what directions were the most promising for tobacco control in their local communities and organizations.

Engaging Communities

Community participation and engagement are critical to interdisciplinary researchers' understanding and ability to solve urban health problems. Yet in many urban communities, residents are frequently overwhelmed by economic, legal, housing, educational, family, or other issues, and they may perceive that the study of isolated health problems is more likely to enhance the researcher's career than improve their lives. Indeed, the recognition that successful public health interventions require knowledge of context for intervention in people's everyday lives has been a major driver for the development of both interdisciplinary and community-based participatory research.

One challenge for interdisciplinary urban health researchers seeking to engage communities is to be able to listen to community needs and perceptions and find common ground, a part of the framing exercise. The cultural competence and sensitivity of researchers become very important when working with the usually diverse urban populations. In Chapter Eleven, Jones and Liburd describe why a deep understanding of the conditions of a particular population's historical and cultural experiences must be integrated with analysis of social inequalities in health status if interventions to improve health, in this case type 2 diabetes in African American populations, are to actually promote the well-being of the population. In Chapter Six, Geronimus and Thompson go another step, insisting that researchers and policymakers must also consider health problems as political and cultural problems that must be addressed in ways well beyond the scope of public health interventions, even sensitive ones.

Several chapters, including Chapters Two, Five, and Eight, illustrate how traditional researcher-community barriers to collaboration (e.g., mistrust, researchers benefiting at the expense of communities, lack of financial ability for community participation) have been overcome over time often through the experience of calling attention to problems as they emerged and then developing processes to solve them. One possible lesson is that researchers may benefit from developing conflict-resolution processes before problems emerge. Developing processes that create a level playing field for all participants can help to build trust. If community residents feel that university researchers dominate the problem-solving processes, they are more likely to mistrust the outcome.

A second very practical challenge arises in trying to develop a work plan that integrates the needs of researchers to control the research process to assure fidelity to the question to be answered and validity and reliability of the data while meeting the needs of and working with the daily life demands of research participants and other community partners. In practice, this can be a formidable problem, and researchers rarely describe in adequate detail how they address this situation, making it difficult to assess the limits of generalizability. Starting from a primary identity of interdisciplinary and participatory researchers, Fuqua and colleagues recount in Chapter Eight some of the problems they encountered and note some efforts that they made to overcome them.

In Chapter Two, Angotti and Sze explain that they began more as partners in community action directed toward a perceived environmental social injustice than as independent researchers. The focus on health and the demands to become interdisciplinary emerged within these partnerships, thus reducing the tension between researchers and actors. For this kind of work to become part of the scholarly literature, the authors were required to move from the frame of collaborative action to that of analysis and representation. At that point, their engagement with the community became separate from the scholarly work. As described in Chapter Seven, Saegert and colleagues faced a serious challenge in gaining access to low- and moderate-income homeowners faced with foreclosure, especially the group they needed to understand best, those who were not seeking help from the nonprofit community-based organizations that were the formal partners of the research. They describe the multiple approaches they used to reach this population as well as their failures to reach the truly linguistically isolated.

Engaging Government and Other Institutions

Many of the applied disciplines relevant to study and intervention on urban health and social problems (public health, social work, nursing, urban planning) have a role in government as well as in other sectors—academia, profit and nonprofit community, and advocacy organizations.

At the individual level, it is not unusual for those engaged in urban health research, intervention, and policy to move between government and other sectors during the course of their careers or for those in different sectors to interact through professional organizations or coalitions. At the institutional level, all three branches of government (executive, legislative, and judicial) at all three levels (national, state, and municipal) play a potential role in urban health research, intervention, and policy. Government agencies often have unique access to individuals, institutions, and data, and they have specific authority to implement and evaluate programs and to initiate policy changes that outside researchers lack, making them very powerful potential partners. At the same time, however, government may be influenced or constrained by legal, political, and economic considerations that make them unreliable or problematic partners. To partner effectively with government, interdisciplinary researchers need to understand the strengths, boundaries, and limits of government entities as partners.

Some of the data used in the chapters of this volume were collected by government sources (e.g., on asthma hospitalizations or levels of pollutants in Chapter Five) but are limited in their utility to answer all the questions about, in this case, the causes, incidence, and prevalence of childhood asthma. In other cases, the capacity of governments to act is critical to the timeliness and success of interventions. In Chapter Nine, Hadley et al. illustrate the sorts of comparative analysis that build knowledge about what conditions must exist within government to provide useful interventions to mitigate or prevent the public health consequences of human or natural disasters. Still a third common role for government and other decision-making institutions addresses policy-related problems of the funder. In Chapter Seven, Saegert et al. briefly describe how the relationships with the advisory board of funders helped them understand the different framings of the foreclosure problem and thus the different views on desirable and successful interventions held by quasi-governmental and private sector financial institutions and low-income households threatened with foreclosure.

Linking with Social Movements

Social movements can be the wave that carries interdisciplinary researchers and their work onto the shores of policy and practice relevance. Social movements seek to frame problems, mobilize communities, get the attention of policymakers, change policies, and improve living conditions.

For interdisciplinary urban health researchers, learning how to interact effectively with social movements can make the difference between a career confined to an isolated ivory tower and one where research results inform policy and are informed by ongoing interactions with players who can make a difference. In Chapters Two and Five, the authors discuss their interactions with the environmental justice movement; in Chapter Six, Geronimus and Thompson emphasize that only broader social and political movements can address the fundamental causes of racial/ethnic health inequities in the United States; and in Chapters Ten and Eleven, the authors acknowledge the importance of, respectively, movements for immigrants' and older people's rights and the civil rights movement in creating healthier policies, environments, and services.

In the last fifty years, the civil rights movement, the labor movement, the environmental justice movement, the women's movement, the gay and lesbian movements, and many smaller health movements have each made important contributions to improved public health, and each has supported (and been supported by) a vigorous research effort.[28, 29, 30, 31, 32]

Social movement activists share some of the perspectives of interdisciplinary urban health researchers. Both often start their engagement with a concern about a problem, and their passion about the problem sustains them over time. Both consider multiple levels of organization (e.g., the women's movement slogan "the personal is political") and are comfortable with thinking and acting on more than one level at a time. Both understand the importance of including multiple voices in defining the problem and devising solutions, an interaction that leads to a better understanding of the issue as well as more active engagement in the process of change. Both focus on praxis, the act of putting knowledge into practice and moving through an ongoing cycle of conceptualizing the meanings of what can be learned from experience to reframe strategic and theoretical models. These commonalities may make it easier for movement activists and health researchers to find common ground and to devise practical strategies for working together on often controversial issues.

INFLUENCING POLICY AND PRACTICE

An important goal of interdisciplinary research is to provide the evidence base that can engage stakeholders to influence health-promoting programs, policies, and practices. Here we consider some of the strategies that interdisciplinary researchers can use to increase the impact of their research and intervention studies on policy and practice.

Policymakers

To increase the likelihood that their studies will have an impact on policy, researchers need to spend time learning what motivates policymakers. At a minimum, this requires understanding their legal mandates, political philosophies, the constituencies on whom they depend for support, the superiors to whom they report, their financial resources, their priorities, and their personal connections to and investment in the issue under investigation. Whether researchers and their partners ultimately choose more collegial or more adversarial strategies to bring their research findings into the policy arenas, they will still need this detailed contextualized knowledge about the relevant policymakers.

One way to learn what moves policymakers is to talk to these officials, as the authors of Chapters Five, Seven, Eight, Nine, and Ten suggest. However, it will not always be possible for researchers to gain access to the relevant policymakers, so other approaches are also needed.

Some research teams include government officials, who can more easily reach other people in government than outsiders. Others, such as the group studying urban food systems described in Chapter Three by Zenk and her colleagues, include knowledgeable community residents who understand some of this policy context based on a lifetime of living in a community.

Considering how best to bring evidence to bear on changing policy is a question to consider early in the research process, not the night before the press release on findings is released. Some policymakers appear to be more moved by anecdotes and personal stories than by quantitative evidence. This provides another argument for using mixed methods of data collection to produce a variety of types of evidence to bring into the policy arena.

In some circumstances, researchers may participate in the process of monitoring policy implementation, a critical task where researchers may have relevant skills. This may include assessing policy or program implementation fidelity, providing evidence to negotiate changes in policy based on new findings, or serving as expert witnesses or court masters in legal cases, court reversals, and other slippages. Researchers often step out of the process once policy is implemented, a withdrawal that can jeopardize the public health impact of the policy change.

Providers and Practitioners

Health providers and other frontline professionals can also play an important role in translating research findings into practice and policy. In Chapter Eight, Fuqua and her colleagues explained that researchers invited school officials to join their consortium in part to give them evidence needed for improving school-based tobacco control policies. Hadley, Galea, and Rudenstine observed in Chapter Nine that mental health professionals can play an important role in alerting the victims of urban disaster to early symptoms and needed resources to reduce the complications of disaster-related stress. By having an ongoing dialogue with providers, researchers can design studies that can answer the questions these practitioners raise and also gain an understanding of the obstacles to successful changes in policy and practice. Moreover, practitioners have the capacity to translate findings into practice, enabling patients or clients to benefit from research findings more immediately.

Universities

Universities can also play a role in applying academic knowledge in the policy arena. Academic institutions and disciplines differ in where they draw the line between the creation of new knowledge and the advocacy and implementation of policy change. The traditional view is that university researchers produce new knowledge and others seek to translate it into policy change. In the field of urban health, however, these distinctions may be less relevant. Public health professionals seek to improve population health, not simply to study it. Some researchers feel an ethical and moral imperative to take their findings to the places where they can actually make a difference, wherever that road may lead. In this view, universities become centers of research, critical investigation, advocacy, and action.

In the field of urban health, universities can take several actions to facilitate stronger research/policy collaboration. These include joining or establishing formal and ongoing partnerships with public agencies, communities, and nonprofit organizations;

developing exchanges where faculty and students as well as policymakers can move between these settings through internships, sabbatical programs, or other arrangements; and inviting policymakers to teach or advise research teams. In many cases, the trust and goodwill developed in one collaborative venture can provide a starting point for subsequent efforts on other topics.

Finally, universities can encourage faculty researchers to engage in interdisciplinary and policy research and to cross the research/advocacy divide by rewarding this work through its promotion and tenure practices, pilot interdisciplinary research grant programs, and the creation of academic spaces for interdisciplinary discussions and research.

EVALUATING IMPACT

The final stage in the cycle for interdisciplinary work shown in Figure 12.1 is evaluating the impact of the changes that the research or intervention stimulated. This assessment can take place at a variety of levels, asking such questions as

- Did the research lead to new understanding of an urban health problem that suggested new directions for further research or for policy or practice?

- Did the intervention contribute to improvements in population health or to more health-promoting environments?

- Did the research lead to new theoretical frameworks, methodological approaches, or analytic strategies that offered researchers new tools or insights?

- Did the process of interdisciplinary collaboration lead to new understanding of how researchers can work together across disciplines, sectors, or institutions?

In several chapters, including Chapters Two, Five, Seven, and Eleven, the authors discuss these questions and offer lessons that their experiences suggest. The heterogeneity of their conclusions reflects both the particulars of the research problems and studies they describe and analyze and the challenges of evaluating interdisciplinary research. In a recent review, Klein enumerated some of the unique issues in evaluating interdisciplinary health research.[33] These included the variability of research goals; the variability of criteria and indicators for quality of research; the necessity of integrating organizational, methodological, and epistemological components of a project; the interaction of social and cognitive factors in collaboration; the challenges of management and coaching an interdisciplinary team; the development of transparent processes for iteration of models, theories, and findings; and the development of flexible but consistent measures of impact and effectiveness that consider both intended and unintended outcomes.

Lest readers become overwhelmed by this daunting list of challenges, it is also true that for the most part evaluators of interdisciplinary research projects or processes face the same scientific and logistical problems that evaluators of other types of interventions face. These include assuring validity, reliability, and generalizability while at the same time acknowledging the importance of context. Several recent reviews provide an overview of these issues.[34, 35, 36, 37]

Some approaches to evaluation may be particularly suitable to interdisciplinary health research. These include portfolio evaluation, in which researchers assess a variety of interventions designed to reduce a problem;[38] health impact assessment, which examines retrospectively or prospectively the health consequences of health and non-health policies and programs;[39] and goal-free evaluation, which allows investigators to consider unintended as well as intended effects.[40] Future work on interdisciplinary health research should carefully examine the value and costs of these emerging approaches to evaluation.

Finally, the results of evaluation studies provide feedback to all the stakeholders involved in the problem under study, providing an opportunity to redefine the problem based on new understanding or changing contexts. This final step begins the cycle again, emphasizing the dynamic and iterative dimensions of interdisciplinary urban health research.

WANTED: INTERDISCIPLINARY RESEARCHERS AND PRACTITIONERS

In our view, more interdisciplinary approaches to public health research and practice hold great promise for better understanding and reducing the complex health problems that face people living in cities. Both neophyte and experienced researchers and students entering the fields that contribute to healthier urban populations will enhance their potential to make contributions if they develop the capacity to use interdisciplinary methods, concepts, and frameworks. In our work as teachers, researchers, and advocates, we are frequently asked, "So how do I become an interdisciplinary researcher? What can I do now to develop my skills and competencies?" We close this volume by offering some suggestions.

First, we encourage aspiring researchers to practice crossing boundaries. Perhaps one defining characteristic of an interdisciplinary researcher is someone who can successfully cross multiple borders. In the previous chapters, the authors describe how they worked across a variety of divides, including institutions, service sectors, levels of social organization, roles, translational stages, and disciplines. Just as the White Queen urged Alice in Wonderland to practice imagining impossible things, we urge readers to practice looking at the problems they study from across one or more borders. Questions that might stimulate such thinking include

- What would this problem look like if I viewed it from another discipline, say, as an epidemiologist rather than as a sociologist or as an urban planner rather than as an anthropologist?

- How would I approach this problem from another role, say, as a community activist or a city official rather than as a health researcher?

- How would I approach it if I were based at a different type of institution, say, a hospital rather than a university or a community organization rather than a health department?

- What if I worked in a different sector, say, housing or education or environmental protection rather than public health? What might look different to me from that perspective?

- What new understanding would I gain from focusing on a different level of organization? For example, what would I gain if I considered the biological pathways that contributed to overeating as well as the food industry practices that have been associated with obesity?

The White Queen encouraged Alice to develop her skills by imagining six impossible things before breakfast. By engaging in similar thought exercises, interdisciplinary aspirants can strengthen their capacity to think and act across the boundaries that often constrain them.

Second, researchers and practitioners would benefit from some study of the methods and theories of another discipline. This need not require earning another graduate degree in another discipline but simply some systematic introduction to the history, theories, and methods of a second discipline. By having a point of comparison, researchers gain insights into the limitations—and strengths—of their own discipline. The goal is not for sociologists to become epidemiologists but rather to understand more deeply and specifically that the world looks different through other disciplinary eyes.

Another way to achieve this goal is to bring together researchers and students from different disciplines to consider a single problem from different perspectives. At City University of New York, for example, we have offered a doctoral level course on interdisciplinary research in urban health that examines the concept of health equity and health disparities from different disciplinary perspectives.

Third, those seeking to move beyond their home discipline can read widely outside their own professional journals and books. With the proliferation of scientific journals and easy electronic access to a variety of information sources, it is hard enough to stay current with one's own discipline. But immersing oneself in a single disciplinary perspective can limit one's ability to think creatively or to consider a problem from another perspective. One obvious starting point for this wider scan is the problem of concern. Thus, nutritionists studying diabetes or political scientists investigating legislative approaches to controlling obesity can read in the medical, sociological, anthropological, and epidemiological literatures to expand their understanding of the problem and the methods used to study and intervene.

Fourth, readers are encouraged to seek placements in interdisciplinary research teams. The best preparation for doing interdisciplinary research is doing it. By completing field placements, fellowships, sabbaticals, or other temporary assignments within existing teams, participants gain the experience and skills of working across disciplines. Several fellowship programs, including those sponsored by the Kellogg Foundation, the Robert Wood Johnson Foundation, and several National Institutes of

Health initiatives, provide support for these placements. Finding a mentor on this team who is experienced in interdisciplinary work or, better yet, finding a few mentors who are trained in different disciplines allows aspiring investigators to analyze their experiences as they live them.

Finally, we encourage students, researchers, and practitioners who want to move toward more interdisciplinary approaches to start that process today. In this book, we have shown that disciplinary/interdisciplinary is not a polarity but rather a continuum. Everyone who is working to improve the health of urban populations can take some steps on that continuum. Perhaps it means inviting someone from another discipline to the next team meeting or expanding an advisory board to include more diverse roles or considering interventions at other levels of organization, even if others will be assigned implementation responsibilities. By taking small steps to move from more disciplinary to more interdisciplinary and assessing the success of these steps as they are carried out, we may be able to create momentum for a more transformative change. Ultimately, these small steps can lead to a "tipping point" where the disciplinary eventually becomes truly interdisciplinary.

The chapters in this book show that it is possible for researchers, practitioners, community residents, public officials, and others to design, implement, and evaluate interdisciplinary studies and interventions that can improve the health of urban populations. We hope readers will join us in this quest.

SUMMARY

In this chapter, we considered the central themes that run through this volume. Our focus is on *doing* interdisciplinary research and practice in urban health. We seek to help readers move from an appreciation of interdisciplinary research to a capacity to do it—to apply the principles, concepts, and skills described in the previous chapters and developed elsewhere in recent years to their roles as urban health professionals and researchers. We examined what we have learned about the practical application of the approaches, methods, and frameworks the authors of previous chapters have described and how our readers can apply these lessons in the settings in which they work. We described several stages of interdisciplinary work—defining the problem, creating and implementing a research process, choosing partners, influencing policy and practice, and evaluating impact—and discussed the key tasks and challenges in each stage. We conclude by urging readers concerned with improving the health of urban populations to begin the process of moving from more disciplinary to more interdisciplinary research and practice.

DISCUSSION QUESTIONS

1. Choose a specific urban health problem that concerns you. What are the advantages and disadvantages of using unidisciplinary versus interdisciplinary approaches to addressing this problem?

2. How did the authors of Chapters Two, Seven, and Eight frame the problems they were studying, and how did these decisions affect how they moved through the various stages of research described in this chapter?

3. Use the stages of interdisciplinary research shown in Figure 12.1 to design an intervention to reduce type 2 diabetes in an African American urban neighborhood. What information would you need to guide this process?

4. How will you use interdisciplinary approaches to urban health research and intervention in your professional career? What obstacles might you encounter in using these methods and how might you overcome them?

NOTES

1. Kessel, F., Rosenfield, P. L., and Anderson, N. B., eds. *Expanding the Boundaries of Health and Social Science: Case Studies in Innovation.* New York: Oxford University Press, 2003.

2. Committee on Facilitating Interdisciplinary Research. *Facilitating Interdisciplinary Research.* Washington, D.C.: National Academies Press, 2005.

3. Kessel, F., and Rosenfield, P. L. Toward transdisciplinary research: Historical and contemporary perspectives. *American Journal of Preventative Medicine,* 35, no. 2, Suppl (August 2008): S225–234.

4. Hirsh-Hadorn, G., Hoffman-Riem, H., Biber-Klemm, S., et al., eds. *Handbook of Transdisciplinary Research.* Springer, 2008.

5. Higginbotham, N., Briceno-Leon, R., and Johnson, N. Africa. In *Applying Health Social Science: Best Practice in the Developing World,* pp. 99–100. London: Zed, 2001.

6. Higginbotham, N., Briceno-Leon, R., and Johnson, N. Latin America. In *Applying Health Social Science: Best Practice in the Developing World,* pp. 183–184. London: Zed, 2001.

7. Higginbotham, N., Briceno-Leon, R., and Johnson, N. Asia and the Pacific. In *Applying Health Social Science: Best Practice in the Developing World,* pp. 15–16. London: Zed, 2001.

8. Rutter, M., and Plomin, R. Pathways from science findings to health benefits. *Psychological Medicine* (2008): 1–14.

9. Dorfman, L., Wallack, L., and Woodruff, K. More than a message: Framing public health advocacy to change corporate practices. *Health Education & Behavior,* 32, no. 3 (2005): 320–336.

10. Entman, R. Framing: Toward a clarification of a fractured paradigm. *Journal of Communication,* 43, no. 4 (1993): 53–57.

11. Narayan, K. M., Boyle, J. P., Thompson, T. J., Sorensen, S. W., and Williamson, D. F. Lifetime risk for diabetes mellitus in the United States. *JAMA,* 290, no. 14 (2003): 1884–1890.

12. Horowitz, C. R., Colson, K. A., Hebert, P. L., and Lancaster, K. Barriers to buying healthy foods for people with diabetes: Evidence of environmental disparities. *American Journal of Public Health,* 94, no. 9 (2004): 1549–1554.

13. Brownson, R. C., Haire-Joshu, D., and Luke, D. A. Shaping the context of health: A review of environmental and policy approaches in the prevention of chronic diseases. *Annual Review of Public Health,* 27 (2006): 341–370.

14. Haire-Joshu, D., and Fleming, C. An ecological approach to understanding contributions to disparities in diabetes prevention and care. *Current Diabetes Reports,* 6, no. 2 (April 2006): 123–129.

15. Saegert, S., and Evans, G. Poverty, housing niches, and health in the United States. *Journal of Social Issues,* 59 (2003): 569–589.

16. Galea, S., Freudenberg, N., and Vlahov, D. Cities and population health. *Social Science & Medicine,* 60, no. 5 (March 2005): 1017–1033.

17. Green, L. W. Public health asks of system science: To advance our evidence-based practice, can you help us get more practice-based evidence? *American Journal of Public Health,* 96 (2006): 403–405.

18. Leischow, S. J., Best, A., Trochim, W. M., Clark, P. I., Gallagher, R. S., Marcus, S. E., and Matthews, E. Systems thinking to improve public health. *American Journal of Preventative Medicine,* 35, no. 2S (2008): S196–S203.

19. Trochim, W. M., Cabrera, D. A., Milstein, B., Gallagher, R. S., and Leischow, S. J. Practical challenges of systems thinking and modeling in public health. *American Journal of Public Health,* 96, no. 3 (2006): 538–546.

20. Freudenberg, N. Jails, prisons and the health of urban populations: Review of the impact of the correctional system on community health. *Journal of Urban Health,* 78 (2001): 214–240.

21. Freudenberg, N., Daniels, J., Crum, M., Perkins, T., and Richie, B. E. Coming home from jail: The social and health consequences of community reentry for women, male adolescents, and their families and communities. *American Journal of Public Health,* 95 (2005): 1725–1736.

22. Stokols, D., Hall, K. L., Taylor, B. K., and Moser, R. P. The science of team science: Overview of the field and introduction to the supplement. *American Journal of Preventative Medicine,* 35, no. 2S (2008): S77–S89.

23. Metzler, M. M., Higgins, D. L., Beeker, C. G., Freudenberg, N., et al. Addressing urban health in Detroit, New York City, and Seattle through community-based

participatory research partnerships. *American Journal of Public Health,* 93, no. 5 (2003): 803–811.

24. Israel, B. A., Eng, E., Schulz, A. J., and Parker, E. A., eds. *Methods in Community-Based Participatory Research for Health.* San Francisco: Jossey-Bass, 2005.

25. Minkler, M., and Wallerstein, N., eds. *Community-Based Participatory Research for Health.* San Francisco: Jossey Bass, 2003.

26. Klein, J. T. *Interdisciplinarity: History, Theory and Practice.* Detroit, Mich.: Wayne State University Press, 1990.

27. Freudenberg, N., and Klitzman, S. Teaching urban health. In S. Galea and D. Vlahov, eds., *Handbook of Urban Health,* pp. 521–538. New York: Springer Verlag, 2005.

28. Piven, F. F., and Cloward, R. A. *Poor People's Movements: Why They Succeed, How They Fail.* New York: Vintage, 1979.

29. Nathanson, C. A. Social movements as catalysts for policy change: The case of smoking and guns. *Journal of Health Politics, Policy and Law,* 24, no. 3 (1999): 421–488.

30. Brown, P., Zavestoski, S., McCormick, S., Mayer, B., Morello-Frosch, R., and Gasior Altman, R. Embodied health movements: New approaches to social movements in health. *Social Health and Illness,* 26, no. 1 (2004): 50–80.

31. Keefe, R. H., Lane, S. D., and Swarts, H. J. From the bottom up: Tracing the impact of four health-based social movements on health and social policies. *Journal of Health & Social Policy,* 21, no. 3 (2006): 55–69.

32. Brown, P., and Zavestoski, S., eds., *Social Movements in Health.* San Francisco: Wiley-Blackwell, 2005.

33. Klein, J. T. Evaluation of interdisciplinary and transdisciplinary research: A literature review. *American Journal of Prev Med,* 35, no. 2, Suppl (2008): S116–123.

34. Butterfoss, F. D. Process evaluation for community participation. *Annual Review of Public Health,* 27 (2006): 323–340.

35. Evans, D. B, Adam, T., Edejer, T. T., Lim, S. S., Cassels, A., and Evans, T. G. WHO: Choosing Interventions That Are Cost Effective (CHOICE) millennium development goals team. Time to reassess strategies for improving health in developing countries. *British Medical Journal,* 331, no. 7525 (2005): 1133–1136.

36. Jackson, N., and Waters, E. Guidelines for systematic reviews in health promotion and public health taskforce. Criteria for the systematic review of health promotion and public health interventions. *Health Promotion International,* 20, no. 4 (2005): 367–374.

37. Ogilvie, D., Egan, M., Hamilton, V., and Petticrew, M. Systematic reviews of health effects of social interventions: 2. Best available evidence: How low should you go? *Journal of Epidemiology and Community Health,* 59, no. 10 (2005): 886–892.

38. Sendi, P., Al, M. J., Gafni, A., and Birch, S. Portfolio theory and the alternative decision rule of cost effectiveness analysis: Theoretical and practical considerations. *Social Science & Medicine,* 58 (2004): 1853–1855.

39. Cole, B. L., and Fielding, J. E. Health impact assessment: A tool to help policy makers understand health beyond health care. *Annual Review of Public Health* (2007): 393–412.

40. Scriven, M. Prose and cons about goal-free evaluation. *American Journal of Evaluation,* 12, no. 1 (1991): 55–62.

GLOSSARY

In this glossary, we define some of the key concepts and terms that are used in this book. Because the book is intended for students and researchers of different disciplines, we have included terms that are basic in some fields but may be unfamiliar to those in other disciplines. Interested readers should consult the endnotes at the end of this section for a more detailed discussion of these terms. Words in italics within definitions are also defined separately.

Action research (or **participatory action research**) is a form of research that seeks to engage researchers and participants in a collective process of reflection, data collection, analysis, and action for the purposes of increasing understanding and improving upon research practices and, in the case of public health, promoting participants' health and reducing disparities and disease.[1]

Advocacy is the application of information and resources to promote institutional, community, and policy changes. Public health advocacy is advocacy that is intended to change policies or practices that influence the occurrence or severity of health problems among groups of people.[2]

Allostatic load refers to the cumulative wear and tear on the body's systems owing to repeated adaptation to stressors.[3, 4]

Analytic strategies describe various approaches to analyzing data. Examples include logistic regression, stratification, and searching for recurrent themes in interview transcripts. *Research methods* usually refer to approaches to collecting data, whereas analytic strategies are used to organize and interpret these data.

Community-based participatory research (CBPR) is a collaborative approach to research that equitably involves all partners in the research process and recognizes the unique strengths that each brings. CBPR begins with a research topic of importance to the community with the aim of combining knowledge and action for social change to improve community health and eliminate health disparities.[5]

Conceptual models are used in research to theorize, explain, and predict complex relationships among variables of interest.[6]

Culture describes the shared characteristics of a group of people, which may include patterns of health and social behavior, beliefs, customs, traditions, artistic expression, and language.

Developmental perspective (see *Life course perspective*)

Disciplines (academic) are branches of scholarly instruction that provide a structure through which successive generations of students are trained and socialized. Faculty carry out research, teaching, and administration within these disciplines. Examples include sociology, psychology, anthropology, biology, and chemistry. Disciplines provide systematic approaches to understanding the world and uncovering new knowledge. Traditionally, disciplines have been considered separate and distinct from each other. Among the elements required for the presence of a discipline are the presence of a community of scholars, a tradition of inquiry, a mode of inquiry that defines how data are collected and interpreted, requirements for what constitutes new knowledge, and the existence of a communications network.[7]

Ecological models consider the interaction and integration of multiple influences at multiple levels of social organization (e.g., individual, interpersonal, organizational, community, and societal) in attempting to understand and improve population health.[8] According to Gebbie and colleagues, the use of ecological models in public health comes out of a recognition that the "health of individuals and the community is determined relatively little by health care per se and far more by multiple other factors, and by their interactions. These factors include biology (e.g., genetics), the social and physical environment, education, employment, and behavior (e.g., healthy behaviors such as exercise and unhealthy ones such as overeating)."[9] Ecological models also consider the way that media, economic systems, historical patterns of discrimination, public policies not related to health, and other societal factors exert influence on health and contribute to midlevel factors such as behavior, employment, and education.

Embodiment describes the biological and social processes by which living conditions and social conditions "get under our skins" and influence our health.[10]

Environment describes the complex of physical, chemical, biological, and social factors that act upon an organism or a population and ultimately determine its form and survival. It also describes the aggregate of conditions that influence the life of an individual or community

Environment, physical refers to the human-built environment as well as the air, water, plants and animals, climate, and geological conditions that influence a population.

Environment, social describes the structure and characteristics of relationships among people within a community. Components of the social environment include social networks, social capital, and social support.

Environmental justice, as defined by the U.S. Environmental Protection Agency, is "the fair treatment and meaningful involvement of all people regardless of race, color, national origin, culture, education, or income with respect to the development, implementation, and enforcement of environmental laws, regulations, and policies."[11]

Essentialism is a philosophical concept that states that certain characteristics of a group are universal and not dependent on context. It is often contrasted with *social constructionism.*

Framing is the process by which we select, emphasize, present, and communicate information in such a way as to promote a particular problem definition, causal interpretation, moral evaluation, and/or treatment recommendation.[12, 13]

Fundamental causes are root or primary explanations of a phenomenon or problem. In public health, many fundamental cause explanations focus on the primacy of social conditions as underlying causes of health inequalities. This line of inquiry comes in part from a recognition that socioeconomic gradients in nearly all health outcomes persist after adjusting for well-established individual-level risk factors.[14] The concept also calls attention to unequal distributions of resources and opportunities that put people "at risk for risk."

Geographic Information Sciences is a discipline grounded in geographic spatial analytic theory that provides the intellectual framework for *geographic information systems.*[15]

Geographic information systems (GIS) are computer applications used to store, view, analyze, and map geographic information.

Health disparities refer to gaps in the health status and quality of health care across racial (see *race*), ethnic, gender, and socioeconomic groups. The U.S. Department of Health and Human Services has defined health disparities as "population-specific differences in the presence of disease, health outcomes, or access to health care." One of the stated goals of Healthy People 2010 is the elimination of health disparities in the United States by 2010.[16]

Health equity describes the goal of reducing disparities in health or, in other words, achieving equity in health among different population groups.

Health promotion is defined by the World Health Organization as the process of enabling people to increase control over, and to improve, their health.[17] In the United States, health promotion is often defined more narrowly as "the science and art of helping people change their lifestyle to move toward a state of optimal health."[18]

Interdisciplinary research has been defined by the National Academy of Sciences as "a mode of research by teams or individuals that integrates information, data, techniques, tools, perspectives, concepts, and/or theories from two or more disciplines or bodies of specialized knowledge to advance fundamental understanding or to solve problems whose solutions are beyond the scope of a single discipline or field of research practice."[19]

Levels (of analysis) describe a hierarchical system of considering the influence of different levels of organization on health. Anderson identified five major levels of analysis in health research: social/environmental, behavioral/psychological, organ systems, cellular, and molecular. A variety of conceptual models exist to address the linkages among these levels.[20]

Levels (of social organization) relate to the classification of forms of social organization ranging from the smallest simplest unit to the largest and most complex. Although there are various typologies or classification systems, those used in public health research and practice generally include the individual, interpersonal, organizational, community, national, and global levels.

Life course perspective refers to how health status at specific ages reflects not only contemporary conditions but the embodiment of prior living circumstances, in utero onward, and their biological and social trajectories over time.[21]

Methods (research methods) are systematic approaches to collecting data to answer a research question. Research methods usually refer to strategies for collecting data, whereas *analytic strategies* are used to organize and interpret these data.

Multidisciplinary research is defined by the National Academy of Sciences as research that involves more than a single discipline in which each discipline makes a separate contribution.[19]

Multilevel analysis refers to statistical methodologies that analyze outcomes simultaneously in relation to determinants measured at different levels such as individual, workplace, neighborhood, nation, or geographic region. If conducted properly, these analyses can potentially assess whether individuals' health is shaped by not only "individual" or "household" characteristics but also "population" or "area" characteristics.[19]

Multisectoral initiatives are those that work in more than one sector (e.g., education, health care, or the environment). Intersectoral is another term used to describe such initiatives.[22]

Participatory action research (see *Action research*)

Policy is a guide to action to change that would not otherwise occur, a decision about amounts and allocations of resources: the overall amount is a statement of commitment to certain areas of concern; the distribution of the amount shows the priorities of decision makers. Policy sets priorities and guides resource allocation.[23] Public policies are promulgated and enforced by governments, public health policy influences the health of populations, and health care policy sets the standards for delivery and financing of health care as well as preventive health measures.

Population health describes the well-being of a defined group of people. It has also been defined as "the health outcomes of a group of individuals, including the distribution of such outcomes within the group."[24]

Practice or public health practice refers to the activities undertaken by public health professionals to promote and protect the health of the public. The term is sometimes used to differentiate these activities from *research activities* that are designed to generate new knowledge. In fact, these two types of activities often overlap.[25]

Professional or public health professional or practitioner refers to an individual with graduate training in public health who follows professional standards and guidelines to promote health and prevent disease.

Proximate causes in public health refer to immediate and often individual-level behaviors, exposures, or other conditions that directly impact health. For example, behaviors such as cigarette smoking, inactivity, and a high-fat diet explain a substantial amount of the world's experience with atherosclerosis.[26] Proximate causes are frequently described as occurring "downstream" along the causal chain of influences that impact upon health, with broader social conditions being conceptualized as "upstream" or "fundamental" influences.[27]

Public health has been defined by the Institute of Medicine as "what we as a society do to collectively assure the conditions in which people can be healthy."[28]

Race is often used as a category for individuals based on their physical features such as skin color and hair texture, which reflect ancestry and geographic origins, as identified by others or as self-identified. More recently, researchers have emphasized the social factors that create and perpetuate racial categories. Some use race as a synonym for ethnicity or use the hybrid term race/ethnicity and include characteristics such as common social and political heritages.[29]

Racism (or institutional racism) describes the belief that some races are superior to others. This ideology is used to justify individual and collective actions that impose and maintain inequality among racial and ethnic groups.[29]

Research is defined by the federal government as a "systematic investigation, including research development, testing, and evaluation, designed to develop or contribute to generalizable knowledge."[30]

Research collaborative describes a team of researchers, often interdisciplinary, who work together across departments, disciplines, and institutions.

Risk factors describe individual- or population-level characteristics that are associated with higher risks of specified health conditions.

Social capital, a term with diverse meanings, has been variously described as the resources to which people have access through their social relationships, the mutual respect and trust among citizens or between citizens and the state, and the connections between people and institutions. Although researchers debate its precise meaning, many agree that social capital has an influence on health and health inequities.[31]

Social construction is a philosophical and sociological position that holds that social—or health—problems are "invented" or "constructed" by the people in a particular place and time. The meaning assigned to such problems therefore depends on the particular social context. The term is often contrasted with *essentialism.*

Social justice describes the goal of changing living conditions, policies, and social arrangements that expose some groups to unhealthier social environments than others. With social justice, the goal is often to bring about change through means that give disadvantaged sectors of the population an equal voice in making political decisions.

Social networks are "the relationships that exist between groups of individuals or agencies, and the resources to which membership of such groups facilitates access."[32] An individual's connections to social networks and the characteristics of the social networks within a population influence health.

Socioeconomic status (SES) describes the position of an individual or population within a hierarchy of social and economic arrangements. Common indicators of socioeconomic status are income, education, and occupation. Socioeconomic status is a powerful influence on individual and population health.

Stress is the biological response of an individual to *stressors.* This response is marked by an increase in adrenaline production as well as immunologic and other biological changes.[33] Long-term exposure to stress is believed to contribute to a variety of health problems, and some investigators propose that exposure to stress is the biological pathway by which socioeconomic status influences health.

Stressors are social, environmental, or psychological conditions that elicit a stress response from an organism or population. Stressors can be chronic or acute.

Systems thinking is a conceptual orientation that considers the interrelationships among parts and their relationship to the whole. Systems modeling is a methodological approach that involves the use of formal models or simulations to increase understanding of complex systems and improve the effectiveness of our actions within them.[34, 35] Public health professionals often use systems thinking to understand the complex influences on a health condition and to plan comprehensive responses.

Team science describes scientific endeavors that bring together groups of researchers from different disciplines, institutions, and methodological approaches to study a problem in a more holistic or comprehensive way.[36]

Theory can be defined as "logically related propositions that aim to explain and predict a fairly general set of phenomena. Theories allow for a systematization of knowledge, explanation, and prediction, as well as generating new research hypotheses."[37] Theories provide a guide for designing research and intervention studies, and they are verified, expanded, or rejected as a result of research.

Transdisciplinary research is an integrative process in which researchers work jointly to create a common conceptual framework that synthesizes and extends discipline-specific theories, concepts, methods to create new models, and language to address a common research problem.[36]

Urban health is a field of inquiry that studies the impact of city living on health and the strategies that can improve the health of urban populations.[38]

NOTES

1. Minkler, M., and Wallerstein, N., eds. *Community-Based Participatory Research for Health.* San Francisco: Jossey-Bass, 2003, p. 5.

2. Christoffel, K. Public health advocacy: Process and product. *American Journal of Public Health,* 90 (2000): 722–726.

3. McEwen, B. S. Protective and damaging effects of stress mediators. *New England Journal of Medicine,* 338 (1998): 171–179.

4. Steptoe, A., Feldman, P. J., Kunz, S., Owen, N., Willemsen. G., and Marmot, M. Stress responsivity and socioeconomic status: A mechanism for increased cardiovascular disease risk? *European Heart Journal,* 23 (2002): 1757–1763.

5. Israel, B. A., Schulz, A. J., Parker, E. A., and Becker, A. B. Review of community-based research: Assessing partnership approaches to improve public health. *Annual Review of Public Health,* 19 (1998): 173–202.

6. Botha, M. E. Theory development in perspective: The role of conceptual frameworks and models in theory development. *Journal of Advanced Nursing,* 14, no. 1 (1989): 49–55.

7. Beyer, J. M., and Lodahl, T. M. A comparative study of patterns of influence in United States and English universities. *Administrative Science Quarterly,* 21 (1976): 104–129.

8. Stokols, D. Translating social ecological theory into guidelines for community health promotion. *American Journal of Health Promotion,* 10, no. 4 (1996): 282–298.

9. Gebbie, K., Rosenstock, L., and Hernandez, L. M., eds. *Who Will Keep the Public Healthy? Educating Public Health Professionals for the 21st Century,* p. 168. Washington, D.C.: National Academies Press, 2003.

10. Krieger, N. Embodiment: A conceptual glossary for epidemiology. *Journal of Epidemiology and Community Health,* 59, no. 5 (2005): 350–355.

11. U.S. Environmental Protection Agency. Frequently asked questions: How does EPA define environmental justice? Available at www.epa.gov/compliance/resources/faqs/ej/#faq2. Accessed October 21, 2008.

12. Entman, R. M. Framing: Toward clarification of a fractured paradigm. *Journal of Communication,* 43, no. 4 (1993): 51–58.

13. Gitlin, T. *The Whole World Is Watching: Mass Media in the Making and Unmaking of the New Left.* Berkeley: University of California Press, 1980.

14. Link, B., and Phelan, J. Social conditions as fundamental causes of disease. *Journal of Health and Social Behavior,* 36, Extra issue (1995): 80–94.

15. McLafferty, S. L. GIS and health care. *Annual Review of Public Health,* 24 (2003): 25–42.

16. U.S. Department of Health and Human Services, *Healthy People 2010: National Health Promotion and Disease Prevention Objectives,* conference ed. Washington, D.C.: U.S. Department of Health and Human Services, 2000.

17. World Health Organization. *Ottawa charter for health promotion.* Available at www.who.int/hpr/NPH/docs/ottawa_charter_hp.pdf. Published 1986. Accessed October 29, 2008.

18. O'Donnell, M. Definition of health promotion: Part III: Expanding the definition. *American Journal of Health Promotion,* 3 (1989): 5.

19. Committee on Facilitating Interdisciplinary Research, Commitee on Science, Engineering, and Public Policy, National Academy of Sciences, National Academy of Engineering, and the Institute of Medicine of the National Academies. *Facilitating Interdisciplinary Research.* Washington, D.C.: National Academies Press, 2005.

20. Anderson, N. B. Levels of analysis in health science: A framework for integrating sociobehavioral and bio-medical research. *Annals of the New York Academy of Sciences,* 840 (1989): 563–576.

21. Krieger, N. A glossary for social epidemiology. *Epidemiology Bulletin,* 23, no. 1 (2002): 7–11.

22. Armstrong, R., Doyle, J., Lamb, C., and Waters, E. Multi-sectoral health promotion and public health: The role of evidence. *Journal of Public Health,* 28, no. 2 (2006): 168–172.

23. Milio, N. Glossary: Healthy public policy. *Journal of Epidemiology and Community Health,* 55 (2001): 622–623.

24. Kindig, D., and Stoddart, G. What is population health? *American Journal of Public Health,* 93, no. 3 (2003): 380–383.

25. Hodge, J. G., Gostin, L. O., and the Council of State and Territorial Epidemiologists. *Public health practice vs. research: A report for public health practitioners.* Available at www.cste.org/pdffiles/newpdffiles/CSTEPHR esRptHodgeFinal.5.24.04.pdf. Accessed October 25, 2008.

26. Beaglehole, R., and Magnus, P. The search for new risk factors for coronary heart disease: Occupational ther-apy for epidemiologists? *International Journal of Epidemiology,* 31, no. 6 (2002): 1117–1122.

27. Kaplan, G. A. Where do shared pathways lead? Some reflections on a research agenda. *Psychosomatic Medicine,* 57, no. 3 (1995): 208–212.

28. Institute of Medicine. *The Future of Public Health.* Washington, D.C.: National Academies Press, 1988.

29. Bhopal, R. Glossary of terms relating to ethnicity and race: For reflection and debate. *Journal of Epidemiology and Community Health,* 58, no. 6 (2004): 441–445.

30. Definitions: Protection of human subjects—federal policy for the protection of human subjects. 45 CFR §46.102 (1991).

31. Moore, S., Haines, V., Hawe, P., and Shiell, A. Lost in translation: A genealogy of the "social capital" concept in public health. *Journal of Epidemiology and Community Health,* 60, no. 8 (2006): 729–734.

32. Hawe, P., Webster, C., and Shiell, A. A glossary of terms for navigating the field of social network analysis. *Journal of Epidemiology and Community Health,* 58, no. 12 (2004): 971–975.

33. Selye, H. *The Stress of Life.* New York: McGraw-Hill, 1956.

34. Trochim, W. M., Cabrera, D. A., Milstein, B., Gallagher, R. S., and Leischow, S. J. Practical challenges of sys-tems thinking and modeling in public health. *American Journal of Public Health,* 96, no. 3 (2006): 538–546.

35. Leischow, S. J., Best, A., Trochim, W. M., et al. Systems thinking to improve the public's health. *American Journal of Preventative Medicine,* 35, no. 2, Suppl (2008): S196–S203.

36. Stokols, D., Hall, K. L., Taylor, B. K., and Moser, R. P. The science of team science: Overview of the field. *American Journal of Preventative Medicine,* 35, no. 2S (2008): S77–S89.

37. Carpiano, R. M., and Daley, D. M. A guide and glossary on post-positivist theory building for population health. *Journal of Epidemiology and Community Health,* 60, no. 7 (2006): 564–570.

38. Galea, S., Freudenberg, N., and Vlahov, D. Cities and population health. *Social Science & Medicine,* 60, no. 5 (2005): 1017–1033.

INDEX

Page references followed by *fig* indicate an illustrated diagram; followed by *t* indicate a table.

A

Action research: early call for, 186–187; transdisciplinary (TD) form of, 186–211
Adolescents: developmentalism model on unwed mothers, 140–141; developmentalism on health problems of Black, 131–135
African American communities: building toward public policy reform for, 144–148; health disparities in, 128–131; low ratio of primary care physicians in, 277; postdisaster vulnerabilities of, 225–226, 228–229; retail food environments implications for health in, 47–56. *See also* Communities of color
African American health disparities: American creed as fueling, 132, 136–137, 147–148; developmentalism ideology explanation on, 131–135, 140–142; economism ideology explanation on, 132, 134–136; implications for public policy, 138–144; movement for reform of public policies on, 144–148; weathering process leading to, 137–138
African Americans: "John Henryism" predisposition among, 136–137; mortality rates of, 128–130 *fig;* postdisaster vulnerability of, 225; type 2 diabetes among, 272–286. *See also* Black middle class; Racial/ethnic differences
Agency for Healthcare Research Quality, CBPR defined by, 95
Aging: conceptual framework for urban, 254–255 *fig;* conditions for healthy urban, 254 *fig;* economic and social influences on health policies related to, 242–245; as process of weathering, 137–138; productive, 245; social and environmental considerations related to, 246–254. *See also* Elderly population; Healthy aging
Aging Nation: The Economics and Politics of Growing Older in America (Schulz and Binstock), 242
Air pollution: Bronx minority population and sources of, 100 *fig;* Bronx (New York) health disparities related to, 94–119; Bronx pollution proximity buffers, 106–109, 107 *fig,* 108 *fig;* specific pollutants of, 106

Alameda County Study, 249
Albert Einstein College of Medicine (AECOM), 100, 101, 118
Allostatic load, 138
American creed ideology: African American health problems interpreted by, 136–137; description of, 132; intolerance fueled by, 147–148
American Planning Association, 25
Angloa humanitarian crisis, 223–224, 229
Angotti, Tom, 33–34
Asian Immigrant Workers Advocates, 36
Asian Pacific Environmental Network (APEN) case study: environmental health and housing focus of, 34–37; introduction to, 21
Asthma: Bronx (New York) health disparities related to air pollution and, 94–119; cases by zip code (NYC), 29 *fig;* OWN's solid waste plan to reduce, 29–34
Asthma hospitalizations: Bronx pollution proximity buffers and, 108 *fig;* five-year Bronx hospitalization rates (1995–1999) in, 99, 104 *fig;* Standardized Incidence Ratio (SIR) on Bronx, 111

B

Baby boomers: aging of the, 240 *fig;* conceptual framework for successful aging by urban, 254 *fig*–255 *fig;* economic and social influences on health policy and aging of, 242–245; public health research and policy agenda for, 255–258; social and environmental considerations for aging immigrants and, 246–254
Baer, Hans, 277
Balkans humanitarian crisis, 223–224, 229
Bautista, Eddie, 32–33
Bay Area Environmental Health collaborative, 28
Behavior. *See* Health-related behavior
Behavioral Risk Factor Surveillance System (BRFSS), 248
Black middle class: economism on, 135–136; health disparities between white and, 136. *See also* African Americans

"Blaming the victim," 131

Bloomberg, Michael, 32

Bronfenbrenner's bioecological model: context of, 68 *fig;* description of, 65; PPCT (process-person-context-time) dimensions of, 65–66 *fig,* 67

Bronx (New York): asthma hospitalization cases (in and out of buffers), 108 *fig;* environmental hazards and pollutants in, 105–106; five-year average asthma hospitalization rates (1995–1999) in, 99, 104 *fig;* major stationary sources of air pollution/minority population in, 100 *fig;* pollution proximity buffers in, 106–109, 107 *fig;* role of asthma and air pollution in health disparities in, 98–99; Standardized Incidence Ratio (SIR) on asthma hospitalization in, 111. *See also* South Bronx Environmental Justice Partnership (SBEJP) study

Built environment: definition of, 24; physical determinism applications to, 24–26

C

Cadastral-based Expert Dasymetric System (CEDS) model, 109

California Air Resources Board, 28

California Environmental Protection Agency (Cal/EPA), 36

Center for Human Environments (City University of New York), 166

Center for Spatially Integrated Social Science (CSISS), 49

Centers for Disease Control and Prevention, 272

Centers for Excellence in Cancer Communications and Research (CECCR), 188

Centers for Population Health and Health Disparities (CPHHD), 188

Chang, Vivian, 35, 36

Children: asthma and NYC hospitalization of, 99; developmentalism on health problems of Black, 131–135; mother's health correspondence to well-being of, 141–142

Children's health: agenda for future research and practice, 78–80; agenda for future research on, 78–80; exosystem factors of, 68 *fig,* 72–73; factors operating across systems, 74–76; influences on urban context of, 68–76; macrosystem factors of, 68 *fig*–72; mesosystem factors of, 68 *fig,* 73; microsystem factors of, 68 *fig,* 73–74; mortality from preventable disease, 64; multilevel analyses of, 76–78; multiple levels of research on, 76–78. *See also* Vulnerable population health

City University of New York (CUNY), 5, 166

Clinical Translational Science Centers (CTSC), 188

Collaborative Activities Index, 193

Collaborative conferences: applying transdisciplinary action research principles to, 192–193; UC Irvine Tobacco Policy Consortium (TPC) origin from, 186

Collaborative research: building essential social capital for, 207; community-based participatory research (CBPR) as, 46–54, 95–96; conflict as inherent feature of, 190–191; factors facilitating or impeding collaboration between partners, 196–205; scientific, community problem-solving, and inter-sectional partnerships in, 186, 305; social and intellectual integration dimensions of, 191*t,* 193–196*t;* social-ecological approach as, 164–176, 218–231; study of antecedents and processes of, 208–209; transdisciplinary (TD) action research as, 186–211; understanding professional or academic jargon issue of, 205–206. *See also* Community partnerships; Interdisciplinary research (IR)

Commonwealth Fund, 175

Communities: Global Age-Friendly Cities Project (WHO) work with, 256; primary care physicians in Black vs. white, 277; South Bronx asthma study data contributions from, 116*t;* translating transdisciplinary research into interventions for, 189–196*t;* varying models of health disparities causation in, 96. *See also* Neighborhood; Urban health

Communities of color: Asian Pacific Environmental Network (APEN) case study on, 21, 34–37; environmental justice on inequalities and, 26–28; health implications of retail food environments in, 47–56; OWN/Consumers Union's solid waste plan for NYC, 29 *fig,* 30–34; postdisaster vulnerabilities of, 225–226, 228–229. *See also* African American communities; Racial/ethnic differences

Community partnerships: building movement for policy reform through, 144–148; choosing institutional and, 305–306; conflict as inherent feature of, 190–191; Detroit retail food environment study, 47–56; engaging communities into, 306–307; factors facilitating or impeding collaboration among, 196–205; scientific, community problem-solving, and intersectional, 186, 305; social and intellectual integration among, 191*t,* 193–196*t;* South Bronx Environmental Justice Partnership (SBEJP), 98–119; transdisciplinary (TD) action research use of, 186–211; UC Irvine Tobacco Policy Consortium (TPC) study, 186, 189–211. *See also* Collaborative research; Government/institutional partnerships; Interdisciplinary research (IR)

Community planning: environmental justice activism role in, 20–21; New Urbanists approach to, 25

Community-based participatory research (CBPR): advantages and rationale for using, 95–96; definition and principles of, 95; on Detroit retail food environment and health, 46–54
Conflict between partnerships, 190–191
Critical medical anthropology, 276–278
Critical social psychology: description of, 273–274; inequality or discrimination and health approach of, 274–275; integrated with medical anthropology to reduce diabetes burden, 284–285; research approach of, 273–274. *See also* Medical anthropology
Cultural differences: Detroit retail food environment study on, 53; medical anthropology consideration of, 275–276; mismatch between local community needs and dominant culture, 143–144; related to modal age for first childbirth, 141; structuring postdisaster outcomes and, 222

D

Dahl, Robert, 132
Data collection: GIS (geographic information system) for, 50, 51–52, 96–97, 101, 102*t*–103*t*, 106–109; mortgage foreclosure crisis focus groups for, 168–173; South Bronx asthma study and community contributions to, 116*t*; UC Irvine Tobacco Policy Consortium (TPC) study schedule of, 195*t*–196*t*; U.S. Census as source of, 112, 113*t*, 129 *fig*
Depression. *See* Mental health
Detroit Community-Academic Urban Research Center, 95
Detroit retail food environment study: using CBPR to understand health implications of, 48–54; determinants of, 47–48; Detroit's economic restructuring impact on, 47–48; directions for future research based on, 54–56; race relations impact on dietary behavior, 47; retail food industry restructuring impact, 48
Developed world noninfectious diseases, 8
Developing world infectious diseases, 8
Developmentalism ideology: African American health problems interpreted by, 132–135; description of, 131–132; on unwed mothers, 140–142
Diabetes. *See* Type 2 diabetes
Dietary behaviors: cultural differences related to, 53; health relationship to, 46. *See also* Urban retail food environments
Disasters: comparing health following Angola and Balkans humanitarian, 223–224, 229; examining health consequences of, 218; health after Hurricane Katrina, 224–226, 229; health after September 11, 2001 terrorist attacks, 226–229; prevention and intervention for health consequences of, 229–231;

social-ecological determinants of health after, 218–223
Discrimination: health issues related to, 274–275; racial housing segregation as, 47. *See also* Social inequalities
Diseases: asthma, 29 *fig*–34, 94–119; dietary behaviors relationship to, 46; HIV/AIDS, 147; myth and reality of increased longevity and degenerative, 244–245; Type 2 diabetes, 49, 272–286

E

East Side Village Health Worker Partnership (ESVHWP), 48–52
Ecological models: Bronfenbrenner's bioecological approach to, 65–68 *fig;* on children's health, family, and neighborhood, 77; on children's health, family, and residential crowding, 76–77; on children's health, family, school, and neighborhood, 77–78
Economic inequalities: communities of color and, 26–28; between municipalities, 24; relationship between race and, 53
Economism: African American health problems interpreted by, 135–136; description of, 132; on socioeconomic status (SES) and health, 134–135
Elderly population: Baby boomers aging adding to the, 240 *fig;* conceptual framework for urban aging by, 254–255 *fig;* conditions for healthy aging by urban, 254 *fig;* economic and social influences on aging and health policies on, 242–245; public health research and policy agenda for, 255–258; social and environmental considerations and health of, 246–254. *See also* Aging
Environmental activism organizing, 36–37
Environmental health: connection between environmental justice and, 117; healthy aging component of, 246–247; postdisaster recovery and related, 218–231. *See also* Urban environment; Urban health
Environmental justice (EJ): Bronx asthma study examination of, 97–117; connection between environmental health and, 117; efforts to define and advance, 94; public awareness of, 22. *See also* Social justice movements
Environmental justice movement: community planning and impact of, 20–21; linking interdisciplinary research with, 308–309; public health impacted by, 22–23
Environmental justice praxis: Asian Pacific Environmental Network (APEN) case study on, 21, 34–37; definition of, 21, 26; NYC Organization of Waterfront

Environmental justice praxis (*continued*)
Neighborhoods (OWN) study as example of,
29 *fig*–34; precautionary principle of, 28; *Street Science:*
study on, 21, 27–34
Environmental Justice Project (UCD), 20
Environmental racism: NIMBY (Not in My
Backyard), 31–32, 33; public awareness of, 22.
See also Race
Environmentalism sustainability, 25
EPA. *See* U.S. Environmental Protection Agency (EPA)
Epi Info, 282
Ethnic identity: as coping mechanism, 280–281;
description and creation of, 278–279; diabetes in
context of, 279–280; health behavior and perceptions
related to, 280; spirituality relationship to, 281. *See
also* Racial/ethnic differences
Ethnography: definition of, 281; qualitative research
using, 282–283

F

Facilitating Interdisciplinary Research (National
Academies Press), 5
Families: developmentalism on health role of,
131–135; mortgage foreclosure crisis impact on,
171–173
Family Support Act (1988), 142
Federal Emergency Management Agency (FEMA),
225
Focus groups: mortgage foreclosure crisis research
using, 168–173; on-site reflection written by
facilitators of, 170
For a Better Bronx (FABB), 99–100, 105, 114, 115,
118–119
Foreclosure crisis. *See* Mortgage foreclosure crisis
Freddie Mac, 166
Fresh Kills landfill (Staten Island), 30
The Future of the Public's Health in the 21st Century
(National Academies Press), 5

G

Gilens, Martin, 136
GIS (geographic information system): Bronx asthma
study use of, 101, 102*t*–103*t*, 106–109; description
and health research use of, 96–97; Detroit's food
environment study using, 50, 51–52
Giuliani, Rudolph, 30
Global Age-Friendly Cities Project (WHO), 256
Goals: collaboration and group member's professional, 198–199; collaboration impeded by lack of
shared intermediate, 199; collaborative outcomes
related to achieved, 201–203

Government/institutional partnerships: examples
of engaging, 307–308; U.S. Census provided
data, 112, 113*t*; 129 *fig*. *See also* Community
partnerships

H

Hazards: definition of, 219; social-ecological model
of health consequences of disaster, 218–223
Health after disasters: comparing Anglo and the
Balkans humanitarian crises and, 223–224, 229;
Hurricane Katrina and, 224–226, 229; implications
for prevention and intervention, 229–231; September
11, 2001 attacks, 226–229; social and economic
determinants of, 218–223
Health care systems: myth and reality of
effectiveness of preventive, 244; myth and reality
of immigrants and, 243; myth and reality of
older adults and, 243
Health disparities: of African American communities,
128–149; between Black and white middle class,
136; "blaming the victim" approach to, 131;
communities of color and, 26–28; extrinsic factors
of, 26; neoliberal policies as increasing, 174–176;
NIEHS Strategic Plan for eliminating, 94; universal
health insurance perceived as eliminating, 143;
weathering process leading to, 137–138, 201. *See
also* Social inequalities
Health impact assessment (HIA), 36, 37
Health public policy. *See* Public policies
Health. *See* Urban health
Health-related behavior: Behavioral Risk Factor
Surveillance System (BRFSS), 248; dietary, 46,
53; ethnic identity and perceptions leading to, 280;
physical activity by elderly, 247–248; study on teen
smoking prevention, 186–211
Healthy aging: conceptual model for, 245,
254 *fig*–255 *fig*; conditions for healthy urban, 254
fig; Global Age-Friendly Cities Project (WHO)
focus on, 256; public health research and policy
agenda for, 255–258; social and environmental
considerations for, 246–254. *See also* Aging
Healthy Eating and Exercising to Reduce Diabetes
(HEED), 49
Healthy Environments Partnership (HEP), 48, 50–53
Hierarchical linear modeling (HLM), 79
Hispanic population: comparing mental health of
U.S.-born and immigrants, 252; neighborhood
effects on health of elderly, 247; project
distribution of elderly, 241 *fig*. *See also*
Racial/ethnic differences
HIV/AIDS public policy, 147
Hochschild, Jennifer, 136

Housing: connections between health and adequate, 162–164; health aging issues related to, 257–258; housing niche model on health interventions related to, 177–178; mortgage foreclosure crisis impact on, 162–178; social-ecological context of health and, 164–170. *See also* Neighborhood

Housing Environments Research Group, 166

Housing niche model: description of, 165–166, 176; focus group analysis using the, 170–173; foreclosure and public health findings of, 173–174; health-foreclosure intervention implications of, 177–178; on neoliberalism, foreclosure, and health, 174–176; research using the, 166–170

Housing segregation: economism approach to racial and, 135–136; research on health and, 21, 34–37, 143; urban food environments and, 47

Hurricane Katrina: destruction and deaths from, 224–225; social-ecological study of health consequences of, 225–226, 229

I

Immigrant population: conceptual framework for successful aging of, 254 *fig*–255 *fig;* economic and social influences on policy and aging of, 242–245; increase of elderly among, 240 *fig*–242; public health research and policy agenda for aging, 255–258; social and environmental considerations for aging, 246–254

Immigration Act (1965), 240

Inclusionary zoning, 35–36

Institute for Local Self Reliance, 32

"Integrating Indicators of Cumulative Impact and Socioeconomic Vulnerability into Regulatory Decision-making" study, 28

Interdisciplinary research (IR): as activist organizing tool, 36–37; Bronx health disparities study lessons learned on, 117–119; community-based participatory research (CBPR), 46–54, 95–96; conundrums in, 10–11; definition of, 9; encouraging researchers and practitioners to use, 312–314; examining multiple levels of intervention using, 14; levels and types of, 8–20; methodological challenges and approaches to, 12; policy and practice influence of, 309–312; qualitative and quantitative methods used in, 281–284; recommended for health research, 6; role definitions in, 13–14; selected recent works on, 297t6; social movements as driving, 28, 308–309; social-ecological approach to, 164–176, 218–231; theories of knowledge interaction with, 11–12; on type 2 diabetes among African Americans, 272–286; when, which, and how to use, 12–13. *See also* Collaborative research; Community partnerships; Research models

Interdisciplinary research (IR) stages: assembling team, 302–304; building supportive environment, 304–305; choosing institutional and community partners, 298 *fig*, 305–309; constructing conceptual models, theories, or frameworks, 301–302; crating process for, 298 *fig*, 302–305; defining/framing the problem, 298 *fig*, 299–302; evaluating impact, 298 *fig*, 311–312; illustrated diagram of, 298 *fig;* influencing policy and practice, 298 *fig*, 309–311; selecting methods and analytic strategies, 304

J

Jacobs, Jane, 33

James, Sherman, 136–137

"John Henryism" predisposition, 136–137

K

Keck Foundation, 188

Korean population. *See* Immigrant population

L

LAHs (limited access highways), 106

Laotian Organizing Project (LOP), 34–35

Legislation: Family Support Act (1988), 142; Immigration Act (1965), 240; Personal Responsibility and Work Opportunity Reconciliation Act (PRWORA), 142. *See also* United States

Lehman College, 101, 118

Lingua franca (professional terminology), 205–206

Loneliness-health relationship, 250–252

M

McEwen, Bruce, 137

Medical anthropology: description and research approach taken by, 275–276; integrated with social psychology to reduce diabetes burden, 284–285; research approach of critical, 276–278. *See also* Critical social psychology

Mental health: dynamic social networks/changing filial expectations impact on, 252–253; isolating conditions of neighborhood and, 248–249; loneliness and isolation impact on, 250–252; mortgage foreclosure crisis impact on, 172–173; posttraumatic stress disorder following disasters, 225; September 11 attacks and related issues of, 227–229; U.S.-born Mexican Americans compared to Mexican immigrants, 252. *See also* Urban health

Metropolitan Service Area (MSA), 169
Mexican American population: comparing mental health of U.S.-born and immigrants, 252; low neighborhood SES and depression in, 249; neighborhood effects on health of elderly, 247; project distribution of elderly, 241 *fig*
Mix methodology approach, 283–284
Montefiore Medical Center (MMC), 100, 101, 114, 118
Mortality rates: African American, 128–130 *fig;* of children from preventable disease, 64; social capital related to, 250
Mortgage Brokers of America, 167
Mortgage foreclosure crisis: early warning signs of the, 162–163; findings and implications of health and, 177–178; focus groups used to study health and the, 168–173; health and housing in social-ecological context, 164–170; housing niche model on health-related interventions for, 177–178; public health issues related to, 173–174; social-ecological examination of, 163–178; United Kingdom research on health impact of, 173–174
Moses, Robert, 33
Moving to Opportunity program, 96
MTRs (major truck routes), 106
Mycobacterium tuberculosis, 12

N

National Academies Press, 5, 9
National Cancer Institute, 188
National Center for Research Resources, 188
National Institute of Environmental Health Sciences Health Disparities Strategic Plan, 50, 94
National Institute on Drug Abuse, 188
National Institutes of Health, 6
National People of Color Conference on Environmental Justice, 22
Neighborhood: aging health status and physical environment of, 246–247; definition and social importance of, 246; impact of *el barrio* on elderly Mexican population, 253; impact of loneliness and isolation in, 250–252; mental health and isolating conditions of, 248–249; social capital of, 226, 249–250; transportation access in, 250. *See also* Communities; Housing; Urban health
Neoliberal policies: examining health inequalities relationship to, 174–175; health consequences of, 175–176; ideology and practices related to, 174–175
New Urbanists, 25
New York Asthma Partnership, 118
New York City: asthma cases by zip code, in, 29 *fig;* health after September 11, 2001 attacks in, 226–229; OWN/Consumers Union's solid waste plan for, 30–34; SWMP (Solid Waste Management Plan) of, 30, 32, 33
NIMBY (Not in My Backyard), 31–32, 33
NO$_2$ (nitrogen dioxide), 106
Nonmarital childbearing. *See* Unwed mothers
NYC Organization of Waterfront Neighboorhoods (OWN) study, 29 *fig–*34

O

O$_3$ (ozone), 106
OECD (Organization for Economic Cooperation and Development), 175

P

Partnership. *See* Community partnerships
Personal responsibility: American creed on, 132, 135–137; developmentalism on, 131–135; economism ideology on, 132, 135–136
Personal Responsibility and Work Opportunity Reconciliation Act (PRWORA), 142
Physical activity, 247–248
Physical determinism: definition of, 24; urban planning applications of, 24–26
Postdisaster health: comparing Angola and Balkans humanitarian, 223–224; Hurricane Katrina and, 224–226, 229; prevention and intervention for consequences of, 229–231; September 11, 2001 terrorist attacks and, 226–229; social-ecological determinants of, 218–223
Power in Asians Organizing (PAO), 35
Pratt Institute Graduate Center for Planning and the Environment, 33
Precautionary principle, 28
Productive aging, 245
Professional or academic jargon, 205–206
Progressive era, 23
Project Liberty, 227
Psychology. *See* Critical social psychology
Public health: early urban planning relationship to, 23–26; environmental justice movement impact on, 22–23; foreclosure crisis and related issues of, 173–174; research and policy agenda for successful aging, 255–258; social-ecological approach to studies of, 164–178. *See also* Research models
Public policies: African American health disparity implications for, 138–144; building a movement for reform of, 144–148; developmentalism impact on unwed mothers and, 140–142; economic and social influences on aging and related, 242–245; health inequalities increased by neoliberal, 174–176; HIV/

AIDS, 147; interdisciplinary research influence on, 309–312; structural interventions of, 142–143; university/academic role in, 310–311; vulnerable population health postdisaster, 229–231

Public policy reform: African American activist working toward, 144–148; interdisciplinary research influence on, 309–312; politics of building solidarity for, 145–148

Q

Qualitative research method: description of, 281; ethnography as, 281–283; mixed with quantitative approach, 283–284; topics and patterns emerging from, 282

Quantitative research method: description of, 281; mixed with qualitative approach, 283–284

R

Race: economism on health and, 135; ethnic identity defense from stressors related to, 280–281; relationship between economics and, 53. *See also* Environmental racism

Racial housing segregation. *See* Housing segregation

Racial/ethnic differences: projected distribution of population age 65 and older, 241 *fig;* social networks/changing filial expectations and, 252–253; type 2 diabetes rates and, 272. *See also* African Americans; Communities of color; Ethnic identity; Hispanic population

Racialized ideologies: American Creed, 132, 136–137; Black health and, 137–138; developmentalism, 131–135; economism, 132, 135–136

Religiosity, 281

Research models: community-based participatory research (CBPR), 46–54, 95–96; housing niche model, 165–178; qualitative and quantitative, 281–284; social-ecological approach, 164–176, 218–231; transdisciplinary (TD) action research, 186–205, 209–211. *See also* Interdisciplinary research (IR); Public health; Urban health

Residential segregation. *See* Housing segregation

Retail food industry: health impact of, 47–56; restructuring in the, 48

Robert Wood Johnson Foundation, 188

S

September 11, 2001 attacks, 226–229

"Smart growth" concept, 25

SO_2 (sulfur dioxide), 106

Social capital: elderly/immigrant elderly populations and, 249–250; postdisaster breakdown of, 226; small-group activities building essential, 207

Social inequalities: communities of color and, 26–28; between municipalities, 24; NIEHS Strategic Plan for eliminating, 94; postdisaster vulnerabilities related to, 225–226, 228–229; psychology approach to health and, 274–275. *See also* Discrimination; Health disparities

Social justice movements: environmental, 20–23; interdisciplinary research (IR) driven by, 28, 308–309; Progressive era and, 23; types of, 308–309. *See also* Environmental justice (EJ)

Social networks: health status of elderly/immigrants and, 252–253; postdisaster vulnerabilities and breakdown of, 225–226, 228–229

Social psychology. *See* Critical social psychology

Social-ecological approach: definition of, 164; effects of neoliberal policies examined using, 174–176; examining health after disasters using, 218–231; focus groups used in, 168–173; health and housing in context of, 164–166; mortgage foreclosure crisis examined using, 166–168; public health research using the, 164–166

Socioeconomic status (SES): Bronfenbrenner's bioecological model consideration of, 67; economism on essential nature of, 134–135; placement of retail food outlets, race, and, 53; postdisaster vulnerabilities related to differences in, 225–226, 228–229; urban child's health and relationship to, 70–71, 72, 74–75

South Bronx Clean Air Coalition (SBCAC), 99–100, 101

South Bronx Environmental Justice Partnership (SBEJP) study: Bronx air pollution sources/minority populations during, 100 *fig;* Bronx economic disadvantages, 97–98; community contributions to data collection/analysis during, 116*t;* community-scale assessment techniques/units of analysis used for, 101, 104; environmental hazards and pollutants investigated during, 105–106; findings and implications of, 110*t*–117; five-year average asthma hospitalization rates (1995–1999), 104 *fig;* formation of SBEJP for, 99, 101; geographic scale and context of, 98; GIS analysis during, 101, 102*t*–103*t*, 106–109, 113*t;* interdisciplinary research lessons learned during, 117–119; limitations of data and analyses of, 112, 113; organizational challenges during, 114–117; research partnership during, 99–101; on role of asthma/air pollution in, 98–99. *See also* Bronx (New York)

Spirituality, 281

SPSS, 282

SPSs (stationary point sources), 106

State of the World's Cities report (2001), 4
Statewide Planning and Research Consortium System (SPARCS) database, 104
"Still Toxic After All These Years: Air Quality and Environmental Justice in the San Francisco Bay Are" report, 27–28
Street Science: Community Knowledge and Environmental Health Justice (Corburn): four studies covered in, 27; interdisciplinary research of, 27–28; NYC Organization of Waterfront Neighborhoods (OWN) study, 29 *fig*–34
Stressors: allostatic load from long-term exposure to, 138; health and race-related, 281; of mismatch between local community needs and dominant culture, 143–144
Successful aging. *See* Healthy aging
Sustainability, 25
SWMP (Solid Waste Management Plan) [NYC], 30, 32, 33

T

Teen mothers: cultural differences and circumstances related to, 141–142; developmentalism impact on public policies on, 140–142
Toxic Release Inventories (TRIs), 105, 110
Trandisciplinary (TD) action research: benefits of using, 189; cycle of, 187–188; expanding the file of, 209–211; factors facilitating or impeding collaboration during, 196–205; origins, development, and phases of, 186–187; translating into community intervention and policy, 189–196*t*
Transdisciplianry Research on Energetics Center (TREC), 188
Transportation-health relationship, 250
Type 2 diabetes: African Americans and risk of, 272–273; ethnic identity and experience of African American with, 278–281; HEED pilot project to prevent, 49; integrating social psychology/medical anthropology to reduce burden of, 284–285; interdisciplinary research methods used to study, 281–284; psychology and medical anthropology approach to study of, 273–278

U

UC Irvine Tobacco Policy Consortium (TPC) study: factors facilitating or impeding collaboration during, 196–205; future directions for additional studies, 207–211; implications and lessons learned from, 205–207; organization and background of, 186; tracking intellectual and social developments of collaboration during, 193–196*t*; translating

research into community intervention and policy, 189–196*t*
UC Irvine TTURC (Transdisciplinary Tobacco Use Research Center): accomplishment of stated goals by, 201–203; disciplinary and professional scope of, 197–198; as TD science and training center, 188; translating TR into community intervention and policy, 189–190, 192
UNITA forces (Angola), 224
United Kingdom: comparing health care access in U.S. and, 175; public health study on foreclosure in the, 173–174
United Nations: Angola humanitarian assistance by, 223–224; Consolidated Inter-Agency Appeal (CAP) of, 223–224; *State of the World's Cities* report (2001) by, 4
United Nations Conference (1987), 25
United States: average annual growth rate of elderly population in the, 240 *fig;* comparing health care access of UK and, 174; Hurricane Katrina and health consequences in the, 224–226; OECD health outcomes data on the, 175–176; projected distribution of elderly population by race, 241 *fig*. *See also* Legislation
Universal health insurance, 143
University of California at David, 20
University of California at Los Angeles, 36
University of New York (CUNY), 101
Unwed mothers: cultural differences and circumstances related to, 141–142; developmentalism impact on public policies on, 140–142
Urban environment: Bronfenbrenner's bioecological model on, 65–68 *fig;* ecological model of, 64–65; exosystem of, 68 *fig,* 72–73; macrosystem of, 68 *fig*–72; mesosystem of, 68 *fig,* 73; microsystem of, 68 *fig,* 73–74. *See also* Environmental health
Urban health: conceptual framework for aging and, 245, 254 *fig*–255 *fig;* connections between housing situation and, 162–164; dietary behaviors relationship to, 46; ecological model of children and, 64–80; examining the problems and issues of, 4–6; health after disasters, 218–231; implications for health by, 6–8; implications of urban life for, 6–8; psychology approach to social inequalities and, 274–275; social environment context of, 26; stages of interdisciplinary research (IR) on, 298 *fig;* urban life implications for, 6–8; urban retail food environment implications for, 47–56. *See also* Communities; Environmental health; Mental health; Neighborhood; Research models
Urban planning: early public health relationship to, 23–26; physical determinism of built environment in, 24–26; zoning regulatory tool of, 24, 35–36

Urban retail food environments: CBPR on health implications of Detroit's, 48–54; determinants of, 47–48; directions for future research on, 54–56. *See also* Dietary behaviors

U.S. Census: morality calculations based on, 129 *fig;* SBEJP study GIS analysis data from, 112, 113*t*

U.S. Environmental Protection Agency (EPA), 105, 110

V

VOC$_s$ (volatile organic compounds), 106

Vulnerable population health: Angola and Balkans humanitarian crises impact on, 223–224; elderly/elderly immigrant, 240 *fig*–258; Hurricane Katrina impact on, 225–226; research implications for prevention/interventions for, 229–231; September 11, 2001 terrorist attacks impact on, 226–229; social and economic determinants of postdisaster, 218–223. *See also* Children's health

W

West Harlem Environmental Action Coalition, 29

Who Will Keep the Public Healthy? (National Academies Press), 5

WHO (World Health Organization) Global Age-Friendly Cities Project, 256

World Trade Center (WTC) attacks, 226–229

Z

Zoning: inclusionary, 35–36; urban planning regulatory through, 24